GALLSTONE
· DISEASE ·
and its Management

GALLSTONE
· DISEASE ·
and its Management

Edited by
Malcolm C. Bateson
Consultant Physician and Specialist in Gastroenterology,
General Hospital, Bishop Auckland, U K

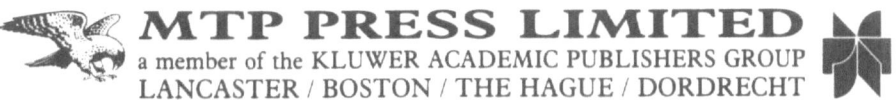
MTP PRESS LIMITED
a member of the KLUWER ACADEMIC PUBLISHERS GROUP
LANCASTER / BOSTON / THE HAGUE / DORDRECHT

Published in the UK and Europe by
MTP Press Limited
Falcon House
Lancaster, England

British Library Cataloguing in Publication Data
Gallstone disease and its management.
   1. Gallstones
   I. Bateson, Malcolm C.
   616.3'65   RC850

   ISBN-13: 978-94-010-8353-9

Published in the USA by
MTP Press
A division of Kluwer Academic Publishers
101 Philip Drive
Norwell, MA 02061, USA

Library of Congress Cataloging-in-Publication Data
Gallstone disease and its management.

   Includes bibliographies and index.
   1. Gallstones.   I. Bateson, Malcolm C. [DNLM:
1. Cholelithiasis.   WI 755 G1735]
RC850.G3   1986   616.3'65   86-20068

ISBN-13: 978-94-010-8353-9   e-ISBN-13: 978-94-009-4173-1
DOI: 10.1007/978-94-009-4173-1

Table of Contents

Authors

A. F. ATTILI MD
Associate Professor of
    Gastroenterology,
L'Aquila, Italy

M. C. BATESON MD, MRCP
Consultant Physician and
    Gastroenterologist,
Bishop Auckland General Hospital,
County Durham, UK

L. H. BLUMGART MD, FRCS
Professor, Hepatobiliary Surgical
    Unit,
Royal Postgraduate Medical School,
Hammersmith Hospital,
London, UK

**D. L. CARR-LOCKE MB, B.Chir,
    DRCOG, MRCP**
Consultant Physician in
    Gastroenterology,
Leicester Royal Infirmary & Glenfield
    General Hospital,
Leicester, UK

**A. CUSCHIERI MD, ChM, FRCS,
    FRCS (Ed)**
Professor of Surgery,
Ninewells Hospital,
Dundee, UK

D. P. MAUDGAL MB, PhD, MRCP
Consultant Physician and
    Gastroenterologist,

Manor House Hospital,
London, UK

T. C. NORTHFIELD MA, MD, FRCP
Consultant Gastroenterologist and
    Reader in Medicine,
St. Georges Hospital & Medical
    School,
London, UK

F. PIXLEY MB, BS
Rhodes Scholar,
Department of Community Medical
    & General Practice,
Oxford, UK

S. A. SADEK MB, FRCS
Senior Registrar,
Department of Surgery,
Ninewells Hospital,
Dundee, UK

R. K. R. SCRAGG MB, BS, MRCP
Senior Lecturer in Epidemiology,
School of Medicine,
Auckland, New Zealand

R. S. STUBBS MD, FRCS
Senior Registrar, Hepatobiliary
    Surgical Unit,
Royal Postgraduate Medical School,
Hammersmith Hospital,
London, UK

Foreword

Exciting major changes have occurred in the understanding and treatment of gallstone disease over the last two decades.

In bygone years, books about gallstones were often based on postgraduate lectures which the author, usually a surgeon of distinction, had given. More recently, many books dealing with this subject have been based upon national or international conferences. The single-author text has the disadvantage that few authors today can authoritatively encompass a whole field: the reports of symposia, conferences or workshops often lack balance and authority. The merits of 'Gallstone disease and its Management' edited by Malcolm Bateson are clear. He has chosen 11 authors, all of whom write on topics relating to their own expertise, and the content of the book has been carefully planned to reflect the most modern ideas about the aetiology and management of cholesterol gallstones.

It is worth repeating that we are experiencing rapid developments in the field of gallstone disease. Disappointingly the least progress has been made in identifying the cause (or causes) of the disease notwithstanding the many data implicating a variety of environmental factors. Most of these affect the chemistry of hepatic bile and the contribution of the gallbladder to lithogenesis remains uncertain and unstudied.

It is when we look at what is known about the natural history and the developments in management that a different scene unfolds. New information abounds, novel techniques are proliferating. The patient is no longer faced solely with the option of a cholecystectomy. The use of ultrasonography and collaboration between gastroenterologists has produced data which widen our understanding of the natural history of cholesterol gallstone disease, although creating at the same time new challenges such as how to define clearly what are silent gallstones and how these should be managed.

There are many therapeutic agents to dissolve gallstones, reflecting the resourcefulness of the pharmacologist. These can be taken orally, instilled into the bile duct or introduced directly in the gallbladder. The endoscopist has a key role, particularly in the management of bile duct stones where he has displaced the surgeon in many instances. The ingenuity of manufacturers and the skill of operators is to be applauded, but the techniques do not end there, for the impact of high technology is manifest in the breaking up of stones using shock-wave therapy and thereby introducing yet another option for removing gallbladder and bile duct stones.

The picture then is one of activity and evolution. This book by Malcolm Bateson and his colleagues actively reflects current thinking. It makes an important contribution to the literature on gallstone disease and the authors are to be congratulated on the quality of their contributions. This book should appeal to physicians, surgeons and epidemiologists, as well as other members of the profession. It deserves to be read widely.

Professor I. A. D. Bouchier
Department of Medicine
University of Edinburgh
1986

1
Epidemiology

F. PIXLEY

HISTORICAL PERSPECTIVES

Much of the recent interest in gallstones stems from the inclusion of this condition in the list of Western Diseases[1]. This label implies that gallstones are a consequence of industrialization and therefore a modern phenomenon. In fact, gallstones have been written about in medical manuscripts for many centuries and paleopathological studies of mummies have revealed gallstones in at least one of the specimens[2].

According to Siegel's translation of Galen's work, *A System of Physiology and Medicine*, neither Galen nor any other physician of this period (AD 130–200) ever mentioned the occurrence of gallstones, although they were quite familiar with stones of the urinary tract[3]. Galen did write about common bile duct obstruction and consequent jaundice as had Erasistratus some centuries earlier, but the diagnosis of gallstones did not become established until the time of the Renaissance. Siegel suggests that physicians of Galen's time would not have overlooked the disorder if it was as frequent then as it is now. He argues plausibly that the Greeks and Romans of antiquity ate a diet similar to underdeveloped nations now with more cereals and vegetables and very few animal products and that they rarely survived even to middle age so gallstones may well have been most uncommon.

Human gallstones began to be mentioned in mediaeval literature. Foligno found a gallstone in the gallbladder of a woman in Padua in 1341 when carrying out an autopsy[4]. Later, according to Muleur[5], Benevenius made the first connection between gallstones and clinical symptoms when he carried out an autopsy on a woman who had presented with symptoms suggestive of either acute cholecystitis or common bile duct occlusion in 1506. Many other notable authors (Vesalius, Fernel, Estienne, Fallopius) began to write of stones in the gallbladder around this time.

Epidemiological associations also began to be noted. Fabricius reported that gallstones were more frequently observed than stones of the urinary bladder. As early as 1755 Haller observed in his *Opuscula Pathologica* that gallstones occurred more frequently in some countries[6]. Estienne had asserted by then that they were found chiefly in older women while Hoffman had said they were rare in young men, more frequent in old men and more frequent still in women[6]. Morgagni had collected information on at least 200 cases of gallstones and had about equal observations in both sexes but he did concur with the effect of increasing age. Haller found stones commonly in prisoners who had been imprisoned for long periods and ascribed this to physical inactivity[6]. Obesity was mentioned by Morgagni as a possible cause. By the time of Crisp's address to the Medical Society of London in 1841 the following associations were regarded as being important: sex (female to male ratio of 3:1), melancholic temperament and mental disquietude, sedentary habits and good living, especially eating[7]. On one major issue Crisp disagreed with other authors at that time, claiming that, 'fat people are not more subject to the disease than those of spare habit'. He thought that stones were most common between the ages of 30 and 60 and that alcohol was not a contributing factor.

The natural history of gallstones was not considered in great detail until surgery became an option in the treatment of gallstones. The first cholecystostomy was performed in 1867 by Stough Hobbs and the first cholecystectomy was carried out by Langenbuch in 1882 in Berlin. Morgagni wrote at length on possible signs that could be used to diagnose gallstones and eventually concluded that he agreed with Fernel who stated, '... (there are) no manifest marks by which the existence of these stones may certainly and easily be known'. Morgagni also recognized that gallstones could lie latent within the gallbladder for many years. Not all authors believed this and Robertson[8] cites Guidetti as having an opposite and more modern view in 1725 when he stated that biliary calculi could not exist without giving rise to symptoms that were, more often than not, severe. Crisp believed that calculi could exist without producing any inconvenience[7].

THE PREVALENCE OF GALLSTONES

Gallstones can be detected in a number of ways: at autopsy, by investigation of a group of symptomatic patients or by screening an asymptomatic population. All three methods may be expected to produce different prevalence rates resulting from the inherent strengths and weaknesses of each.

Autopsy studies

The vast majority of studies, especially those of the first half of this century, have attempted to determine the prevalence of gallstones from data obtained postmortem. Any autopsy survey must present certain difficulties when used to estimate the frequency of the disease in the general population. Spurious results may arise as most autopsies are carried out on hospital patients who differ from the general population in several important respects. Age and sex are the most important factors known to affect prevalence. Hospital patients tend to be older, more men come to autopsy than women and the studies must contain large numbers of autopsies to be useful so need to be carried out over a number of years and time trends may be obscured. Moreover, previous cholecystectomy and cholecystostomy patients are sometimes difficult to discern and many autopsy studies therefore ignored this pool of cases. Another problem which plays a more important role in determining clinical associations with gallstones is that of the bias of associated disease as it has been shown that the occurrence of two disorders in the same person gives an increased possibility of hospital admissions[9]. The major advantage of the autopsy method is that it detects both symptomatic and asymptomatic stones. As a result prevalence figures in these studies are greater than in other studies.

Clinical studies

Clinical studies are much fewer in number than autopsy studies and have been carried out relatively recently. Cases are either identified as symptomatic cases having been diagnosed by oral cholecystography or ultrasonography or as surgical patients undergoing cholecystectomy. Therefore the prevalence rates are underestimated by the exclusion of asymptomatic stones. Evidence of this is provided by the comparison of the results of these studies with autopsy studies in similar countries. Friedman *et al.*[10] in Boston found a prevalence rate of 8.2% in 1966 compared with the rate of 24.3% quoted in an autopsy study of New York[11]. Variable diagnostic criteria of gallstones in clinical studies also affect prevalence rates and the results tend to be about half those of autopsy rates.

Cholecystectomy rates are also used to determine the prevalence of gallstones as at least 98% of all cholecystectomies are carried out for gallstones. However, bias is an even greater problem in these studies because many factors apart from the prevalence of a disorder influence surgery rates. Supply variables are crucial factors in the production of surgical rate variations. A marked difference was found in cholecystectomy rates between North America and England and Wales which was not accountable for by different disease prevalence[12].

Prevalence surveys

Prevalence surveys number even fewer than clinical studies and most have studied selected populations known to be at high risk of developing gallstones such as American Indian tribes[13]. The first study that screened an unselected population was carried out by Bainton *et al.* in a South Wales industrial town using oral cholecystography[14]. Recent studies have used real-time ultrasonography as the screening technique[15-17]. These surveys are less likely to be biased as they study unselected populations and allow inclusion of both symptomatic and asymptomatic cases. A common problem is that of poor response rates.

INTERNATIONAL DIFFERENCES

Important geographical and racial variations in the prevalence of gallstones have been observed by several workers. Brett and Barker in 1976 summarized all published autopsy data to determine the world distribution of gallstones[18].

3

Their results should be interpreted with caution as the included studies varied in sex and age distributions which in some cases were not even known. Nevertheless they calculated the mean prevalence of gallstones in Europe after 1940 to be 18.5%. Rates varied within Europe from Ireland (the lowest at 5%) to Sweden (the highest at 38%). Other western nations such as the United States and Australia showed prevalence rates similar to those of Great Britain and several other European countries whose rates lay between the

Table 1.1 The autopsy prevalence of gallstones in western and other communities

Place	Year	Age	Prevalence Male %	Female %	Total %
London	1969	>20	9.5	19.2	15.5
London	1941–50	>25	6.2	12.1	8.6
Malmo	1971	>20	26.5	46.8	36.2
Oslo	1952–57	>20	13.5	28.6	20.1
New York	1959	>20	16.0	32.5	24.3
Melbourne	1945–59	all	11.3	20.3	14.9
American Indian	1962	>15	16.6	40.0	29.9
Santiago	1960–71	>20	20.5	50.0	35.2
Ibadan	1964	all	—	—	0.8
Kampala	1950–62	all	—	—	0.9
Johannesburg	1936–50	all	(w) 10.0	19.5	14.7
			(b) 1.0	3.8	2.4
Japan	1955–61	all	—	—	4.4
Singapore	1962–66	>20	6.4	7.9	6.6

w = white population, b = black population

two extremes. See Table 1.1 for a summary of the international differences described both above and on following pages.

International variation becomes much more marked when African rates are compared to those in western nations. Gallstones are so uncommon in Africa that in some areas they are virtually never seen and most recorded rates are less than 1%. The degree of urbanization appears to be very important in disease patterns in Africa. Studies of urbanized blacks in Johannesburg show that western influences result in an increased risk of gallstones but these rates are still well below those of the white population living in Johannesburg[19].

Not many studies have been carried out in Asia but in those that have, low prevalences are found except in Singapore opium addicts[20]. Japanese studies present an interesting epidemiological feature. In western civilization most gallstones are composed mainly of crystalline cholesterol while Asian stones are almost always pigment. Japan occupies an intermediate position in that both types of stones occur. Nakayama and Miyake[21] confirmed that the composition of gallstones in Japan is gradually changing from the once predominant pigment stone (55% in 1927) to cholesterol (85% in 1968). The prevalence of gallstone disease has increased over a similar period from 1.7% to 6.7%. The increasing urbanization and changing food habits that had taken place in Japan since the Second World War were blamed for the changes in character of gallstone disease[21].

The American Indian is particularly prone to developing cholesterol stones.

4

Clinical evidence suggested this in earlier studies but a prevalence survey using oral cholecystography confirmed the relationship in 1971[13]. They found that the Pima Indian tribe of Arizona had an overall prevalence of gallbladder disease of 48.6% and the rate rose rapidly in females to 73% in the group aged 25–34 years and remained around this figure in the older age groups. As more epidemiological research is being carried out in South America, it is becoming evident that cholesterol gallstones are very common there also. A Chilean study in 1960–71 showed that 35.2% of people over 20 in Santiago had gallstones[22]. Figure 1.1 illustrates on a world map the international differences mentioned above.

As well as noting international variations in the prevalence of gallstones, within-nation variations have been shown to occur. Malhotra showed that railway workers from the north of India had a seven times greater risk of developing gallstones than did their counterparts in southern India[23]. This risk was blamed on the diet of the northern population as they ate much more fat, much of it being animal in origin. Barker *et al.* in their autopsy survey of nine towns in England and Wales showed wide regional variations in the prevalence of gallstones[24]. The variations in gallstone prevalence did not follow those for all-cause mortality which showed a trend towards the highest mortalities occurring in the north and west of Great Britain. If anything, the prevalence of gallstones appeared to be negatively correlated with the prevalence of ischaemic heart disease despite the two disorders both being classified as western diseases. The significance of these variations has been disputed on the basis that the study looked at too few autopsies over a very short period of time. Regional variation has also been reported when different British studies have been compared. The autopsy prevalence of stones in women in Leeds before 1929 was about twice that in Birmingham despite the fact that the study in Birmingham was carried out some 25 years later[25,26]. Moreover, a national autopsy survey showed that cholelithiasis was twice as common in elderly people in Glasgow compared with those in London[27].

WESTERN TRENDS

The prevalence of gallstones appears to have risen quite markedly in the western world during the past century. Dessau[28] reported an increase in Boston from 18.9% in 1900–22 to 22.2% in 1923–42 and Cleland[29] showed an increase of 10–15% in Adelaide, Australia between 1920 and 1948. The increase is even more clearly evident if early autopsy surveys are compared with recent ones as was done by Brett and Barker in 1976[18]. Comparisons between studies that are not standardized for age, sex or race can lead to difficulties but, looking at Table 1.2 which has adapted the two tables given by Brett and Barker[18], an increase can be seen in the gallstone prevalence of western nations. Holland and Heaton[30] gave support to this impression when they reported that gallbladder operations had become significantly more common in Bristol. This increase was particularly large in the younger age groups and appeared to be essentially a post-war phenomenon. Similar increases had been found by Plant and his co-workers[31] who showed that cholecystectomy rates had doubled in Canada, France and England between

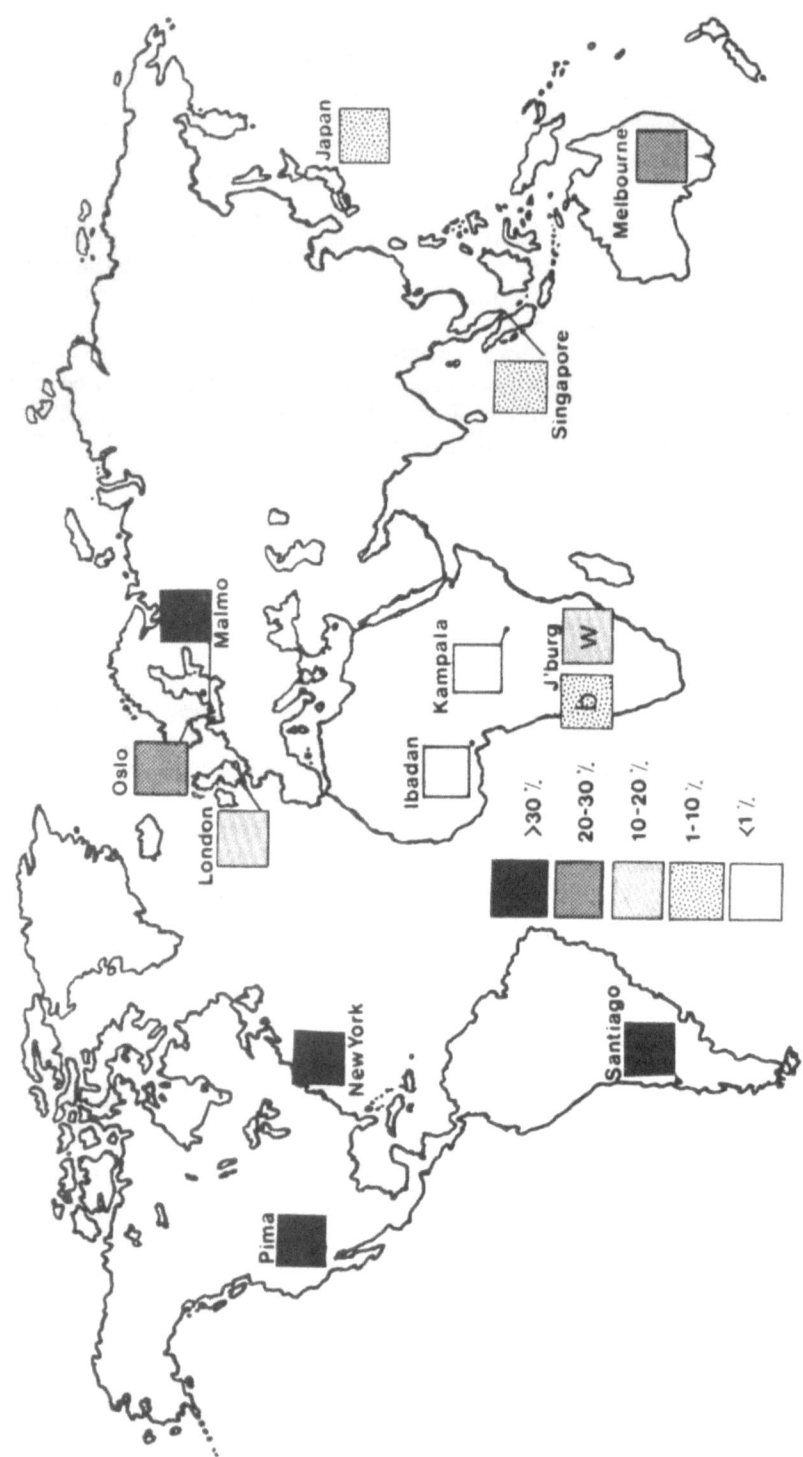

Figure 1.1 The autopsy prevalence of gallstones in women

Table 1.2 Western trends in the autopsy prevalence of gallstones

| Place | Year | Age | Prevalence | | |
			Male %	Female %	Total %
Copenhagen	1911	>20	10.1	21.7	14.8
Oslo	1952–57	>20	13.5	28.6	20.1
Stockholm	1925–34	all	12.0	27.0	19.6
Malmo	1971	>20	26.5	46.8	36.2
London	1911–12	?	—	—	4.1
London	1969	>20	9.5	19.2	15.5
New York	1903–12	?	—	—	7.4
New York	1959	>20	16.0	32.5	24.3
Adelaide	1920–48	>20	10.1	19.4	13.3
Melbourne	1945–59	all	11.3	20.3	14.9

1961 and 1971. Such increases cannot be fully explained by better diagnostic or surgical techniques or by service availability. Unfortunately, studies based on autopsy figures and surgical statistics can be confounded by influences such as the age structure of the population being studied. Bateson, in an analysis of autopsies in Dundee, detected an increase in the age – standardized rates in 1974–83 compared with 1953–73 figures from an earlier study[32,33]. He also showed that cholecystectomy rates had trebled in Dundee between 1961 and 1981, a very much greater increase than could be explained by changes in prevalence[33].

Less confusion surrounds the nature of increases reported in non-western areas such as Japan and Africa. The documented increase in gallstone prevalence in these areas is attributed to lifestyle changes, specifically those associated with western cultures[21,34]. It is not unreasonable to extrapolate these observations to our own communities which have also undergone enormous lifestyle and dietary changes, especially with industrialization. The influence of lifestyle and diet on increasing the prevalence of gallstone disease in western nations may well have taken effect earlier than the recent attempts to quantify these changes.

GALLSTONE PATHOGENESIS

The pathogenesis of cholesterol gallstones can be looked at in terms of three main stages.

Cholesterol supersaturation

Cholesterol supersaturation is a necessary step in the process of gallstone formation. Gallstone patients have been shown to have supersaturated gallbladder and hepatic bile almost without exception[35]. There are a number of ways to form abnormal bile. Many normal people will produce supersaturated hepatic bile during their overnight fast as fasting reduces bile salt secretion rates and increases the concentration of cholesterol accordingly. This supersaturated bile mixes with large amounts of unsaturated gallbladder bile in normal people to give an unsaturated mean composition. Pathophysiological mechanisms that may produce abnormal bile include:

(1) Excessive bile salt loss which may occur with diseases that affect the terminal ileum where most of the bile salts are actively reabsorbed from the intestines. Such diseases include ileectomy, extensive Crohn's disease and ileal bypass surgery. Losses can be greater than hepatic synthetic capacity resulting in low bile salt secretion rates and subsequent cholesterol supersaturation. Drugs such as cholestyramine and lignin can cause excessive loss by chelating bile salts in the gut and preventing reabsorption but they only tend to cause severe loss when given in association with terminal ileal disease.

(2) Oversensitive bile salt feedback appears to be a possible mechanism where certain patients have a small bile salt pool but hepatic synthesis does not increase to compensate. Patients with gallstones have significantly smaller bile salt pools than normal controls. Overactivity of the normal feedback inhibition results in depression of bile acid synthesis by low rates of bile salt return. Alternatively, a small bile salt pool can be sustained by increased enterohepatic cycling.

(3) Inadequate bile acid synthesis is probably very uncommon but is found in the rare disease cerebrotendinous xanthomatosis which has, as one of its features, a greatly increased risk of cholesterol cholelithiasis.

(4) Excessive cholesterol secretion has been shown to be the cause of bile supersaturation in the face of normal or even increased bile salt pools. Bennion and Grundy[36] have reported that obesity is associated with an increase in the biliary secretion of cholesterol. This observation has been confirmed by Mabee et al.[37]. In their comprehensive investigation, Bennion and Grundy showed that weight reduction in obese patients resulted in a significant reduction of cholesterol output but not of bile salt or phospholipid output. The exact mechanisms responsible for increased cholesterol synthesis in obesity are not known but Bennion and Grundy have hypothesized that HMG CoA reductase activity is increased, perhaps by insulin stimulation as insulin levels are chronically elevated in the obese[36].

(5) Phospholipid synthesis reduction is another possibility but little is known about it except for one study that has shown that gallstone patients have a greatly diminished phospholipid secretion[38]. This diminution is thought to be a result of the relationship where phospholipid secretion is directly linked to the availability of bile salts in the enterohepatic circulation.

(6) A combination of reduced bile salt pools and increased cholesterol secretion has been documented in the American Indians of the southwestern areas[39]. The authors postulated that a defect in the conversion

of cholesterol to bile acids may be present, curtailing the production of bile acids and allowing an increase in unmetabolized cholesterol.

(7) Other factors than the relative concentrations of the three components of mixed micelles can influence the capacity of bile to hold cholesterol in secretion. These include the water content and ionic strength of bile. Dilute bile is less able to solubilize cholesterol than concentrated bile of the same relative lipid proportions.

The liver is mainly responsible for the production of abnormal bile while the gallbladder is the reservoir that stores, concentrates and expels bile. Thus, it plays no part in the essential first step of gallstone pathogenesis but makes its contribution during the next two steps: the nucleation of cholesterol crystals and the growth of macroscopic gallstones.

Cholesterol crystal nucleation

Nucleation of cholesterol can occur by homogeneous nucleation if the cholesterol concentration is high enough to allow spontaneous coalescence of the cholesterol molecules. However, it is most uncommon to have gallbladder cholesterol concentrations within this range. Heterogeneous nucleation can occur at lower cholesterol concentrations as precipitation starts around some other substance such as mucus, calcium bilirubinate, bacterial fragments or epithelial slough from the gallbladder wall. Bile that is supersaturated to the extent that heterogeneous nucleation is possible in the presence of appropriate nucleating agents is said to be 'metastable' while bile that allows homogeneous nucleation is called 'labile'. The boundary between the two concentration zones has been labelled the 'metastable/labile' limit[35].

Many people secrete supersaturated bile yet do not go on to form gallstones. Sedaghat and Grundy[40] showed that the supersaturated bile of people without gallstones did not contain cholesterol monohydrate crystals while patients with gallstones almost always had cholesterol crystals. Moreover, these crystals were shown to have formed *de novo* in the bile rather than arising from crystal shedding from the gallstone surface. Cholesterol in gallstones forms clumps of cholesterol monohydrate crystals and cholesterol monohydrate precipitation seems to be an essential prerequisite of gallstone formation. This suggests that gallstone patients are either lacking a factor in their bile that normally prevents cholesterol crystallization or they have factors present in their bile that promote crystal nucleation. Recent research has provided substantial evidence for the existence of a potent nucleating factor in the bile of gallstone patients. Whiting and Watts[41] demonstrated that supersaturated bile from obese subjects without gallstones would not form cholesterol crystals *in vitro* unless small seed crystals of cholesterol monohydrate were added. In the absence of seed crystals the bile of patients with gallstones showed a much greater tendency to form cholesterol crystals *in vitro* although biliary cholesterol saturation levels were similar in both groups. Another study has been carried out to specifically determine whether the rapid nucleation time of gallbladder bile obtained from gallstone patients is due to the presence of a nucleating factor or the absence of a protective factor. Burnstein *et al.*[42]

9

mixed the bile of normal controls with that of gallstone patients and showed that the mixtures had rapid nucleation times, similar to those of the gallbladder bile from gallstone patients. This indicated the presence of a nucleating factor in the abnormal bile and further investigations using decreasing amounts of abnormal bile in the mixtures revealed that the factor was extremely potent. Microfiltration at a level that would be expected to remove microcrystals of cholesterol did not eliminate the nucleating potency of the abnormal bile. Thus, some other nucleating factor that promotes the initial nucleation of cholesterol seems to be present in the bile of people who have gallstones. High cholesterol levels in the bile may also initiate excess secretion of gallbladder mucus which, in turn, acts as a nucleating agent for cholesterol gallstone formation.

Gallstone growth

The microscopic crystals need time to grow to macroscopic size and people without gallstones occasionally have been shown to have microliths in their bile. Sluggish gallbladder contraction and stratification of the bile within the gallbladder influence gallstone growth. Pregnancy and diabetes mellitus have been associated with impaired gallbladder contraction. Incomplete emptying of the gallbladder with a large residual volume has been shown in late pregnancy and diabetics were thought to be prone to gallstones as a result of atony secondary to autonomic neuropathy. However, the importance of the influence of gallbladder tone on the growth of gallstones has been disputed. On the one hand gallstone patients have been shown to have gallbladder stasis. In contrast to this it has been suggested that gallbladder atony may lead to an increase in the bile salt pool size by decreasing the enterohepatic circulation of bile salts and thereby decreasing intestinal losses and negative feedback inhibition[43]. This would theoretically reduce the risk of developing gallstones and therefore counteract the direct effect of gallbladder stasis on gallstone growth. The concentrations of counter ions such as calcium are thought to be important also in determining the aggregate growth of crystals. Each of the three steps in gallstone pathogenesis is a necessary step in the evolution of a gallstone. The importance of gallstone nucleating and growth factors has only recently been realized and physicochemical research into gallstone formation has ironically been brought through something of a full circle as the role of infection and stasis is again being considered as it was much earlier this century.

ASSOCIATED RISK FACTORS

Well before theories were evolved on the physicochemical aspects of gallstone formation, opinions were formed on the type of person most likely to harbour gallstones. By Naunyn's time a number of autopsy series had already been published enabling him to evaluate possible risk factors[44]. He showed that gallstones were less frequent in younger populations (2–3% in people less than 30 years) than older populations (25% in 'old' people). This was one of the first attempts at quantifying the effects of ageing. After looking more closely at one particular study he pointed out the preponderance in women – 20.6% of women had gallstones compared with 4.4% of men. These two influences had been implicated by Morgagni[6]. 90% of the affected women in the collection of series were parous so parity was thought to play an important role despite the fact that cases were never compared with controls to see if 90% of the normal population of women were also parous. Women were also thought to be at risk of developing gallstones because of their style of dress. The tight corsets that women wore then certainly restricted abdominal move-ment and often left rib markings on the liver. A sedentary lifestyle was also blamed as a risk factor because decreased body activity was thought to cause decreased biliary flow but Naunyn did not believe that obesity or diet were at all important as possible risk factors[44].

Osler in 1901[45] listed the associated risk factors as age, with nearly 50% of all cases occurring in people over 50 years old, sex, parity and any condition which favoured the stagnation of bile in the gallbladder such as 'corset-wearing, occupations requiring a leaning-forward position, lack of exercise, sedentary occupations, an overindulgence in food, constipation and depress-ing mental emotions'. There was a lack of agreement about the importance of diet with some authors believing that meat predisposed least to gallstones while vegetable foodstuffs provided the greatest risk and others believing that animal foodstuffs and alcohol were to blame for inducing gallstones.

The opinions outlined above show that the understanding of associated risk factors in the aetiology of gallstones had not developed much further in the 60 years since Crisp's address to the Medical Society in London (1841)[7] when he stated that the following associations were important: sex, mel-ancholic temperament and mental disquietude, sedentary habits and good living, especially eating. This state of affairs continued well into the twentieth century. Littler and Ellis' review of 1952[46] quotes writers as recently as 1944 blaming sedentary habits and tightly fitting garments for gallstones. By this time, though, an hereditary predisposition had been recognized. Even with the increase in epidemiological studies of gallstones in the last 30 years or so, only a few risk factors have been established as confirmed influences and many more are disputed. Yet the misleading aphorism of the 'fair, fat, fertile, 40-year-old female who is flatulent' being the most likely sufferer of gallbladder disease is still commonly taught in our medical schools.

A great number of clinical associations with gallstones have been made, too many to mention them all individually. This chapter will attempt to describe the more important or more controversial associations only and is meant to be read in conjunction with the next chapter.

Age

The frequency of gallstones increases with age as has been shown by the overwhelming majority of epidemiological surveys. Studies do vary, however, in the constancy of the increase with age.

Metabolic studies investigating the underlying causes of increased preva-lence with age are very uncommon but there is one of interest, a study carried out on two groups of Chilean women – 12 young and 12 elderly women with recent normal oral cholecystograms – showed that the older group had a higher biliary saturation index than the younger group[47]. This was believed to be due to an increase in the canalicular secretion of cholesterol as the study also showed that the bile acid pool sizes and the metabolism of cholic acid were the same in the two groups.

The increase is due, in part at least, to the cumulative effect of age but there are no studies of incident cases categorized by age to allow analysis of the different risks faced by each age group of developing gallstones. A prospective survey would be necessary to reveal such information.

Sex

Gallstones are also very clearly associated with sex. The exact strength of the relationship varies from study to study but most give a ratio of about 2 or 2.5:1, female to male. Several surveys have shown that the disparity between women and men diminishes in the older age groups and this has been related to a relatively reduced risk in postmenopausal women.

Specific metabolic studies designed to investigate physicochemical differences in the bile of women compared with men have shown that both the bile salt pool size and the total amount of chenodeoxycholic acid are reduced in women[48]. The total bile salt pool and chenodeoxycholic acid pool size decreases in Pima Indian girls at the menarche. This is accompanied by a slight rise in the biliary cholesterol saturation[49]. Puberty in the Pima Indian boys is also associated with an increase in their biliary cholesterol concentration but to a lesser degree than the girls[50]. Bennion also looked at changes in the bile of a woman undergoing surgical menopause and demonstrated an expansion of her bile salt pool size with a simultaneous decrease in her biliary cholesterol saturation[51].

The exact mechanism behind the contraction of the bile salt pool size in women of reproductive years is not known but it seems logical that endogenous female sex hormones mediate some change in the pathway of cholesterol metabolism.

Obesity

Obesity is the other condition that has been clearly associated with gallstones. Numerous epidemiological investigations have confirmed the clinical impression that gallstones are more frequent in obese people although findings in a few studies were limited to the younger age groups.

In support of these descriptive surveys, metabolic studies have demonstrated that bile is lithogenic in overweight individuals. Excess hepatic secretion of cholesterol appears to be the basic mechanism in this lithogenicity and is almost certainly a consequence of increased hepatic synthesis of cholesterol as bile salt and lecithin output are unchanged or even increased in obesity. It has been hypothesized that the underlying cause is increased acitivity of the enzyme, HMG CoA reductase. Weight reduction resulted in a significant lessening of cholesterol output in the subjects studied by Bennion and Grundy[36] with no change in the output of the other biliary constituents.

Obesity may be a stronger influence in younger women. Those overweight women who develop gallstones could be considered as being more susceptible than women of normal weight and therefore liable to developing them early on in their adult life.

Diet

The question of dietary influence on gallstone pathogenesis is a much more difficult one to evaluate than the preceding factors. Descriptive epidemiological studies have emphasized that factors related to lifestyle, and more specifically diet, are involved in the causation of gallstones. The wide international variations, especially between developed and developing nations, and the increase in prevalence within developed countries throughout the course of the last 100 years or more support a role for lifestyle and diet in the aetiology of gallstones. The major changes are an increase in animal protein consumption with little change in the overall protein intake, a great reduction in complex starch intake and therefore in fibre intake with an increase in simple sugars and sizeable increase in the intake of fat, this increase occurring in animal fats only. The greatest alterations in diet association with a change from rural to urban life in South Africa are an increase in sugar and meat consumption with a fivefold decrease in the consumption of fibre[34]. The changing nature of gallstone disease in Japan has been attributed to dietary changes occurring since the Second World War[21]. Observations such as these plus the increasing prevalence of a number of other diseases typical of western countries including ischaemic heart disease, diabetes mellitus, diverticular disease and cancer of the large bowel led Cleave, Burkitt, Painter, Trowell and others to the hypothesis that many of the diseases of western civilization were due to the consumption of highly refined and fibre-depleted carbohydrate diets. A recent prevalence survey of non-vegetarian and vegetarian women supports this theory in that the vegetarian women were significantly less likely to have gallstones[17]. The vegetarian women in this study consumed a diet that was higher in carbohydrate and fibre intake and much lower in fat intake than their non-vegetarian counterparts.

However, descriptive studies cannot give any specific details about which dietary components might be causative as they provide information about the total population, not diseased individuals within that population. They generate useful hypotheses that are subsequently more carefully examined using clinical metabolic studies and analytical epidemiological studies. The next chapter describes in detail the metabolic and analytical studies that have implicated specific dietary nutrients in the aetiology of gallstones.

Pregnancy

When Naunyn published his work[44] on gallstones in 1896 he relied heavily on the findings of his student, Schroder, who had analysed the autopsy series of Von Recklinghausen. In the analysis, Schroder had calculated the number of women with gallstones who had had at least one pregnancy and found it to be exactly 90%. However, no attempt had been made to determine the proportion of gallstone-free women who were also parous. Osler[45] adopted this figure for the later editions of his text, as did William Mayo[52] and many other authors throughout the first half of this century. So it was a well-accepted risk factor in the aetiology of gallstones without being statistically proven in the first place. A few autopsy surveys carried out during this period looked carefully for evidence of a positive association of pregnancy with gallstones and were unable to find one. Gross[25] reported that 89.8% of women with gallstones in Leeds were married compared with 86.6% without gallstones. Robertson and Dochat, in a meticulous review in 1944[53], came to the conclusion that pregnancy could not account to any great extent for the prevalence of gallstones in women compared with men. In a combined series of autopsy studies, where they grouped the results of their autopsy survey with those of a number of other authors, 79.6% of women with gallstones were parous and they estimated that about 79.2% of the female population become pregnant at some stage. Unfortunately the compiled series was not separated according to race and a large proportion were black and more likely to be parous yet less likely to have gallstones.

The studies carried out more recently do not provide any confirmatory evidence either. Studies which report a positive association of gallstones with pregnancy include the Framingham study[10] which showed risk with increasing pregnancies. The statistical significance of this trend, though, was not very strong. In a clinical survey by Wheeler et al.[54], parous women were more likely to have presented to hospital with symptomatic disease than nulliparous women. A highly statistically significant association of parity with clinical gallbladder disease was reported in an Appalachian community[55]. In the large study by Layde et al.[56], a trend was reported for increasing parity and surgically confirmed gallbladder disease but this was not significant when standardized for other risk factors.

Two important factors need to be taken into consideration when considering the effect of parity on the development of gallstones. Firstly, the age of the study population may influence the significance of the results. Horn reported in 1956[26] that there appeared to be a transitional age when the effect of parity changed. In his autopsy series, gallstones occurred more commonly in parous women up to the age of 50 after which nulliparous women had more gallstones. In the clinical study by Bernstein et al.[57], women with a history of gallbladder disease had a significantly higher average number of live births than women without such a history. This result was found in each age group from 30 to 62 but the relationship was strongest in the youngest age group. In Chippewa Indian women, pregnancy was associated with an increased risk of gallstones, especially in women less than 30 years old[58]. In a recent case–control study[59], the risk of developing gallstones was shown to increase in association with increasing parity, particularly among younger women. The risk was also negatively correlated to the age at first pregnancy, independent of parity. These results suggest that there may be a group of women who are susceptible to the early formation of gallstones and are selected out. The effect of parity, therefore, cannot be detected in the older, less susceptible age groups.

The other influence that appears to be important is the presence of symptoms. Virtually all the studies that found a positive relationship between gallbladder disease and parity were clinical studies of people who had either undergone surgery for symptomatic gallstones or had had some diagnostic procedure to confirm the presence of gallstones after complaining of symptoms. Autopsy surveys provide conflicting but usually negative evidence for the effect of parity on the development of gallstones. In a careful autopsy study and review by Van der Linden in 1961, his results showed a positive association between parity and symptomatic gallbladder disease[60]. This association was not seen in women with atypical symptoms of gallstones and asymptomatic stones and the author concluded that parity did not influence the development of gallstones, only the development of symptoms associated with gallstones. Studies of American Indians illustrate this effect well. In 1962 Sievers and Marquis[61] reported that early and frequent childbearing was associated with an increased risk of developing gallstones in Indian women of the southwestern areas of the United States although no figures were given in evidence of this claim. Their cases were derived from both surgical and autopsy data so included some asymptomatic cases. A clinical study of the Pima Indians supported the association[62] but a later prevalence survey of the same tribe using oral cholecystography failed to show any association[13]. It is evident that prevalence surveys are necessary to be able to determine the nature of the association of parity with gallstone risk as asymptomatic cases will also be included. As these studies are still few in number it is difficult to draw any conclusions from their results. In the ultrasonographic study of female office workers in Rome[15], the mean age-corrected number of pregnancies was significantly higher in women with gallstones. There was a slight 'dose–response' effect as women with three or more pregnancies had a higher risk than women with one or two pregnancies. In contrast, an ultrasonographic survey of women aged 45–70 in Oxford showed no effect of parity on the prevalence of gallstones[17] as did a similar survey in a Tyrolean village[16].

Metabolic studies do not provide consistent results either. One study has shown that there is incomplete emptying of the gallbladder after eating in the second and third trimester of pregnancy[63]. Gallbladder stasis may result and could influence the growth of gallstones provided that supersaturation and crystal nucleation has already occurred. Increased bile saturation during pregnancy has been reported recently as being associated with a decrease in the amount of chenodeoxycholic acid in the bile[64].

Thus, evidence for an association between pregnancy and the formation of new gallstones is weak. However, pregnancy may lead to the development of symptoms associated with previously quiescent gallstones.

Drugs

Oral contraceptives and exogenous oestrogens

The first report to identify an association between oral contraceptive use and gallstones was published in 1973[65]. The relative risk of developing gallstones for women who used the oral contraceptive was calculated to be 2.0. In the following year, similar findings for the effects of hormone replacement therapy were published by the same group[66]. The relative risk estimate for conjugated oestrogen therapy was 2.5. In both studies the result was highly statistically significant and was not confounded by other risk factors such as age or obesity. The oral contraceptive users appeared to have a greater risk of developing symptoms after 6–12 months of use compared with longer term use although the risk was still increased for long-term users compared with controls. Another study carried out around the same time reported that 32% of women undergoing biliary tract surgery had used the oral contraceptive pill compared with 19% of the controls[67]. It also yielded a relative risk of 2.0.

However, more recent studies do not confirm the above findings. A preliminary report of the Royal College of General Practitioners' Oral Contraception Study showed that pill-users were 1.32 times more likely to develop symptomatic gallstones than controls[68]. The result was not statistically significant and was even less so when the results of the full study were published in 1982[69] and the relative risk was calculated as 1.12. When the figures were analysed for duration of contraceptive use it was evident that there was an initial rise in incidence during the first 4 years of use followed by a decline over the next 6 years to a rate below that of the controls. The authors concluded that there was a positive association between oral contraceptive use and gallbladder disease that diminished with long-term use. They also pointed out that if this was the case then oral contraceptives do not probably cause the formation of new gallstones but encourage the development of symptoms associated with previously asymptomatic gallstones. Another study, which had earlier published evidence of a positive effect of oral contraceptives, reported similar findings to the RCGP study[56]. In this study the use of oral contraceptives had little overall effect on the risk of surgically confirmed gallbladder disease. Scragg *et al.*[59] reported an age-dependent variation in the risk associated with oral contraceptive use. The risk was greatest for women aged 29 years or less and decreased to below unity for all other age groups. However, their numbers were very small in these groups and were not significant, yet the authors conclude that there is a subpopulation of women who are susceptible to the formation of gallstones and who are likely to develop stones soon after exposure to oral contraceptives.

It is important to note that the above clinical studies analysed the effects of oral contraceptives on the prevalence of clinically apparent gallbladder disease. Further analysis is possible from data on asymptomatic populations that have been screened for evidence of gallstones. Both the Roman study[15] and the Oxford study[17] reported no significant difference in gallstone prevalence between women using the oral contraceptive pill and those who were not.

Lipid-lowering drugs

Clofibrate has been used widely in the treatment of hyperlipidaemia. The net effect is a mobilization of cholesterol from tissue stores and, as the excretory pathway, bile becomes relatively more lithogenic. Several studies have shown an increased prevalence of gallstones in patients taking clofibrate[70,71]. The authors in both studies admitted to the possibility that clofibrate may have induced symptoms from previously formed stones rather than inducing gallstone formation.

Bile acid sequestrants such as cholestyramine and colestipol are used as lipid-lowering agents because they are anion-exchange resins and bind bile salts in the intestines, preventing reabsorption of the bile salts. The reduced bile acid pool leads to enhanced conversion of cholesterol to bile acids in the liver. Theoretically, depletion of bile acids can lead to increased cholesterol saturation of bile but, in practice, this rarely happens, presumably because the compensatory hepatic synthesis of bile acids is always sufficient to prevent cholesterol supersaturation of bile.

Thiazide diuretics

Thiazide diuretics have been associated with an increased risk of acute cholecystitis. In a case–control study of lifetime drug histories, subjects who had taken thiazide diuretics in the month before admission were found to have twice the incidence of acute cholecystitis[72]. Van der Linden and his group estimated a relative risk of 2.1 for developing acute cholecystitis in patients who had purchased thiazides in the year before admission compared with those who had not[73]. No significant risk was associated with past purchase of thiazides and in Rosenberg's study the relative risk dropped to unity only 1 month after thiazides had been stopped. The finding of such a quick reversion to normality after thiazide cessation implies that gallstones themselves are not induced by thiazide therapy but that thiazides increase the risk of acute cholecystitis developing in a patient with gallstones.

ASSOCIATED CLINICAL CONDITIONS

A large number of clinical conditions have been associated with gallstones at one time or another. Some conditions have been thought to be causative while others were considered to be complications of gallstones. The same confusion and controversy surrounds clinical associations with gallstones as surrounds dietary and drug associations. There are some conditions which are undoubtedly caused by or which predispose to gallstones but these confirmed risks or complications are in the minority. Failure to allow for age, sex, parity, race, diet and obesity combined with observations being made on selected populations at autopsy have led to a wide variety of associations with gallstones, many being inaccurate and ill-founded. The discovery of the clinical coexistence of multiple gastrointestinal diseases is often due to a thorough gastrointestinal examination which reveals otherwise clinically silent disorders. The more definite associations along with several tenuous ones will be briefly outlined below.

Ileal disorders

Bile salts undergo most of their active reabsorption in the terminal section of the ileum and any disruption to this portion of the small bowel will affect the enterohepatic circulation of bile salts. Significant bile salt malabsorption can occur due to extensive small bowel loss as a consequence of a number of conditions: Crohn's disease, ileal resection and ileal bypass surgery for obesity. However, recent research into the composition of gallstones induced by ileal dysfunction has shown that the majority of stones are pigment gallstones[74].

Cystic fibrosis

Children with cystic fibrosis have an increased risk of developing gallstones due to abnormal mucus either interfering with bile flow or allowing gallstone nucleation. Cystic fibrosis is also associated with bile acid malabsorption. Pancreatic enzyme replacement therapy returns the bile saturation to normal.

Diabetes mellitus

Autopsy studies have suggested an association between gallstones and diabetes mellitus for a number of years. The risk was originally thought to be a result of the hypercholesterolaemia found in diabetes together with the high fat diet once recommended for diabetics. Autonomic neuropathy leading to atony of the gallbladder and gallstone formation due to stasis were also implicated. More recently the saturation index of bile has been shown to be significiantly elevated in maturity onset diabetics and not in juvenile diabetics[75]. The mechanism behind the cholesterol supersaturation of bile in these diabetics is uncertain.

Pancreatitis

Gallstones are more common in patients with pancreatitis as pancreatitis commonly results from the impaction of a gallstone in the lower end of the common bile duct.

Hepatic cirrhosis

Bouchier[76] reported that cirrhotics coming to autopsy had twice the frequency of gallstone disease compared with non-cirrhotics. These findings were not in complete agreement with those of Lieber[77] who recorded only slightly higher frequencies in cirrhotics while Newman and Northup[11] found no consistent association of gallstones with cirrhosis. Bouchier also found that pigment stones accounted for a much higher proportion of stones in cirrhotics than in the normal population implying a disturbance of the excretion of bilirubin rather than cholesterol[76].

Carcinoma of the gallbladder

An association between gallstones and carcinoma of the gallbladder is well established. Numerous autopsy studies have found that gallstones are present in 60–95% of gallbladder cancer cases although gallbladder cancer itself is a rare tumour found in less than 1% of gallstone cases. The main controversy surrounding the association between gallstones and gallbladder cancer has been the nature of the association in terms of causality. The idea that gallstones may play a causal role in the pathogenesis of carcinoma of the gallbladder is supported by a number of observations. Gallstones are present in the vast majority of patients with gallbladder cancer and the female to male ratio of the cancer is similar to that of gallstone disease, although gallstones are found in a similar percentage of men and women with cancer of the gallbladder. However, direct evidence of any causal link is not available and indirect evidence such as that given above implies only that the two conditions may have common causes.

Since only a small fraction of people with gallstones develop gallbladder cancer (< 1%) and approximately 20% of cancer cases do not have associated gallstones, even if gallstones are causal, it would have importance only in subpopulations of people identified as having a high risk of developing gallbladder cancer. Subpopulations such as these have been identified. American Indians, Mexicans and Mexican-Americans have been shown to have an incidence of carcinomatous change of 4–5% of gallbladders removed for stones[78].

Hyperlipidaemia

An increased risk of developing gallstones has been reported in certain types of hyperlipoproteinaemias. Type II hyperlipoproteinaemia is associated with hypercholesterolaemia, probably as a result of reduced hepatic conversion of cholesterol to cholic acid. The cholesterol-rich low density lipoprotein is increased in this disorder. Type IV hyperlipoproteinaemia is associated with an increase in triglyceride-rich very low density lipoprotein levels and an increase in bile acid pool size. The results of studies determining the importance of hyperlipoproteinaemias in the aetiology of gallstones are conflicting. Despite the abnormal biliary lipid metabolism seen in type II hypercholesterolaemia, there does not appear to be an increased tendency to form gallstones, yet, in the face of increased bile acid pools in type IV disease, gallstones are more likely to occur. Serum triglyceride appears to be more important in the determination of biliary lipid levels than serum cholesterol and serum triglyceride levels have been shown to be higher in gallstone patients.

Ischaemic heart disease

The problem of spurious associations with gallbladder disease becomes an even more complex one when an association with ischaemic heart disease is considered. Both conditions are extremely common in western communities so it is not surprising that the two have been considered to be related. Many studies have addressed the question of an association between gallstones and ischaemic heart disease but no consensus has been agreed upon. One study has shown an inverse relationship between the prevalence of gallstones and the prevalence of ischaemic heart disease[24].

Haemolytic anaemia

Gallstone prevalence is increased, but the mechanism is unclear, and the excess is composed at least in part of cholesterol stones, so the problem is not just one of raised bilirubin secretion.

GENETIC AND ETHNIC FACTORS

The evidence for genetic factors being important in the aetiology of gallstones is quite strong. The American Indian tribes, particularly those in the south-west such as the Pimas, show extremely high prevalence rates of cholesterol gallstones while gallstones very rarely develop in some ethnic groups such as the Masai. These ethnic variations correlate roughly with the biliary cholesterol concentration of the different races. Studies of the Pima Indians have shown that they have a dual genetic defect leading to the formation of supersaturated bile. They also secrete deficient amounts of bile acids[39].

Additional evidence for genetic influences is given by reports of familial aggregations of gallbladder disease. A positive family history of gallstones is commoner in people with gallstones compared with controls. Furthermore, sisters of women with cholesterol gallstones were shown to have bile that was more highly saturated with cholesterol than the controls[79].

References

1. Burkitt, D. P. and Trowell, H. (1975). *Refined Carbohydrate Foods and Disease: Some Implications of Dietary Fibre.* (London: Academic Press)
2. Cockburn, A. and Cockburn, E. (1983). *Mummies, Disease and Ancient Cultures* (Abridged version). (Cambridge: Cambridge University Press)
3. Siegel, R. E. (1968). Translation of Galen's *System of Physiology and Medicine.* (Basel)
4. Mani, N. (1959). *Die Historischen Grundlagen der Leberforschung.* (Basel)
5. Muleur, G. (1884). *Essai historique sur l'affection calculeure du fois depuis Hippocrate jusqu'a Fourcroy et Piajet (1801–1802).* No. 320, pp. 258. Paris
6. Morgagni, G. B. (1761). *The Seats and Causes of Diseases. Book III – Of Diseases of the Belly.* Translated by Alexander, B., Millar, A. and Caddell, T. 1769. (London: Johnson and Payne)
7. Crisp, E. (1841). On gallstones. *Lancet,* 365–70
8. Robertson, H. E. (1945). Silent gallstones. *Gastroenterology,* **5,** 345–71
9. Mainland, D. (1953). The risk of fallacious conclusions from autopsy data on the incidence of diseases with applications to heart disease. *Am. Heart J.,* **45,** 641–54
10. Friedman, G. D., Kannel, W. B. and Dawber, T. R. (1966). The epidemiology of gallbladder disease: observations in the Framingham study. *J. Chron. Dis.,* **19,** 273–92
11. Newman, H. F. and Northup, J. D. (1959). The autopsy incidence of gallstones. *Int. Abstr. Surg.,* **109,** 1–13
12. McPherson, K., Strong, P. M., Epstein, A. and Jones, L. (1981). Regional variations in the use of common surgical procedures: within and between England and Wales, Canada and U.S.A. *Soc. Sci. Med.,* **15,** 273–88
13. Sampliner, R. E., Bennett, P. H., Comess, L. J., Rose, F. A. and Burch, T. A. (1970). Gallbladder disease in Pima Indians. *N. Engl. J. Med.,* **283,** 1358–64
14. Bainton, D., Davies, G. T., Evans, K. T. and HuwGravelle, I. (1976). Gallbladder disease –

prevalence in a South Wales industrial town. *N. Engl. J. Med.*, **294**, 1147–9
15. Rome Group for the Epidemiology and Prevention of Cholelithiasis (GREPCO) (1984). Prevalence of gallstone disease in an Italian adult female population. *Am. J. Epidemiol.*, **119**, 796–805
16. Rhomberg, H. P., Judmair, G. and Lochs, A. (1984). How common are gallstones? *Br. Med. J.*, **4**, 1002 (letter)
17. Pixley, F., Wilson, D., McPherson, K. and Mann, J. (1985). Effect of vegetarianism on the development of gallstones in women. *Br. Med. J.*, **291**, 11–12
18. Brett, M. and Barker, D. J. P. (1976). The world distribution of gallstones. *Int. J. Epidemiol.*, **5**, 335–41
19. Becker, B. J. P. and Chatgidakis, C. B. (1952). Carcinoma of the gallbladder and cholelithiasis on the Witwatersrand; autopsy survey of racial incidence. *S. Afr. J. Clin. Sci.*, **3**, 13–22
20. Hwang, W. S. (1970). Cholelithiasis in Singapore. *Gut*, **11**, 141–52
21. Nakayama, F. and Miyake, H. (1970). Changing state of gallstone disease in Japan. *Am. J. Surg.*, **120**, 794–9
22. Marinovic, I., Guerra, C. and Larach, G. (1972). Incidencia de litiasis biliar en material de autopsias y analisis de composicion de los calculos. *Revista Medica de Chile*, **100**, 1320–7
23. MaPhotra, S. M. (1968). Epidemiological study of cholelithiasis among railroad workers in India, with special reference to causation. *Gut*, **9**, 290–5
24. Barker, D. J. P., Gardner, M. J., Power, C. and Hutt, M. S. R. (1979). Prevalence of gallstones at necropsy in nine British towns: A collaborative study. *Br. Med. J.*, **4**, 189–92
25. Gross, D. M. B. (1929). A statistical study of cholelithiasis. *J. Pathol. Bacteriol.*, **32**, 503–26
26. Horn, G. (1956). Observations on the aetiology of cholelithiasis. *Br. Med. J.*, **2**, 732–7
27. Watkinson, G. (1966). The autopsy incidence of gallstones in England and Scotland. *Proceedings of the III World Congress in Gastroenterology*, Tokyo, **4**, 157–62
28. Dessau, F. I. (1943). The incidence of gallstones in the higher age groups. *N. Engl. J. Med.*, **229**, 464–6
29. Cleland, J. B. (1953). Gallstones in seven thousand post-mortem examinations. *Med. J. Aust.*, **2**, 488–9
30. Holland, C. and Heaton, K. W. (1972). Increasing frequency of gallbladder operations in the Bristol clinical area. *Br. Med. J.* **3**, 672–5
31. Plant, J. C., Percy, I., Bates, T., Gastard, J. and Hita de Nercy, Y. (1973). Incidence of gallbladder disease in Canada, England and France. *Lancet*, **2**, 249–51
32. Bateson, M. C. and Bouchier, I. A. D. (1975). Prevalence of gallstones in Dundee: a necropsy study. *Br. Med. J.*, **4**, 427–30
33. Bateson, M. C. (1984). Gallbladder disease and cholecystectomy rate are independently variable. *Lancet*, **2**, 621–4
34. Burkitt, D. P. (1973). Some diseases characteristic of modern western civilization. *Br. Med. J.*, **1**, 274–8
35. Carey, M. C. and Small, S. M. (1978). The physical chemistry of cholesterol solubility in bile – relationship to gallstone formation and dissolution in man. *J. Clin. Invest.*, **61**, 998–1026
36. Bennion, L. J. and Grundy, S. M. (1975). Effects of obesity and caloric intake on biliary lipid metabolism in man. *J. Clin. Invest.*, **56**, 996–1011
37. Mabee, T. M., Meyer, P., DenBesten, L. and Mason, E. E. (1976). The mechanism of increased gallstone formation in obese human subjects. *Surgery*, **79**, 460–8
38. Swell, L., Bell, C. C. Jr. and Vlahcevic, Z. R. (1971). Relationship of bile acid pool size to biliary lipid excretion and the formation of lithogenic bile in man. *Gastroenterology*, **61**, 716–22
39. Grundy, S. M., Metzger, A. L. and Adler, R. D. (1972). Mechanisms of lithogenic bile formation in American Indian women with cholesterol gallstones. *J. Clin. Invest.*, **51**, 3026–43
40. Sedaghat, A. and Grundy, S. M. (1980). Cholesterol crystals and the formation of cholesterol gallstones. *N. Engl. J. Med.*, **302**, 1274–7
41. Whiting, M. J. and Watts, J. McK. (1984). Supersaturated bile from obese patients without gallstones supports cholesterol crystal growth but not nucleation. *Gastroenterology*, **86**, 243–8
42. Burnstein, M. J., Ilson, R. G., Petrunka, C. N., Taylor, R. D. and Strasberg, S. M. (1983).

Evidence for a potent nucleating factor in the gallbladder bile of patients with cholesterol gallstones. *Gastroenterology*, **85**, 801–7
43. Low-Beer, T. S. and Pomare, E. W. (1973). Regulation of bile salt pool size in man. *Br. Med. J.*, **2**, 338–40
44. Naunyn, B. (1896). *A Treatise on Cholelithiasis*. Translated by Garrod, A. The New Sydenham Society
45. Osler, W. B. (1901). Diseases of the digestive system. VI. Cholelithiasis. *Osler's Principles and Practices of Medicine*. 4th Edn., pp. 568–75. London
46. Littler, T. R. and Ellis, G. R. (1952). Gallstones: a clinical survey. *Br. Med. J.*, **1**, 842
47. Valdivieso, V., Palma, R., Wunkhaus, R., Antezana, C., Severin, C. and Contreras, A. (1978). Effect of aging on biliary lipid composition and bile acid metabolism in normal Chilean women. *Gastroenterology*, **74**, 871–4
48. Bennion, L. J., Mott, D. M., Spagnola, A. M. and Bennett, P. H. (1978). A biochemical basis for the higher prevalence of cholesterol gallstones in women. *Clin. Res.*, **26**, 496
49. Bennion, L. J., Drobny, E., Knowler, W. C., Ginsberg, R. L., Garnick, M. B., Adler, R. D. and Duane, W. C. (1978). Sex differences in the size of bile acid pools. *Metabolism*, **27**, 961–9
50. Bennion, L. J., Knowler, W. C., Mott, D. M., Spagnola, A. M. and Bennett, P. H. (1979). Development of lithogenic bile during puberty in Pima Indians. *N. Engl. J. Med.*, **300**, 873–6
51. Bennion, L. J. (1977). Changes in bile lipids accompanying oophorectomy in a premenopausal woman. *N. Engl. J. Med.*, **297**, 709–11
52. Mayo, W. (1911). 'Innocent' gallstones a myth. *J. Am. Med. Assoc.*, **56**, 1021–4
53. Robertson, H. E. and Dochat, G. R. (1944). Pregnancy and gallstones. *Int. Abstr. Surg.*, **78**, 193–204
54. Wheeler, M., Loftus Hills, L. and Laby, B. (1970). Cholelithiasis: a clinical and dietary survey. *Gut*, **11**, 430–7
55. Richardson, J. D., Scutchfield, F. D., Proudfoot, W. H. and Benenson, A. S. (1973). Epidemiology of gallbladder disease in an Appalachian community. *Health Ser. Rep.*, **88**, 241–6
56. Layde, P. M., Vessey, M. P. and Yeates, D. (1982). Risk factors for gallbladder disease: a cohort study of young women attending Family Planning Clinics. *J. Epidemiol. Commun. Health*, **36**, 274–8
57. Bernstein, R. A., Werner, L. H. and Rimm, A. A. (1973). Relationship of gallbladder disease to parity, obesity and age. *Health Ser. Rep.*, **88**, 925–36
58. Thistle, J. L., Eckhart, K. L., Nensel, R. E., Norbrega, F. T., Poehling, G. G., Reimer, M. and Schoenfield, L. J. (1971). Prevalence of gallbladder disease among Chippewa Indians. *Mayo Clin. Proc.*, **46**, 603–8
59. Scragg, R. K. R., McMichael, A. J. and Seamark, R. F. (1984). Oral contraceptives, pregnancy and endogenous oestrogen in gallstone disease: a case–control study. *Br. Med. J.*, **288**, 1795–9
60. Van der Linden, W. (1961). Some biological traits in female gallstone-disease patients. *Acta Chirurgica Scand.*, suppl. 269
61. Sievers, M. L. and Marquis, J. R. (1962). The Southwestern American Indian's burden: biliary disease. *J. Am. Med. Assoc.*, **182**, 570–2
62. Commess, L. J., Bennett, P. H. and Burch, T. A. (1967). Clinical gallbladder disease in Pima Indians – its high prevalence in contrast to Framingham, Mass. *N. Engl. J. Med.*, **277**, 894–8
63. Braverman, D. Z., Johnson, M. L. and Kern, F. (1980). Effects of pregnancy and contraceptive steroids on gallbladder function. *N. Engl. J. Med.*, **302**, 363–4
64. Everson, G. T., McKinley, C., Lawson, M., Johnson, M. and Kern, F. Jr. (1982). Gallbladder function in the human female: effect of the ovulatory cycle, pregnancy and contraceptive steroids. *Gastroenterology*, **82**, 711–9
65. Boston Collaborative Drug Surveillance Programme (1973). Oral contraceptives and venous thromboembolic disease, surgically confirmed gallbladder disease and breast tumours. *Lancet*, **1**, 1399–404
66. Boston Collaborative Drug Surveillance Programme (1974). Surgically confirmed gallbladder disease, venous thromboembolism and breast tumours in relation to postmenopausal oestrogen treatment. *N. Engl. J. Med.*, **290**, 15–19

67. Stolley, P. D., Tonascia, J. A., Tockman, M. S., Sartwell, P. E., Rutledge, A. H. and Jacobs, M. P. (1975). Thrombosis with low-oestrogen oral contraceptives. *Am. J. Epidemiol.* **102**, 197–208

68. Royal College of General Practitioners (1974). Oral contraceptives and health. (London: Pitman Medical)

69. Royal College of General Practitioners: Oral Contraception Study (1982). Oral contraceptives and gallbladder disease. *Lancet*, **2**, 957–9

70. Coronary Drug Project Research Group (1977). Gallbladder disease as a side effect of drugs influencing lipid metabolism. *N. Engl. J. Med.*, **296**, 1185–90

71. Cooper, J., Geizerova, H. and Oliver, M. F. (1975). Clofibrate and gallstones. *Lancet*, **1**, 1083

72. Rosenberg, L., Shapiro, S., Slone, D., Kaufman, D. W., Miettinen, O. S. and Stolley, P. D. (1980). Thiazides and acute cholecystitis. *N. Engl. J. Med.*, **303**, 546–8

73. Van der Linden, W., Ritter, B. and Edlund, G. (1984). Acute cholecystitis and thiazides. *Br. Med. J.*, **289**, 654–5

74. Pitt, H. A., Lewinski, M. A., Muller, E. L., Porter-Fink, V. and DenBesten, L. (1984). Ileal resection-induced gallstones: altered bilirubin or cholesterol metabolism? *Surgery*, **96**, 154–60

75. Ponz de Leon, M., Murphy, G. M. and Dowling, R. H. (1978). Physiological factors influencing serum bile acid levels. *Gut*, **19**, 32–9

76. Bouchier, I. A. D. (1969). Postmortem study of the frequency of gallstones in patients with cirrhosis of the liver. *Gut*, **10**, 705–10

77. Lieber, M. M. (1952). The incidence of gallstones and their correlation with other diseases. *Ann. Surg.*, **135**, 394–405

78. Weiss, K. M. and Hanis, C. L. (1984). All 'silent' gallstones are not silent. *N. Engl. J. Surg.*, **310**, 657–8

79. Danzinger, R. G., Gordon, H., Schoenfield, L. J. and Thistle, J. L. (1972). Lithogenic bile in siblings of young women with cholelithiasis. *Mayo Clin. Proc.*, **47**, 762–6

2
Aetiology of Cholesterol Gallstones

R.K.R. SCRAGG

INTRODUCTION

The epidemiology of gallstone disease suggests that the commonly occurring causes of cholesterol gallstones can be divided into two major categories: dietary and hormonal. The large international variations in gallstone prevalence, with gallstones being common in developed countries but rare in underdeveloped countries, suggest that factors related to lifestyle, in particular diet, have an important role in gallstone aetiology. Secondly, the well-documented increased gallstone prevalence in women, compared with men, supports a role for factors associated with the female sex, such as pregnancy and oral contraceptives. Other important risk factors, such as obesity and hypertriglyceridaemia, may themselves possibly be the results of altered dietary and hormonal risk profiles.

Studies of gallstone aetiology can be divided into three major categories:

(1) Descriptive epidemiological studies, mainly of gallstone prevalence at autopsy, which, by comparing international and temporal variations in gallstone prevalence, have drawn attention to the importance of lifestyle factors, such as diet, in gallstone aetiology, and by comparing prevalence rates between the sexes have emphasized a role for hormonal factors.

(2) Clinical experimental studies of the effects of dietary nutrients or sex hormones on bile cholesterol saturation in small selected groups of patients which have attempted to elucidate the dietary and hormonal mechanisms involved in gallstone aetiology.

(3) Analytical epidemiological studies (e.g. case–control, prospective or intervention studies) which have compared the dietary intake or hormonal exposure of persons with and without gallstones, and thus provide an empirical test of the results and conclusions of the previous two categories. This is not to suggest that these research categories follow a temporal sequence, but rather to emphasize the role of each category. In fact, these three areas of research have continued simultaneously, with each stimulating and complementing the other.

In the following discussion greatest attention will be given to the analytical epidemiological studies. Less emphasis will be given to clinical experimental studies because their often discordant results do not provide a clear picture, particularly of the effect of diet on biliary metabolism, although they can offer biological insights into the results of the analytical epidemiological studies. Little or no reference is made to animal studies for two reasons. Firstly, they are rendered superfluous by the many studies carried out on humans. Secondly, it cannot be assumed that the biliary lipid metabolism of animals responds to dietary or hormonal factors in a similar way to that of humans[1]. To include a systematic review of animal studies would open up a Pandora's box of studies carried out on many species which would only confuse an already complex issue.

DIET

The notion that diet is involved in the aetiology of gallstones has existed since the time of Paracelsus (AD 1493–1541), who in the sixteenth century proposed that digestive disturbances produce an 'acidulation of the blood' which acted on the bile to form gallstones[2]. During the ensuing centuries many theories were published by medical practitioners which attempted to explain a role for diet in gallstone aetiology. But it was not until the unexpected finding by Dam and Christensen in 1952, that feeding sucrose produced cholesterol gallstones in hamsters[3], that medical researchers begin to systematically study the dietary aetiology of cholesterol gallstones.

International variations in gallstone prevalence

The large variations in gallstone prevalence between countries provide some of the strongest evidence that lifestyle factors, of which diet is one of the most important, are involved in gallstone aetiology. Populations living in the Americas, such as Pima Indians, Chileans and United States whites, have the highest gallstone prevalence rates in the world. For example, the prevalence rates in adult female Pimas[4] are about 70% and about 50–60% in adult female Chileans[5]. Northern and central European countries, such as Sweden, Czechoslovakia, Germany and Austria also have very high gallstone prevalence rates, followed by other westernized populations such as New Zealand, Australia, England, Scotland, Ireland and Norway[6]. Asian countries (e.g. Singapore and Thailand) have intermediate gallstone prevalence rates, while in underdeveloped populations, such as in Africa and New Guinea, cholesterol gallstones are extremely rare[7]. Furthermore, American blacks have much higher gallstone prevalence rates than do African blacks[8], despite their common ancestry.

International comparisons have shown that per capita intake of calories, animal protein and animal fats are each positively correlated with gallstone prevalence[9]. However, in this particular study it was not possible to decide which of these dietary factors was causing gallstones since the dietary factors were also highly correlated with each other.

26

Temporal variations in gallstone prevalence

Progressive increases in the gallstone prevalence rate during this century in several countries also support a role for lifestyle and dietary factors in gallstone aetiology. The gallstone prevalence rate in Helsinki increased more than tenfold[10] from the 1860s to the 1930s. Over this period, food consumption changed from a subsistence diet, based on bark and bread, to a typical modern western diet as a result of increased intakes of meat, dairy products and sugar. In Athens, the crude gallstone prevalence rate for both sexes combined increased by threefold[11] from the 1920s to the 1970s. The authors of this report attributed the changes to an increased consumption of sugar and white flour. In Tokyo, the gallstone prevalence doubled during a 15 year period beginning in 1949[12]. During this time in Japan, per capita consumption of fat, animal protein, cholesterol and sugar all greatly increased, vegetable intake decreased, while, surprisingly, consumption of calories changed little[13].

The descriptive epidemiological studies described above have shown conclusively that the prevalence of gallstones varies between cultures and over time. Their findings strongly support a role for lifestyle factors, including diet, in gallstone aetiology. However, descriptive studies are not able to identify which lifestyle factors (dietary or otherwise) are causative, since they provide information about the total population and not specifically the persons with gallstones in that population. Any dietary components which may have a role in causing gallstones can only be identified from analytical epidemiological studies which compare the diets of persons with or without gallstones.

Experimental studies

Experimental studies are defined here as studies of humans which measure in a clinical setting the effect produced on the cholesterol saturation of bile by varying the intake of dietary nutrients. They are important because of their contribution in elucidating the biological mechanisms associated with those dietary nutrients which the descriptive epidemiological studies have suggested may be important in causing gallstones.

The nutrients which have been investigated in metabolic studies are fat (saturated and unsaturated), cholesterol, fibre, refined carbohydrate, alcohol and total caloric intake. (Theoretically, total caloric intake is not a specific nutrient but represents the energy taken in from all nutrients combined.) There exists a strong interrelationship between some of these nutrients such that variation in the intake of one is often accompanied by a changed intake of another. For instance, diets containing high quantities of refined carbohydrates usually contain less fibre, and vice versa. Because refined carbohydrates, particularly sucrose, are an efficient source of energy, increasing their intake usually results in an increased caloric intake. Also, saturated fats and cholesterol occur in the same types of foods, especially red meats, so that variations in their intake are often in the same direction.

In reviewing the effects of the various dietary intakes on bile acid metabolism, evidence is presented primarily from studies of bile, in which measurements have been made of secretion rates and concentrations of the three major biliary lipids – cholesterol, bile acids and phospholipids – in addition to the cholesterol saturation index. Sterol balance studies are also referred to, mainly to illustrate the phenomenon of cholesterol homoeostasis. The results of these experimental studies are summarized in Table 2.1.

Table 2.1 Summary of experimental studies which have investigated the effect of *increased* intake of a nutrient on biliary cholesterol saturation – study reference numbers listed

Nutrient	Cholesterol saturation		
	Increase	*No change*	*Decrease*
Calories	14, 16, 17		
Fats			
(1) polyunsaturated (vs. unsaturated)	20	18, 19	21, 22
(2) total fat	24, 25	19, 23	
Cholesterol	27, 28, 29	30, 31, 32	
Refined carbohydrates	49	48, 50	
Fibre		56, 57, 58 61, 62	53, 54, 55
Alcohol		70	66, 69, 71

Total caloric intake

The well-recognized observation that obesity increases the risk of gallstones has led some researchers, perhaps on the assumption that there is a positive correlation between caloric intake and obesity, to postulate an increased risk of gallstones amongst those who eat high calorie diets[14,15].

In a study on cholecystectomized patients with T-tubes in the common bile duct, postoperative bile was collected over a period of 3–37 days, during which dietary intakes of protein, carbohydrate, fat and total calories were varied every 3–6 days. For the total period of the study, there was a significant positive correlation between mean caloric intake and mean biliary cholesterol concentration for gallstone subjects ($r = 0.81$, $p < 0.001$), but not for controls[16]. A second study by the same research group on four patients with gallstones found that a change from a low calorie diet (range 900–1300 kcal/day) to a high calorie diet (range 2200–2800 kcal/day) caused an elevation in the biliary cholesterol saturation in each subject[14].

The effects of caloric restriction are the opposite to the findings described above. When obese subjects were put on a low calorie diet, in which the proportions of the major nutrients were unchanged, both the secretion of cholesterol into bile, as well as the saturation index, were reduced, although these changes were simultaneous with a lowering of body weight[17].

Dietary fats

The studies which have investigated the effect of dietary fat on biliary metabolism are of two types, those comparing the effect of polyunsaturated fats
with saturated fats, and studies comparing high and low intakes of fat.

Studies which have compared the effects of saturated versus polyunsaturated fats on biliary lipids show that there is variability in response to
the type of fat, which may be associated with the presence of hypertriglyceridaemia in study subjects. For instance, substituting margarine for
butter in the diets of healthy normolipidaemic volunteers did not significantly
alter the ratio of cholesterol to bile acids in their bile[18], while the median
cholesterol saturation index of healthy young males was the same either on
a saturated fat diet of olive oil or a polyunsaturated diet of sunflower oil[19].
However, patients with hypertriglyceridaemia who changed from a saturated
fat diet after 1 month to a polyunsaturated fat diet for another month, were
found to have an increased biliary cholesterol saturation[20], although earlier
studies of gallstone patients reported that unsaturated fats lowered liver
cholesterol secretion[21] or increased the cholesterol holding capacity of bile[22],
compared with saturated fats. The latter two changes would be theoretically
associated with a lowered cholesterol saturation.

With regard to the level of fat intake, rather than the type of fat, nearly all
of these studies have substituted fat for carbohydrate or vice versa, and have
reported results which are inconsistent. Patients with hyperlipidaemia, who
changed their fat intake from 5% to 40% of calories, were observed to
increase the liver secretion of all three bile lipids (cholesterol, bile acids
and phospholipids), so it is unlikely that their biliary cholesterol saturation
changed[23]. Healthy young males who changed to a low fat–high carbohydrate
diet did not alter their median cholesterol saturation[19].

In contrast, a low fat–high carbohydrate diet was found to lower the molar
cholesterol concentration and increase the molar bile acid concentration of
bile in patients with hyperlipidaemia[24], while in another study a low fat and
protein diet, supplemented with sugar, increased the bile acid pool in gallstone
patients and healthy subjects[25]. These latter two studies suggest that a low
fat–high carbohydrate diet lowers biliary cholesterol saturation. However,
one cannot conclude which of the two nutrients is responsible for the alterations to biliary metabolism since the proportions of fat and carbohydrate
intake have been changed simultaneously.

Dietary cholesterol

Dietary cholesterol has often been thought to have a role in the aetiology of
gallstones ever since Aschoff and Bacmeister first proposed in 1909 that
cholelithiasis was a metabolic disorder due to excess cholesterol in bile[26].
Three studies have found that increasing dietary cholesterol increases or
produces changes consistent with an increased cholesterol saturation. The
daily addition of 750 mg of cholesterol over a period of 3 weeks to the diets
of young healthy men without gallstones caused a statistically significant
($p < 0.01$) lowering in the ratio of phospholipids and bile acids to cholesterol,

and in gallstone patients a relatively greater increase in the liver secretion of cholesterol compared with phospholipids and bile acids[27]. Gallstone subjects and normal controls who ate diets which contained 500 mg, 750 mg and 1000 mg of cholesterol per day for three consecutive periods of 3 weeks, had successive increases in their mean bile saturation index[28]. Gallstone patients taking chenodeoxycholic acid, who were given a normal diet containing 600 mg of cholesterol per day for 1 month, followed by a low-cholesterol diet of 100 mg per day for a further month, had a significant ($p < 0.01$), although small, lowering of their cholesterol saturation index[29].

In contrast, another three studies have reported that increases in dietary cholesterol do not alter the cholesterol saturation of bile. In healthy volunteers who increased their dietary cholesterol from 1 g to 2 g per day, the ratios of the concentrations of total bile acids/cholesterol and phospholipid/cholesterol were not significantly altered[30]. An increased dietary intake of 1.5 g of cholesterol per day for 6 days did not increase the cholesterol saturation of a 60-year-old female gallstone patient[31]. A study of postmenopausal nor-molipidaemic and hyperlipidaemic women found that a diet of five eggs per day for 2 weeks did not alter their mean cholesterol saturation index[32].

It is difficult to reconcile the opposite findings from those studies which have examined the effect of dietary cholesterol on cholesterol saturation. There is evidence that individuals respond differently to increased dietary cholesterol either by suppressing liver cholesterol synthesis; by increasing faecal excretion of cholesterol or bile acids; or by decreasing the percentage of dietary cholesterol absorbed from the gut[33]. The effect of these cholesterol homoeostatic mechanisms is to limit the body pool of cholesterol. Individuals may use these mechanisms singly or in combination in response to increased cholesterol consumption[34,35]. This individual variation in response may be one explanation for the inconsistent results from studies of dietary cholesterol and its effect on bile. It is also possible that gallstone patients as a group respond by a different homoeostatic mechanism to increased dietary cholesterol compared to persons without gallstones. Some evidence for this is provided by Lee et al.[28]. While they observed that increased dietary cholesterol increased the biliary saturation index of both gallstone patients and healthy controls, they also reported a different response of biliary bile acids and phospholipids to increased dietary cholesterol between controls and gallstone subjects. With increasing dietary cholesterol the molar percentage of bile acids fell in gallstone patients, but remained unchanged in controls, while the molar percentage of phospholipids increased in gallstone subjects and was unchanged in controls.

The other important implication of cholesterol homoeostasis is that it may act to limit the effect of dietary cholesterol on biliary cholesterol saturation. Furthermore, only about 300 mg per day of cholesterol are absorbed on a typical western diet, yet liver synthesis is approximately 1 g per day[36]. Thus, as a source of cholesterol entering the bile, the liver is likely to be of much greater importance than diet.

Refined carbohydrates

Following on from Cleave's hypothesis that many of the modern diseases of western civilization were due to the overconsumption of refined carbohydrates, Heaton suggested that gallstones may be similarly caused[37]. Two mechanisms have been put forward to explain a possible association between refined carbohydrates and the risk of gallstones.

Firstly, a diet rich in refined carbohydrates lacks the bulking and satiating effect of a fibre-replete diet, so that caloric overconsumption, and consequently obesity, which increases the risk of gallstones, are more likely to occur. This has been observed in gallstone subjects who increased their dietary energy intake and weight by eating freely a refined carbohydrate diet for 6 weeks, compared with the 6-week period when they ate an unrefined carbohydrate diet[38].

The second mechanism (which has been developed more fully by Cleave[39] in relation to diabetes) is that the rapid absorption by the gut of refined carbohydrates stimulates the pancreas to secrete more insulin, which in turn stimulates the liver to secrete cholesterol-saturated bile[40]. The evidence concerning the acute effects of simple and complex carbohydrates (from single meals) on postprandial responses in blood insulin concentration is conflicting[41-43]. However, studies of longer term increases (over several weeks) in sucrose intake show a consistent increase in fasting plasma insulin and glucose concentrations and an increase of insulin response to sucrose[44-47].

At least three studies have examined the effect of refined carbohydrates on biliary metabolism. A Swedish study found no difference in the biliary concentrations of cholesterol, bile acids and phospholipids when normolipidaemic gallstone patients on a normal diet were compared with the same type of patients who had eaten a high sucrose diet for 2 weeks[48]. However, this study also reported that gallstone patients with pre-beta hyperlipoproteinaemia on the high sucrose diet had a decreased concentration of bile acids, particularly chenodeoxycholic acid, when compared with normolipidaemic gallstone patients on the high sucrose diet.

A Bristol study, in which gallstone subjects acted as their own controls found that 6 weeks of eating a diet high in refined carbohydrates caused the mean cholesterol saturation index to significantly rise from 1.20 to 1.50 while on a diet low in refined carbohydrates, but also low in dietary fibre[49]. Because it was not possible to decide whether the changes in the saturation index observed in this study were due to fibre or refined carbohydrates, the same group carried out a further study on gallstone patients of similar design in which biliary and blood lipid factors were compared after 6 weeks each on diets which contained high or low sucrose intakes[50]. This study found no changes in biliary metabolism between the two diets, but did observe a significant increase in triglyceride and decrease in high density lipoprotein (HDL) cholesterol on the high sucrose diet; changes which are known to be associated with an increased risk of gallstone formation. However, the study also reported a significantly increased caloric intake, body weight and decreased fibre intake on the high sucrose diet, each of which may have contributed to the changes in lipid metabolism.

Dietary fibre

A role for dietary fibre in the aetiology of gallstone disease was first put forward independently by Heaton[37], and Burkitt[51]. Burkitt's epidemiological observations on the rarity of gallstones amongst black Africans led him to Cleaves's hypothesis that many of the western diseases, including gallstones, were the result of overconsumption of refined carbohydrates. Burkitt's contribution was to shift the emphasis away from an excess of refined carbohydrates to a deficiency in dietary fibre[52].

Since the publication of the hypothesis associating gallstones with a deficiency in fibre intake, a number of studies have been carried out to examine the effect of fibre on biliary metabolism. Most of these studies have used wheat bran.

Bran, which is composed mainly of hemicelluloses, appears to lower the cholesterol saturation of bile in those with supersaturated bile, but not in those whose bile is unsaturated or who have colonic disease. The mean saturation index in gallstone subjects decreased from 1.49 to 1.29 after eating an average of 57 g of bran per day for 4–6 weeks[53]. Another group of gallstone subjects also lowered their mean saturation index from 1.43 to 0.76 after 4 weeks on a diet which was supplemented by 50 g of wheat bran per day[54]. People without gallstones who consumed 30 g of wheat bran per day for 2 months were also able to lower their saturation index only if it was initially[55] above 1.0.

Other studies have found that the addition of bran to the diet has no effect on biliary cholesterol saturation. The mean saturation index in a group of young healthy men remained at about 0.6 after the addition of 30 g of wheat bran per day to the diet for 6 weeks[56]. Another group of young healthy males was also unable to change its saturation index away from an average initial level of about 1.0 after adding approximately 30 g per day of wheat bran to the diet for 4–8 weeks[57]. People with diverticular disease were also unable to alter their bile saturation index by adding wheat bran for a period of 12 months[58]. The lack of any change in the mean saturation index of subjects in this last study may be because their colonic disease interfered with the action of bran which is thought to occur in the right colon[56].

All the studies which reported a bran-induced fall in the saturation index also reported a fall in the deoxycholate proportion of total bile acids[53-55]. This suggests that bran may protect against gallstones by altering the metabolism of deoxycholate. The fall in the deoxycholate proportion is most likely due to decreased formation of deoxycholate by bacteria in the colon[59], possibly because of a lowered colonic pH. That bran does not alter the halflife for cholate and chenodeoxycholate further supports the notion that bran does not act by binding bile acids to increase their excretion[53,60].

Two studies have reported that the ingestion of other types of dietary fibre does not alter biliary cholesterol saturation. Morbidly obese subjects who were given a combination of vegetable and cereal fibre for 6 weeks slightly increased their saturation index[61]. The second study found that neither psyllium hydrocolloid nor lignin given to gallstone subjects had any effect on the saturation index or the proportions of the major bile acids[62].

32

It appears that in the same way some types of dietary fibre lower serum cholesterol while others do not[63], so it seems that only certain types of dietary fibre can lower the saturation index in persons with supersaturated bile. It is possible that fibre which acts by inhibiting the bacterial formation of deoxycholate (e.g. bran) is protective against the formation of gallstones, while those fibres which strongly bind bile acids may actually increase the saturation index of bile (and the risk of gallstones) by depleting the bile acid pool. The latter possibility is supported by the finding that prolonged administration of cholestyramine, which strongly binds to bile acids in the gut, induces the formation of gallstones in baboons[64].

Alcohol

The effect of alcohol ingestion on biliary metabolism and cholesterol saturation has been little studied by clinicians or laboratory scientists. This perhaps reflects a lack of awareness of the epidemiological literature which shows that alcohol appears to protect against the formation of cholesterol gallstones. However, the metabolic studies of alcohol ingestion which have been carried out, as well as studies of patients with cirrhosis, do support the epidemiological literature.

In a sterol balance study in which alcohol was given to hyperlipidaemic patients and healthy volunteers for periods of up to 48 days, faecal acidic sterol excretion increased while neutral sterol excretion was unchanged[65]. The authors concluded that the increased bile acid excretion could be due to decreased bile acid reabsorption or to increased conversion of cholesterol to bile acids. If the latter explanation is correct, then alcohol should theoretically increase bile acid secretion and lower the saturation index. In support of this conclusion, patients with alcoholic pancreatitis, but normal plasma liver enzymes, were found to have an increased secretion of bile acids compared with healthy volunteers[66]. Thus chronic ingestion of alcohol appears to increase liver bile acid secretion which would theoretically lower the cholesterol saturation index. This is opposite to the effects of acute alcohol ingestion which reduces liver bile acid secretion[66].

Cirrhosis patients have been described as having an increased prevalence of pigment stones, but not cholesterol stones[67,68]. In agreement with this, the cholesterol saturation index in cirrhosis is either reduced[69] or normal[70].

In apparently the only study of alcohol and cholesterol saturation in healthy adults to date, a moderate 39 g daily increase in alcohol intake by subjects with a normally low consumption of alcohol (range 0–6 g/day) over 6 weeks, significantly lowered[71] the bile cholesterol saturation index by 20%. More similar studies are required before firm conclusions can be made about the effect of alcohol on the saturation index in healthy subjects.

Summary of experimental studies

By and large, the results of studies which have investigated the effect of the major dietary nutrients on bile metabolism and the saturation index are inconsistent (Table 2.1). The only area of consistency is the effect of increased caloric intake in raising cholesterol saturation index by bran.

A possible reason for the inconsistency in the results of the studies listed in this table is variation between individuals in their response to dietary variables, for which there is strong evidence contained within some of these studies. For instance, Sarles and co-workers[16] found, for the total period of their study, that there was a significant positive correlation between mean caloric intake and mean biliary cholesterol concentration for gallstone subjects, but not for controls. Patients with hypertriglyceridaemia[20], which itself is associated with an increased risk of gallstones, respond differently to polyunsaturated fats from healthy young volunteers[18,19]. Individual variation exists for the mechanisms used to maintain cholesterol homoeostasis[34,35]. Also, bran appears only to lower the saturation index of those whose bile is already supersaturated[53-55]. However, the inconsistent results of these studies may also be due, in part, to the poor precision associated with the measurement of biliary cholesterol saturation[72].

To find out whether gallstone subjects respond differently to dietary nutrients from controls, controlled studies comparing diseased and disease-free persons are required. So far, only three such studies appear to have been carried out. Two research groups have reported differences between gallstone subjects and healthy controls in their biliary response to changes in caloric[16] and cholesterol intake[28]. In contrast one report[25] found no difference between cases and controls in the frequency of bile acid cycling when dietary fat, protein and carbohydrate were changed. There is clearly a need for further studies to compare the responses of gallstone patients and controls to changes in the intakes of the dietary nutrients.

Case–control studies

The importance of the case–control studies is that they comprise observations on representative samples of diseased and disease-free persons, and thus provide an empirical test for the relevance of the dietary hypotheses developed by the descriptive epidemiological and clinical metabolic studies. Case–control studies have been carried out in Marseilles[73-76], Paris[77], Brisbane[78], Melbourne[79], Edmonton[80], Nova Scotia[81], Rome[82] and Adelaide[83]. A case–control study has also been carried out on Pima Indians[84], while the prospective Framingham study is also included in this list because its dietary analysis, in part, was along the lines of a case–control study[85].

Before examining their results, some comments about their respective study designs are worthwhile. Firstly, the statistical power of most of these studies to exclude a type II error is small. Based on data from those studies which published standard errors with their means[77,79-81,83,84], the median required number of cases is in the region of 150–200 to detect a 10% case–control difference in mean caloric intake with a two-tail type I error of 0.05 and a type II error of 0.10. Thus, only the Adelaide study with 267 cases[83] and the Rome study with 160 cases[82] have case numbers equal to or above the required sample size. The next largest study had 101 cases[75], while all others, including the Framingham study[85], measured the diets of less than 100 gallstone cases.

The selection of cases and controls is also important. Ideally, cases and controls should be representative of all gallstone patients and gallstone-free persons, respectively, in the total population. Only the Framingham[85], Pima Indian[84], Nova Scotia[81] and Adelaide[83] studies had community selected controls. Two studies carried out in Marseilles[75,76] used controls from healthy working populations to avoid the selection biases associated with hospital-selected controls. The remaining studies all used hospital controls exclusively[73,74,77-79,82]. The use of hospital controls is fraught with danger as they all have some symptom or disease which may be related to, or the result of, the study variable (e.g. diet). The possibility always remains high that they are not representative of all gallstone-free persons, such that their mean levels of dietary consumption may be biased up or down.

The method of dietary assessment is also important. Most studies used methods currently considered acceptable for measuring dietary intake[86]: specifically the food-frequency method[83,84]; the diet-history method[79,82,85] or similar type of interview by a dietitian[73-78]; or the diet-record method[81]. The Edmonton Study used the diet-recall method[80], which may under-report dietary intake[86], although with the case–control study design it can be assumed that the degree of any under-reporting is likely to be equal for cases and controls if the interview is standardized for both groups.

However, the period of dietary assessment is also important. A number of studies measured current intake of cases months or years after cholecystectomy[80,81,84,85]. The diets recorded for cases in these latter studies may not be the same as that eaten prior to the onset of gallstone disease, since there is evidence that gallstone cases lower their caloric intake after the onset of symptoms or after cholecystectomy[75].

The nutrients which have been most reported in the case–control studies are total caloric intake, fats, carbohydrate, protein, cholesterol and alcohol. Except for protein, these nutrients, in addition to fibre, are those which have been investigated in clinical experimental studies. As mentioned earlier, the case–control studies provide an empirical test for the hypotheses and mechanisms derived from the experimental studies. This is important and necessary since the dietary intakes used in experimental studies may not reflect those in everyday life.

Total calories, fats and carbohydrates

The results of mean daily caloric intake found in all case–control studies, except for the Adelaide study, are listed in Table 2.2. It is apparent from the column of the ratios of mean intake for cases and controls that there is no consistent increase or decrease in the caloric consumption of cases compared to controls. The same studies found a similar pattern in case–control differences for intake of total fat, total carbohydrates and protein, which suggests that these major nutrients are highly correlated with each other.

A critical analysis of Table 2.2 suggests that factors associated with study design may explain these differences. Firstly, an examination for consistent trends within each sex is negative since the case–control ratios of intake within each sex are both above and below 1.00. Of the studies which meas-

Table 2.2   Mean daily intakes of calories (kcal) reported in case–control studies

Study*	Calories		p-value (difference in means)	Ratio: cases/ controls
	Cases (n)	Controls (n)		
Males				
Marseilles, 1957 (73)	3263 (9)	3437 (12)	?	0.95
Paris, 1979 (77)	3244 (32)	3117 (32)	n.s.	1.04
Melbourne, 1970 (79)	2670 (19)	2840 (22)	n.s.	0.94
Edmonton, 1979 (80)	2357 (14)	2967 (12)	n.s.	0.79
Females				
Marseilles, 1957 (73)	2932 (42)	2470 (30)	<0.05	1.19
Marseilles, 1966 (74)	3062 (46)	2537 (46)	<0.00005	1.21
Marseilles, 1969 (75)	2495 (101)	2163 (101)	<0.0005	1.15
Marseilles, 1978 (76)	2324 (30)	2302 (30)	n.s.	1.01
Paris, 1979 (77)	2226 (69)	2180 (69)	n.s.	1.02
Melbourne, 1970 (79)	2140 (52)	2160 (50)	n.s.	0.99
Pima Indians, 1971 (84)	3055 (48)	3238 (16)	n.s.	0.94
Edmonton, 1979 (80)	1566 (59)	1856 (65)	<0.05	0.84
Nova Scotia, 1980 (81)	3905 (20)	2828 (76)	<0.001	1.38
Males and females combined				
Brisbane, 1968 (78)	2538 (79)	2931 (79)	<0.05	0.87

n.s. = not significant (p > 0.05)
?   = p-value not reported
*   = study reference number in brackets for this column

ured sex-specific intakes, only the Marseilles study carried out in 1957[73] found a difference in the ratio between the sexes. All the others found the case–control intake ratio to be in the same direction for both sexes[77,79,80]. For these last three studies, the finding of a similar within-study ratio of intake for the sexes, along with a difference in the ratios between the studies, suggests the presence of bias associated with study design.

The factors associated with study design which are most likely to bias the results are selection of controls and method of dietary measurement, particularly the period of dietary measurement. However, it is not possible to identify which of these factors is responsible for the inconsistent results found for caloric intake. For example, amongst females those studies which selected their controls from hospital or occupational populations have caloric intake ratios well above 1.00[73-75], well below 1.00[78,80], or near to 1.00[76,77,79]. Similarly, for those studies which measured caloric intake after the onset of symptoms (or treatment), the caloric intake ratio is either above 1.00[81] or below 1.00[80,84].

An alternative explanation for these discordant results is provided by the Adelaide study[83]. Because of the relatively large number of subjects in this study, it was possible to examine for a possible interaction between age and dietary intake by comparing the mean nutrient intake of cases and controls within age-strata. Table 2.3 shows the mean caloric intake for cases and controls in the Adelaide study by decade of age. For both sexes, cases ate

Table 2.3 Mean (SE) daily intake of calories (kcal) by cases and matched community controls in the Adelaide case–control study

Age group (years)	Females			Males		
	Cases(n)	Controls(n)	Pairs	Cases(n)	Controls(n)	Pairs
< 30	2009(103)*	1559(73)	38	2374(257)	2169(232)	5
30–39	2197(122)*	1727(97)	37	2643(488)	2166(127)	8
40–49	1730(101)	1629(63)	32	2140(212)	1979(158)	11
50–59	1794(102)	1860(113)	42	1976(155)	2447(217)	17
≤ 60	1508(102)	1719(112)	27	1984(191)	2434(177)	16

* Cases significantly different from matched controls: $p < 0.005$

more calories than community controls in the age groups below 50 years, but less than their community controls in the age groups above 50 years. There was a similar age-related pattern for intake of fats, total carbohydrates (complex plus simple) and protein. Three other case–control studies which included women aged < 55 years also found that cases ate significantly more calories than controls[75,76,81], although another study with subjects whose mean age was 38 years found the opposite[80].

The observation in the Adelaide study that cases aged < 50 years ate more than their controls, while older cases ate less than their controls, suggests that there is a subpopulation of persons who are prone to gallstone formation, perhaps because of a genetic or lifestyle-related metabolic susceptibility. Among such a 'stone-prone' population, there may be an inverse relationship between the extent of caloric (or fat) intake and the age of onset of gallstone disease. This notion of gallstone susceptibility is discussed below in relation to oral contraceptives.

Cholesterol

It is commonly believed by medical practitioners that increased dietary cholesterol increases the risk of gallstone disease. However, the evidence from epidemiological studies does not support this.

The Adelaide study found no differences in cholesterol intake between male cases and controls; while in women intake was significantly ($p < 0.05$) greater among cases aged < 50 years, and lower among cases above age 50 years, than controls in the respective age groups[83]. This age-related case–control difference in women was also observed for most other nutrients, including total caloric intake, which suggests that cholesterol intake merely reflected total dietary intake. In multivariate analyses, dietary cholesterol was inversely associated with gallstone risk in women after controlling for calories (or fat). This observation must be treated with caution as a similar relation was not found in men.

Only three other case–control studies have compared cholesterol intakes between cases and controls (Table 2.4). All three studies found no significant difference in mean daily cholesterol intake between cases and controls[78,84,85]. The results of the case–control studies, combined with the equivocal findings

Table 2.4   Mean daily intakes of cholesterol (mg) reported in case-control studies

Study*	Cholesterol		p-value (difference in means)	Ratio: cases/ controls
	Cases (n)	Controls(n)		
Females				
Framingham, 1966 (85)	482 (44)	497 (405)	n.s.	0.97
Pima Indians, 1971 (84)	483 (48)	511 (16)	n.s.	0.95
Males				
Framingham, 1966 (85)	724 (23)	701 (407)	n.s.	1.03
Males and females combined				
Brisbane, 1968 (78)	536 (79)	581 (79)	n.s.	0.92

n.s. = not significant ($p > 0.05$)
*   = study reference number in brackets for this column

from the experimental studies, suggest that dietary cholesterol does not have an important role in the aetiology of cholesterol gallstones.

Sugar

The Adelaide study found in both men and women that an increased intake of simple sugars (mono- and disaccharides) in drinks (tea, coffee, cordial and aerated soft drinks) and sweets (jam, honey, chocolate and other confectionery), mostly sucrose, was associated with an increased risk of gallstone disease[83]. This was in contrast to intakes of simple sugars in cereals, fruit and dairy products, which were similar for cases and controls (Table 2.5). This result is supported by the Rome case–control study in which gallstone patients were found to eat significantly ($p < 0.05$) more refined sugar than controls[82], although a further recent Italian cross-sectional study reported that sugar intake was lower in women with gallstones than those who were stone-free[87]. In contrast, the Brisbane study found no significant difference between cases and controls for mean consumption of sucrose (and fructose) for the largest of its dietary groups[78], while the Pima Indian study also found similar intakes of sucrose by cases and controls[84].

Fibre

The role of fibre has been little studied in gallstone case–control studies, probably because most were carried out prior to the publication of the dietary fibre hypothesis in the early 1970s. Only three studies have measured fibre intake.

The Edmonton study found that crude fibre intake was lower amongst cases of both sexes, the differences being significant ($p < 0.05$) for females[80]. A decreased daily intake of bread and bakery products by cases was mainly responsible for the difference. However, the intake of crude fibre per 1000 calories of total dietary intake was the same in cases and controls. This suggests that there were no percentage differences in fibre intake between

Table 2.5 Mean daily intake of sugar (g) (mono- and disaccharides), categorized by food source: Adelaide case–control study

Food source of sugar	Age < 50 years		Age > 50 years		All ages	
	Cases	Community controls	Cases	Community controls	Cases	Community controls
Females						
(matched pairs)		(107)		(69)		(176)
Cereals	12	10	14	16	13	12
Fruit						
raw†	30	28	32	38	31	32
sweetened	19	22	19	22	19	22
Dairy products						
unsweetened	8	6	5	6	7	6
sweetened†	18	15	17	16	18	15
Drinks and sweets†	53 ***	28	36 **	23	46 ***	26
Total‡	147 ***	113	128	126	140 **	118
Males						
(matched pairs)		(24)		(33)		(57)
Cereals	16	14	17	25	17	21
Fruit						
raw†	19	17	21 *	34	20	27
sweetened	23	20	17	22	20	21
Dairy products						
unsweetened	5	6	7	2	6	5
sweetened†	25	20	21	20	23	20
Drinks and sweets†	58 *	40	46	40	51	40
Total‡	160 *	121	135	153	146	140

* $p < 0.95$; ** $p < 0.01$; *** $p < 0.001$
‡ Total includes sugar in other food groups not listed above
† All carbohydrates, although > 95% simple sugars

cases and controls, and that the quantitative differences described above may have reflected differences in the absolute total dietary intake.

In contrast, the Rome study did not find a significant difference between cases and controls in intake of total dietary fibre, nor of cereal fibre; although intake of dietary fibre from fruit and vegetables was significantly lower for cases than controls[82]. In the Adelaide study, intake of dietary fibre by cases, compared to controls, was significantly decreased among females aged > 50 years, but similar for cases and controls among women aged < 50 years and among men in both age groups[83]. Increased dietary fibre was found to be inversely associated with gallstone risk in the Adelaide study only after controlling for dietary fat (or calories) and cholesterol. However, fibre was inversely correlated with sugar in drinks and sweets and had no significant association with gallstone risk when included in multivariate statistical models with this sugar variable.

While experimental studies have shown that increased intake of dietary fibre lowers a pre-existing raised cholesterol saturation index, the role of dietary fibre in the aetiology of gallstone disease, and whether its effects are independent of the above-mentioned effects of sugar remains to be defined.

Alcohol

In contrast with other nutrients (especially calories and fats), the results for alcohol intake reported by case–control studies are more consistent and

Table 2.6 Mean daily intakes of alcohol reported in case-control studies

Study*	Cases (n)	Controls (n)	p-value	Ratio: cases/ controls
Females				
Marseilles, 1966 (74)	232 kcal (46)	228 kcal (46)	n.s.	1.02
Marseilles, 1969 (75)	17 g (101)	18 g (101)	n.s.	0.94
Marseilles, 1978 (76)	63 kcal (30)	81 kcal (30)	n.s.	0.78
Paris, 1979 (77)	13 g (69)	13 g (69)	n.s.	1.00
Melbourne, 1970 (79)	20 kcal (52)	30 kcal (50)	?	0.67
Adelaide, 1984 (83)	2.9 g (176)	5.3 g (176)	<0.001	0.55
Males				
Paris, 1979 (77)	57 g (32)	64 g (32)	n.s.	0.89
Melbourne, 1970 (79)	110 kcal (19)	140 kcal (22)	?	0.79
Adelaide, 1984 (83)	10.4 g (57)	11.7 g (57)	n.s.	0.89

n.s. = not significant (p > 0.05)
? = p-value not reported
* = study reference number in brackets for this column

suggest that alcohol may protect against gallstone disease. Table 2.6 shows that the case–control ratio for mean alcohol intake is below 1.00 in all studies in which it was measured except for females in studies in Marseilles[74] and Paris[77], and even in these latter two studies the ratio is 1.00 or only just above it. The lack of significant case–control differences in alcohol intake in some of these studies is possibly due to their small sample sizes. However, when the proportion of abstainers is compared, both the Melbourne and Adelaide studies found this was significantly increased among cases compared with controls[79,83]. In the Adelaide study, most of the reduced risk of gallstone disease among drinkers, compared with abstainers, occurred in subjects who drank less than 30 g of alcohol per day, while increased consumption beyond that level carried a negligible further reduction in gallstone risk[83].

The Framingham study found an inverse, albeit non-significant, relationship between alcohol intake and the risk of gallstones, more so for women than men[85]. The gallstone morbidity ratio used in this study provides a conservative measure of the association between gallstones and alcohol, since the comparison was with all study subjects, and not just with non-drinkers. Further, the Kaiser-Permanente study has observed an inverse relation between alcohol intake and admission to hospital for gallstone disease[88].

Table 2.6 also shows that women consume much less alcohol than men. If future epidemiological studies confirm the above results that alcohol appears to protect against gallstone formation, this sex difference in alcohol intake may partly explain the greater prevalence of gallstones in women than men.

Dietary studies of populations with different gallstone prevalences

At least two studies have compared the dietary intake of North American Indians, who have the highest gallstone prevalence in the world, with North American Caucasians.

Firstly, at the same time that the case–control study of Pima Indians was carried out, the researchers also examined the dietary intakes of all Pima Indian women aged 25–44 years living on a section of the Gila River Indian Reservation, Arizona[84]. Compared with the general (male and female) United States population, the Indian women had similar intakes of total calories and all major nutrients except for absolute intakes of protein and sucrose, which were both decreased amongst the Indians. However, this study does not provide a good comparison as the two groups did not have the same method of dietary assessment, or the same age and sex distribution.

A better comparison is provided by a study of Micmac Indian and Caucasian women in Canada[89]. Both populations in this study were of similar age (15–50 years) and sex, lived in communities close to each other, and had the dietary intakes of their individuals measured by the same method (4-day diary). For Indian women compared to Caucasians, absolute intakes of protein and fibre were decreased, while percentage intakes of carbohydrates and alcohol were increased and decreased, respectively. Absolute intakers of total calories, carbohydrates, fat and cholesterol, as well as the ratio of polyunsaturated/saturated fats, were the same for both groups.

A recent cross-sectional study from England found that the gallstone prevalence in vegetarian women was about half that in non-vegetarian women[90]. The authors attributed this to a lower saturated fat and higher fibre intake in vegetarians compared with non-vegetarians.

Dietary intervention studies

Intervention studies, which have used variations in diet to lower cardiovascular risk factors such as serum cholesterol, have also provided information on the relationship of diet and gallstone prevalence.

The first of these studies to be reported has often been cited as evidence in the medical literature that polyunsaturated fats increase the risk of gallstone disease[91]. It was a prospective study of United States veterans living in an institution, who were randomly assigned to either an experimental or normal diet group. The experimental diet differed from the normal diet because of its lower cholesterol and higher plant sterol contents, and higher polyunsaturated/saturated fat ratio. The veterans ate only the study diets when eating in the institution, where the diets were prepared for a period of 10 years. After completion of the study period, the records of those study subjects who had autopsies were reviewed and the gallstone prevalence for each dietary group was calculated. The major finding was a raised gallstone prevalence amongst the group eating the experimental diet, which was only significantly different from the control group when subjects who ate more than a third of the study meals during their period in the study were compared. The authors also found a dose–response relationship in the experimental group between the number of study meals eaten and gallstone prevalence.

However, a second intervention study, carried out on mental inmates in two hospitals in Finland, did not confirm the results of the American study[92]. In the Finnish study, the experimental diet differed from the normal diet (as it did in the American study) by its lower cholesterol content and raised polyunsaturated/saturated fat ratio. A crossover design was used with the two diets being administered for 6 years each to the total male and female population aged over 15 years in each mental hospital. For males and females, separately, the researchers found no differences in the gallstone prevalence between the experimental and control groups. There was also no dose–response relationship.

A possible explanation offered by the Finns for the disparate findings between these two studies, which used almost similar study methods, is that the sample sizes used to measure gallstone prevalence in both studies were small, and that the positive result for the American study may have been due to chance. As evidence, the Finns compared the relative risk from each study and found that they were not significantly different[92].

Summary of dietary studies

Since most of the analytical epidemiological studies, in particular the case–control studies, can be faulted because of poor study design, any conclusions made from their results must be tentative.

However, the results do suggest the following. Firstly, dietary cholesterol does not appear to have an important role in gallstone aetiology, and the evidence implicating polyunsaturated fats as a causative factor is inconsistent. Secondly, increased intake of calories (or total fat which is highly correlated with calories) appears to increase gallstone risk, particularly in people aged less than 50 years. Thirdly, either increased intake of sucrose or decreased fibre intake, or both, may increase gallstone risk. Finally increased intake of alcohol appears to lower the risk of gallstone disease.

OBESITY

Epidemiological studies of the role of obesity in gallstone disease include case–control, prospective, and cross-sectional studies, and also autopsy series which have typically been analysed in case–control fashion. These studies have used a variety of methods to define obesity and to analyse its association with gallstones. Therefore, to simplify the following discussion, emphasis has been given to the results and conclusions of these studies, rather than to their methods.

Among females of all ages combined, several studies have found a significant ($p < 0.05$) positive association between obesity and gall-stones[5,79,80,83,85,90,93-96]; while non-significant, although positive, associations between obesity and gallstones have also been reported by a number of studies[4,75,77,97]. Thus, among females, the evidence from epidemiological studies is strongly in favour of a positive relation between obesity and gall-stones.

However, there is also evidence among females that age interacts in the association between obesity and gallstones. An English study concluded that female cases < 50 years of age were heavier compared with a population sample published in a separate study[98]. A cross-sectional study of weight-conscious women found that obesity was associated with an increased gall-stone incidence amongst women aged 20–29 years and 30–39 years, but not among older women[99]. An autopsy series in America observed that the association between obesity and gallstones was strongest among women aged 20–39 years, compared with the older age groups[8]. Case–control differ-ences in obesity (with cases being heavier) were greater among females aged < 50 years than among older females in the Adelaide study[83]. The same study also reported that the increase in the level of obesity since age 21 years was significantly ($p < 0.05$) greater for cases aged < 50 years than their controls, while the increase was similar for cases and controls aged > 50 years. Also, in case–control studies which examined young women exclusively, significant ($p < 0.05$) positive associations between obesity and gallstones were found in women aged 15–50 years[81] and in female adolescents aged 14–20 years[100], although a study of women aged 20–55 years failed to find a significant positive association between gallstones and obesity[75].

Among males, the evidence is less clear with several studies finding significant ($p < 0.05$) positive associations between obesity and gall-stones[5,8,79,93,94], while a similar number of studies found no significant association[4,77,80,83,85]. Neither is there sufficient evidence of an interaction between age and obesity on the risk of gallstone disease in men as appears the position in women.

The studies described above show that the evidence supporting a role for obesity in gallstone formation is more conclusive for females than males, particularly young females. The conclusion that obesity appears to be a risk factor primarily among premenopausal females suggests a role for repro-ductive or hormonal factors, or both, in the association between obesity and gallstones.

The mechanism by which obesity increases the risk of gallstone formation has been clarified in metabolic studies. Obesity is associated with increased cholesterol synthesis[101,102], primarily by the liver, which results in increased cholesterol secretion into bile[17,103,104] and an increased biliary cholesterol concentration and saturation index[17,104,105].

A further phenomenon, related to obesity, is that moderate to massive weight-loss, which follows gastric bypass surgery in morbidly obese persons is associated with an increased risk of gallstone formation. It is thought that removal of part of the jejunum and ileum results in decreased bile acid synthesis or resorption, and consequently a reduced bile acid pool[106,107]. The role of dietary-induced weight-loss in gallstone formation is unclear at present, although subjects who lost an average of 25 kg over several weeks as a result of caloric restriction, were reported to have increased cholesterol saturation indices during the weight reduction period[17].

SEX

The increased gallstone prevalence among women compared to men has been well documented in autopsy studies[6]. The female increase first occurs during the second decade of life around the time of puberty and persists into old age. Hormonal and reproductive factors, such as pregnancy and oral contraceptives, are thought to be primarily responsible for the increased gallstone prevalence in women, although other non-hormonal lifestyle factors – for example, a decreased alcohol consumption, which may protect against gallstone formation, by women compared with men – may also contribute. However, epidemiological studies have mostly investigated a role for pregnancy and oral contraception in gallstone formation, and each of these is discussed more fully below.

Pregnancy

A positive association between gallstone disease and pregnancy has been described by epidemiological studies in England[98,108], Sweden[97,109], Italy [110], Australia[78,79,111], and of North American Indians[112-114] and Caucasians[85,99,110]. No association was found in living subjects by three North American studies[4,80,95] and an English study[90], nor in two series of postmortem examinations[93,115]. Thus, the evidence is weighted in favour of an increased risk of gallstone disease associated with pregnancy.

There is also evidence that the gallstone risk associated with pregnancy varies inversely with age. Studies of Chippewa Indians[113], weight-conscious women[99], the Adelaide case–control study[111], and the GREPCO study in Rome[110] all found that the gallstone risk associated with pregnancy was strongest for women aged <30 years. Further, an English study observed that parous women aged < 50 years showed a greater prevalence of gallstones than did nulliparous women of the same age, but that in women aged over 50 the prevalence was greater in nulliparous women[98].

A relation between the relative risk of gallstone disease and number of exposures to pregnancy, which is maximal among younger women, has been described in a number of studies. The study by Horn[98] and the Adelaide case–control study[111] both found such a relationship in women aged < 50 years, but not in older women; while a study of weight-conscious women observed a relation only in women aged < 30 years[99]. An English study of women aged 25–39 years also found a correlation[108]. Other studies have investigated women over a broad age range (20–60 years) – some of these have described a correlation of the gallstone risk with pregnancy[75,85,113], and others have not[79,97].

The age dependence of the risk of developing gallstones associated with pregnancy, with the increased risk being strongest in premenopausal women, suggests that the effect of pregnancy on gallstone risk is immediate and temporary, and not long-term. This conclusion would be consistent with the known immediate and temporary effect of pregnancy on the contraction of the gallbladder[116], itself a probable risk factor, and on the cholesterol saturation of bile[117].

Oral contraceptives and oestrogens

Epidemiological studies carried out in the late 1960s and early 1970s found an approximate twofold increase in gallstone risk associated with exposure to oral contraceptives[118-120], and oestrogens in women[121] and in men[122]. An explanation as to how oral contraceptives increased gallstone risk was readily forthcoming from experimental studies, which regularly showed that oral contraceptives increased bile cholesterol saturation[123-125]. Thus, the impression was quickly gained by the medical community that oral contraceptives increase the risk of gallstone formation.

However, subsequent epidemiological studies have been published which found no association between oral contraceptive exposure and gallstone disease[80,81,90,95,108,110,126]. A possible explanation for these discordant epidemiological results is provided by observations in the Royal College of General Practitioners' oral contraception study[127] and the Adelaide case–control study[111].

Both of these studies provide evidence which suggests that there is a susceptibility to gallstone formation associated with oral contraceptives. The general practitioners' study found among women taking oral contraceptives, that after an initial rise in the incidence of gallstone disease for those taking oral contraceptives for 3 years or less, the gallstone incidence rate then progressively declined with further use to levels below that for women not taking oral contraceptives[127]. The Adelaide case–control study found an age–dependent variation in the risk of gallstone disease associated with exposure to oral contraceptives, with the risk being above unity for young subjects and below unity for older subjects[111]. The results from these two studies suggest that there is a subpopulation of women who are susceptible to gallstone disease after exposure to oral contraceptives. In these women the onset of gallstone disease is accelerated so that gallstones develop soon after initial exposure to oral contraceptives. This conclusion is consistent with evidence that the most common duration of oral contraceptive exposure in gallstone subjects is 6–12 months[118,128].

Those epidemiological studies which found a positive association between gallstone disease and oral contraceptive use were carried out in the late 1960s and early 1970s, soon after oral contraceptives became widely used. They were likely to have included women who were susceptible to gallstone formation and in whom recent first use of oral contraceptives had accelerated this formation. That subgroup of susceptible women would not, therefore, have been available for inclusion as new cases among the older age groups in later studies. If this explanation is correct, future epidemiological studies can be expected to find a positive association between oral contraceptive use and gallstone disease only among women recently exposed to oral contraceptives for the first time. Such women are typically teenagers or in their twenties.

Other possible reasons for the failure of later studies to confirm the observations of a positive association between gallstones and oral contraceptives described in the earlier studies are: firstly, the women in the earlier studies may have taken, on average, a stronger dose oral contraceptive than women in more recent studies, who were more likely to be taking the 'minipills'[129]; and secondly, oral contraceptives may have a positive association with cholecystitis but not gallstones[130].

BLOOD LIPIDS AND INSULIN

Because cholesterol gallstones are known to be the result of an altered lipid metabolism, information on the role of blood lipids in gallstone disease may provide indirect clues as to the changes in lipid metabolism that are associated with their formation. Most of the case–control studies on blood lipids have examined triglyceride and total cholesterol, while the roles of insulin, which stimulates triglyceride synthesis by the liver[131] and of HDL-cholesterol have been little studied.

Studies of blood *triglyceride* have found that it is raised in gallstone cases compared with controls[109,110,132–134], except for the Brisbane case–control study[78]. The Adelaide case–control study observed that increased triglyceride levels occurred only in cases aged < 50 years, compared with similarly aged controls, and not in older cases who had levels similar to their controls[134]. It is tempting to speculate from this result of an age-related variation in the case–control difference of triglyceride levels found in the Adelaide study, that a raised triglyceride level early in adult life may be a marker for the above-mentioned gallstone susceptibility, thought to be associated with oral contraceptives and calories.

Furthermore, the presence of gallstone disease is positively associated with type IV hyperlipoproteinaemia[109,133,135], an association that has also been reported to decrease with increasing age[135], and also with type IIb hyperlipoproteinaemia[109]. An increase in the blood level of pre-beta lipoprotein is the common characteristic of each hyperlipoproteinaemia. In studies on the relationship between blood triglyceride and biliary cholesterol, most have found a positive association[136–138]; although no association was found in patients eligible for the National Cooperative Gallstone Study[139].

Studies on the role of blood total *cholesterol* in gallstone disease have mostly found no relationship between blood cholesterol and the presence of gallstones[4,78,85,95,109,133,140]. In contrast, one study found a raised plasma cholesterol in cases[132] while an earlier Swedish study reported lower serum cholesterol levels in female cases compared with controls[97].

The observations in the latter study are supported by recent epidemiological studies which have used multivariate analyses to control for the confounding effect of other lipids. Both the Adelaide case–control study[134] and the GREPCO study in Rome[110] found that an increased plasma total cholesterol was associated with a decreased risk of gallstones after controlling for plasma triglyceride level. Further, gallstone patients in the National Cooperative Gallstone Study who took chenodeoxycholic acid, used to reverse the process of gallstone formation, had a greater increase in serum cholesterol than patients who took the placebo[141]. Additional evidence that increases in serum total cholesterol are negatively associated with gallstone risk comes from studies of Pima Indians, who while they have the highest documented gallstone prevalence in the world, also have lower serum cholesterol levels than North

American Caucasians[142,143].

Three studies have found no correlation between blood and bile cholesterol[136,139,144]; another paper reported a positive correlation between non-HDL-cholesterol and bile cholesterol saturation[138]; while in contrast, studies on Pakistani gallstone cases have shown that serum cholesterol is inversely correlated with bile and stone cholesterol concentrations[137,145].

The role of blood *HDL-cholesterol* in gallstone disease has not been extensively studied. Gallstone cases have been reported to have lower mean levels of HDL-cholesterol than controls[134,146] and an inverse association between HDL-cholesterol and gallstone risk has been described[134,147]. The results from the last two studies do not give a consistent indication as to whether this association is independent of triglyceride, which varies inversely with HDL-cholesterol[148]. An inverse relationship between plasma HDL-cholesterol and biliary cholesterol saturation has been reported in healthy women[138], although a more recent study of selected gallstone patients has not confirmed this[139]. Collectively, the studies on HDL-cholesterol in gallstone disease are reasonably consistent and suggest an inverse association between gallstone risk and HDL-cholesterol. This suggests that the free cholesterol in high density lipoprotein is preferentially metabolized to bile acids rather than secreted into bile as cholesterol.

Insulin is relevant to gallstone disease because it stimulates liver triglyceride synthesis[131]. The only epidemiological study of insulin with a sample size of sufficient statistical power is the Adelaide Study[134]. It found that gallstone cases had significantly increased fasting plasma insulin levels compared with controls. Also, increased plasma insulin was associated with an increased gallstone risk, independent of plasma triglyceride and obesity, which suggests that all three are independent risk factors of gallstone disease. An earlier hospital-based case–control study reported that cases had a raised fasting plasma insulin level, compared with controls, although the case–control differences were not significant ($p > 0.05$), probably because of the small sample sizes[149].

Studies of bile metabolism also support a role for insulin in gallstone disease. Maturity onset diabetics, who typically have raised blood insulin values[150] due to obesity-related insulin resistance[151], also have a bile cholesterol saturation index higher than that of controls[152,153], although this was not confirmed in another study which matched diabetics and controls by age, sex and level of obesity[154]. The administration of insulin to maturity onset diabetics has also been observed to significantly ($p < 0.05$) raise their bile saturation index[40].

In summary, the literature suggests that gallstone disease is associated positively with triglyceride and insulin, and negatively with HDL-cholesterol, although the associations of gallstone disease with triglyceride and HDL-cholesterol may be different manifestations of the same phenomenon, given the inverse correlation that exists between triglyceride and HDL-cholesterol. In contrast, the evidence suggests that there is no association between the presence of gallstone disease and total cholesterol, and perhaps even a negative association.

INTEGRATED MODEL OF GALLSTONE DISEASE

The dietary and hormonal risk factors of gallstone disease may act through the pathways described in Figure 2.1 to produce alterations in blood lipid and

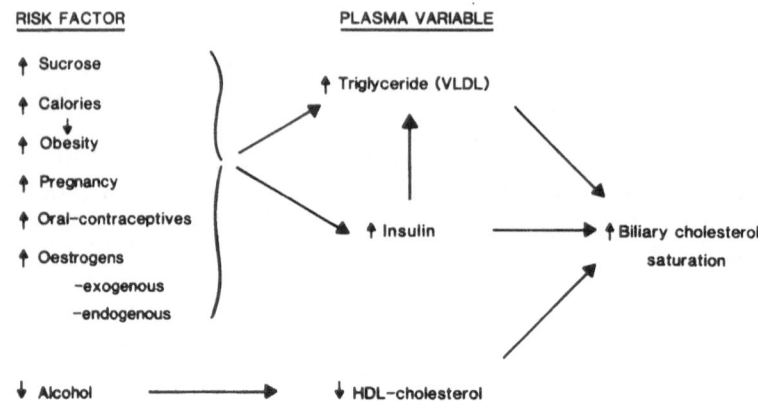

Figure 2.1   A suggested integrated model of gallstone formation

insulin levels that are associated with increased biliary cholesterol saturation and, consequently, gallstone disease. It must be stressed that this proposition is somewhat speculative; nevertheless it provides a unifying model of gallstone aetiology that integrates the various empirical observations discussed above.

Increased sucrose intake, which can increase caloric intake[38], increases both fasting plasma insulin[44-47] and triglyceride[50] levels, particularly in subjects who already are hypertriglyceridaemic and thought to be carbohydrate-sensitive[45]. Obesity is also known to cause raised blood insulin and triglyceride levels through the phenomenon of insulin resistance[131]. By contrast, alcohol's effect on biliary cholesterol saturation and gallstone risk may be reflected by changes in blood levels of HDL-cholesterol[155].

The effect of hormonal factors on gallstone risk may also be manifested through changes in blood insulin and triglyceride levels. Oral contraceptives can induce hypertriglyceridaemia and affect (variably) insulin secretion[156]. The third trimester of pregnancy is associated with hyperinsulinaemia[157] due to insulin resistance and hypertriglyceridaemia[158]. Oestradiol, the most biologically active premenopausal sex hormone in women, has been reported to increase insulin secretion[159] and fasting plasma insulin concentrations[160] in the rat.

The age interrelations between the relative risk of gallstone disease and the aetiological variables described above also provide clues as to how the metabolic disorders involved in gallstone disease may change with age. The observation in the Adelaide case–control study that caloric intake, obesity and plasma triglyceride are all increased in young cases only, compared with controls[83,134], suggests that young cases typically form gallstones because of an increased liver cholesterol synthesis, since other studies have shown that these three factors are positively associated with cholesterol synthesis[17,102,161]

In contrast, the finding in the Adelaide study that older cases do not have increased levels of obesity or plasma triglyceride, compared with their controls, suggests that they typically develop gallstones because of a reduced bile acid pool, which has been observed in non-obese gallstone patients[162].

The epidemiological evidence that gallstone risk factors vary with age suggests that the aetiology of gallstones is more complex than we have hitherto assumed. The recent findings that there may be a susceptibility to gallstone formation associated with oral contraceptives, and possibly with caloric intake, which may be marked by a raised blood triglyceride level early in adult life, has important implications with regard to our understanding of the gallstone disease process and its possible future prevention. These conclusions need to be confirmed by further epidemiological studies, particularly of diet, the results of which may have potential to be used as a basis both in the prevention of gallstone disease and also as an adjuvant to the medical therapy of existing disease.

References

1. Dam, H. (1971). Determinants of cholesterol cholelithiasis in man and animals. *Am. J. Med.*, **51**, 596–613
2. Hoppe-Seyler, H. (1903). Cholelithiasis. In Nothnagel's *Encyclopedia of Practical Medicine.* Vol. 6, pp. 525–607. (American Edition: W. B. Saunders)
3. Dam, H. and Christensen, F. (1952). Alimentary production of gallstones in hamsters. *Acta Path. Microbiol. Scand.*, **30**, 236–41
4. Sampliner, R. E., Bennet, P. H., Comess, L. J. and Rose, F. A. (1970). Gallbladder disease in Pima Indians. Demonstration of high prevalence and early onset by cholecystography. *N. Engl. J. Med.*, **283**, 1358–64
5. Marinovic, I., Guerra, C. and Larach, G. (1972). Incidencia de litiasis biliar en material de autopsias y analisis de composicion de los calculos. *Rev. Med. Chile*, **100**, 1320–7
6. Brett, M. and Barker, D. J. P. (1976). The world distribution of gallstones. *Int. J. Epidemiol.*, **5**, 335–41
7. Burkitt, D. P. and Tunstall, M. (1975). Gallstones: geographical and chronological features. *J. Trop. Med. Hyg.*, **78**, 140–4
8. Newman, H. F. and Northup, J. D. (1959). The autopsy incidence of gallstones. *Int. Abst. Surg.*, **109**, 1–13
9. Sarles, H., Gerolami, A. and Cros, R. C. (1978). Diet and cholesterol gallstones. A multicentre study. *Digestion*, **7**, 121–7
10. Ehrstrom, R. (1942). The prevalence of gallstones and the standard of living in Finland, 1836–1939. *Nordisk. Med.*, **14**, 1559–65
11. Kalos, A., Delidou, A., Kosdosis, Th., Archimandritis, A., Gaganis, A. and Angelopoulos, B. (1977). The incidence of gallstones in Greece: an autopsy study. *Acta Hepato-gastroenterol.*, **24**, 20–3
12. Kameda, H. (1966). Gallstones: compositions, structural characteristics and geographic distribution. Third World Congress of Gastroenterology, Tokyo. *Rec. Adv. Gastroenterol.*, **4**, 117–24
13. Insull, W., Oiso, T. and Tsuchiya, K. (1968). Diet and nutritional status of Japanese. *Am. J. Clin. Nutr.*, **21**, 753–77
14. Sarles, H., Crotte, C., Gerolami, A., Mule, A., Domingo, N. and Hauton, J. (1971). The influence of calorie intake and of dietary protein on the bile lipids. *Scand. J. Gastroenterol.*, **6**, 189–91
15. Shaffer, E. A. (1980). Gallstones: current concepts of pathogenesis and medical dissolution. *Can. J. Surg.*, **23**, 517–32, 557
16. Sarles, H., Hauton, J., Lafont, H., Teissier, N., Planche, N. and Gerolami, A. (1968). Effect of diet on the biliary cholesterol concentration in normals and gallstone patients. *Clin. Chim. Acta*, **19**, 147–55

17. Bennion, L. J. and Grundy, S. M. (1975). Effects obesity and caloric intake on biliary lipid metabolism in man. *J. Clin. Invest.*, **56**, 996–1011
18. Dam, H., Kruse, I., Jensen, K. and Kallehauge, H. E. (1967). Studies on human bile. II. Influence of two different fats on the composition of human bile. *Scand. J. Clin. Lab. Invest.*, **19**, 367–78
19. Schlierf, G., Nikolaus, T., Stiehl, A. *et al.* (1979). Zur wirkung lipidspiegelsenkender kostforman auf gallenlipide und plasmalipoproteine bei normalpersonen. *Schweiz Med. Wschr.*, **109**, 1743–7
20. Grundy, S. M. (1975). Effects of polyunsaturated fats on lipid metabolism in patients with hypertriglyceridemia. *J. Clin. Invest.*, **55**, 269–82
21. Lewis, B. (1958). Effect of certain dietary oils on bile-acid secretion and serum cholesterol. *Lancet*, **1**, 1090–2
22. Watanabe, N., Gimbel, N. S. and Johnston, C. G. (1962). Effect of polyunsaturated and saturated fatty acids on the cholesterol holding capacity of human bile. *Arch. Surg.*, **85**, 136–41
23. Grundy, S. M. and Metzger, A. L. (1972). A physiological method for estimation of hepatic biliary lipids in man. *Gastroenterology*, **62**, 1200–17
24. Andersen, E. and Hellstrom, K. (1980). Influence of fat-rich versus carbohydrate-rich diets on bile acid kinetics, biliary lipids, and net-steroid balance in hyperlipidemic subjects. *Metabolism*, **29**, 400–9
25. Hepner, G. W. (1975). Effect of decreased gallbladder stimulation on enterohepatic cycling and kinetics of bile acids. *Gastroenterology*, **68**, 1574–81
26. Aschoff, L. and Bacmeister, A. (1909). *Die Cholelithiasis.* (Jena: Fischer)
27. DenBesten, L., Conner, W. E. and Bell, S. (1973). The effect of dietary cholesterol on the composition of human bile. *Surgery*, **73**, 266–73
28. Lee, D. W. T., Gilmore, C. J., Bonorris, G. *et al.* (1985). Effect of dietary cholesterol on biliary lipids in patients with gallstones and normal subjects. *Am. J. Clin. Nutr.*, **42**, 414–20
29. Maudgal, D. P., Bird, R., Blackwood, W. S. and Northfield, T. C. (1978). Low-cholesterol diet: enhancement of effect of CDCA in patients with gallstones. *Br. Med. J.*, **2**, 851–3
30. Dam, H., Prange, I., Jensen, K., Kallehauge, H. E. and Fenger, H. J. (1971). Studies on human bile. IV. Influence of ingestion of cholesterol in the form of eggs on the composition of bile in healthy subjects. *Z. Ernaehrungswiss.*, **10**, 178–87
31. Sarles, E., Crotte, C., Gerolami, A., Mule, A., Domingo, N. and Hauton, J. (1970). Influence of cholestyramine, bile salt, and cholesterol feeding on the lipid composition of hepatic bile in man. *Scand. J. Gastroenterol.*, **5**, 603–8
32. Andersen, E. and Hellstrom, K. (1974). The effects of cholesterol feeding on bile acid kinetics and biliary lipids in normolipidemic and hypertriglyceridemic subjects. *J. Lipid Res.*, **20**, 1020–7
33. Wilson, J. D. and Lindsey, C. A. (1965). Studies on the influence of dietary cholesterol on cholesterol metabolism in the isotopic steady state in man. *J. Clin. Invest.*, **44**, 1805–14
34. Quintao, E., Grundy, S. M. and Ahrens, E. H. (1971). Effects of dietary cholesterol on the regulation of total body cholesterol in man. *J. Lipid Res.*, **12**, 1233–47
35. Nestel, P. J. and Poyser, A. (1976). Changes in cholesterol synthesis and excretion when cholesterol intake is increased. *Metabolism*, **25**, 1591–9
36. Harper, H. A., Rodwell, V. W. and Mayes, P. A. (1977). *Review of Physiological Chemistry.* 6th Edn. (Los Altos: Lange Medical)
37. Heaton, K. W. (1972). *Bile Salts in Health and Disease.* (Edinburgh: Churchill Livingstone)
38. Heaton, K. W., Emmett, P. M., Henry, C. L., Thornton, J. R., Manhire, A. and Hartog, M. (1983). Not just fibre – the nutritional consequences of refined carbohydrate foods. *Human Nutr.: Clin. Nutr.*, **37C**, 31–5
39. Cleave, T. L. (1974). *The Saccharine Disease.* (Bristol: John Wright and Sons)
40. Bennion, L. J. and Grundy, S. M. (1977). Effects of diabetes mellitus on cholesterol metabolism in man. *N. Engl. J. Med.*, **296**, 1365–71
41. Swan, D. C., Davidson, P. and Albrink, M. J. (1966). Effect of simple and complex carbohydrates on plasma non-esterified fatty acids, plasma sugar, and plasma insulin during oral carbohydrate tolerance tests. *Lancet*, **1**, 60–3
42. Wahlqvist, M. L., Wilmshurst, E. G., Murton, C. R. and Richardson, C. N. (1978). The effect

of chain length of glucose absorption and the related metabolic response. *Am. J. Clin. Nutr.,* **31,** 1998–2001

43. Crapo, P. A., Scarlett, J. A. and Kolterman, O. G. (1982) Comparison of the metabolic responses to fructose and sucrose sweetened foods. *Am. J. Clin. Nutr.,* **36,** 256–61

44. Szanto, S, and Yudkin, J. (1969). The effect of dietary sucrose on blood lipids, serum insulin, platelet adhesiveness and body weight in human volunteers. *Postgrad. Med. J.,* **45,** 602–7

45. Reiser, S., Handler, H. B., Gardner, L. B., Hallfrisch, J. G., Michaelis, O. E. and Prather, E. S. (1979). Isocaloric exchange of dietary starch and sucrose in humans. II. Effect on fasting blood insulin, glucose and glucagon and on insulin and glucose response to a sucrose load. *Am. J. Clin. Nutr.,* **32,** 2206–16

46. Reiser, S., Bohn, E., Hallfrisch, J., Michaelis, O. E., Keeney, M. and Prather, E. S. (1981). Serum insulin and glucose in hyperinsulinemic subjects fed three different levels of sucrose. *Am. J. Clin. Nutr.,* **34,** 2348–58

47. Coulston, A., Greenfield, M. S., Kraemer, F. B. *et al.* (1981). Effect of differences in sources of dietary carbohydrates on plasma glucose and insulin responses to meals in patients with impaired carbohydrate tolerance. *Am. J. Clin. Nutr.,* **34,** 2716–20

48. Cahlin, E., Jonsson, J., Nilsson, S. and Schersten, T. (1973). Biliary lipid composition in normolipidemic and prebeta hyperlipoproteinemic gallstone patients. Influence of sucrose feeding of the patients on the biliary lipid composition. *Scand. J. Gastroenterol.,* **8,** 449–56

49. Thornton., R. R., Emmett, P. M. and Heaton, K. W. (1983). Diet and gallstones: effects of refined and unrefined carbohydrate diets on bile cholesterol saturation and bile acid metabolism. *Gut,* **24,** 2–6

50. Werner, D., Emmett, P. M. and Heaton, K. W. (1984). Effects of dietary sucrose on factors influencing cholesterol gallstone formation. *Gut,* **25,** 269–74

51. Burkitt, D. P. (1973). Some diseases characteristic of modern western civilization. *Br. Med. J.,* **1,** 274–8

52. Trowell, H. (1978). The development of the concept of dietary fiber in human nutrition. *Am. J. Clin. Nutr.,* **31,** S3–S11

53. Pomare, E. W., Heaton, K. W., Low-Beer, T. S. and Espiner, H. J. (1976). The effect of wheat bran upon bile salt metabolism and upon the lipid composition of bile in gallstone patients. *Am. J. Dig. Dis.,* **21,** 521–6

54. McDougall, R. M., Yakymyshyn, L., Walker, K. and Thorston, O. G. (1978). Effect of wheat bran on serum lipoproteins and biliary lipids. *Can. J. Surg.,* **21,** 433–5

55. Watts, J. McK., Jablonski, P. and Toouli, J. (1978). The effect of added bran to the diet on the saturation of bile in people without gallstones. *Am. J. Surg.,* **135,** 321–4

56. Wicks, A. C. B., Yeates, J. and Heaton, K. W. (1978). Bran and bile time-course of changes in normal young men given a standard dose. *Scand. J. Gastroenterol.,* **13,** 289–92

57. Huijbregts, A. W. M., Van Berge-Henegouwen, G. P., Hectors, M. P. C., Van Schaik, A. and Van der Werf, S. D. J. (1980). Effects of a standardized wheat bran preparation on biliary lipid composition and bile acid metabolism in young healthy males. *Eur. J. Clin. Invest.,* **10,** 451–8

58. Tarpila, S., Miettinen, T.A. and Metsaranta, L. (1978). Effects of bran on serum cholesterol, faecal mass, fat, bile acids and neutral sterols, and biliary lipids in patients with diverticular disease of the colon. *Gut,* **19,** 137–45

59. Thornton, J. R. and Heaton, K. W. (1981). Do colonic bacteria contribute to cholesterol gallstone formation? Effects of lactulose on bile. *Br. Med. J.* **282,** 1018–20

60. Pomare, E.W. and Heaton, K. W. (1973). Alteration of bile salt metabolism by dietary fibre (bran). *Br. Med. J.,* **4,** 262–4

61. Meyer, P. D., DenBesten, L. and Mason, E. E. (1979). The effects of a high-fibre diet on bile acid pool size, bile acid kinetics and biliary lipid secretory rates in the morbidly obese. *Surgery,* **85,** 311–6

62. Brydon, W. G., Borup-Christensen, S., Van der Linden, W. and Eastwood, M. A. (1979). The effect of dietary psyllium hydrocolloid and lignin on bile. *Z. Ernaehrungswiss.,* **18,** 77–80

63. Kelsay, J. (1978). A review of research on effects of fiber intake on man. *Am. J. Clin. Nutr.,* **31,** 142–59

64. Redinger, R. N. and Grace, D. M. (1976). Cholestyramine induced cholesterol gallstones in the baboon. *Clin. Res.,* **24,** 666A

65. Nestel, P. J., Simons, L. A. and Homma, Y. (1976). Effects of ethanol on bile acid and cholesterol metabolism. *Am. J. Clin. Nutr.*, **29**, 1007–15
66. Marin, G. A., Ward, N. L. and Fischer, R. (1973). Effects of ethanol on pancreatic biliary secretions in humans. *Am. J. Dig. Dis.*, **18**, 825–33
67. Bouchier, I. A. D. (1969). Postmortem study of the frequency of gallstones in patients with cirrhosis of the liver. *Gut*, **10**, 705–10
68. Nicholas, P., Rinaudo, P. A. and Conn, H. O. (1972). Increased incidence of cholelithiasis in Laennec's cirrhosis. *Gastroenterology*, **63**, 112–21
69. Vlahcevic, Z. R., Yoshida, T., Juttijudata, P., Bell, C. C. and Swell, L. (1973). Bile acid metabolism in cirrhosis. III. Biliary lipid secretion in patients with cirrhosis and its relevance to gallstone formation. *Gastroenterology*, **64**, 298–303
70. Schwartz, C. C., Almond, H. R., Vlahcevic, Z. R. and Swell, L. (1979). Bile acid metabolism in cirrhosis. V. Determination of biliary lipid secretion rates in patients with advanced cirrhosis. *Gastroenterology*, **77**, 1177–82
71. Thornton, J., Symes, C. and Heaton, K. (1983). Moderate alcohol intake reduces bile cholesterol saturation and raises HDL cholesterol. *Lancet*, **2**, 819–22
72. Whiting, M. J., Down, R. H. L. and Watts, J. McK. (1981). Precision and saturation index of duodenal bile. *Gastroenterology*, **80**, 533–8
73. Sarles, H., Chalvet, H., Ambrosi, L. and D'Ortoli, G. (1957). Etude statistique des facteurs dietetiques dans la pathogenie de la lithiase biliare humaine. *Sem. Hop. Paris*, **58**, 3424–8
74. Hauton, J. (1966). Cholelithiasis. Third World Congress of Gastroenterology, Tokyo. *Rec. Adv. Gastroenterol.*, **4**, 109–16
75. Sarles, H., Chabert, C., Pommeau, Y., Save, E., Mouret, H. and Gerolami, A. (1969). Diet and cholesterol gallstones. A study of 101 patients with cholelithiasis compared to 101 matched controls. *Am. J. Dig. Dis.*, **14**, 531–7
76. Sarles, H., Gerolami, A. and Bord, A. (1978). Diet and cholesterol gallstones. A further study. *Digestion*, **17**, 128–34
77. Coste, T., Karsenti, P., Berta, J. l., Cubeau, J. and Guilloud-Bataille, M. (1979). Facteurs dietetiques de la lithiase biliare: comparaison de l'alimentation d'un groupe temion. *Gastroenterol. Clin. Biol.*, **3**, 417–24
78. Burnett, W. (1971). The epidemiology of gallstones. *Tijdschr. Gastroenterol.*, **14**, 79–89
79. Wheeler, M., Hills, L. L. and Laby, B. (1970). Cholelithiasis: a clinical and dietary survey. *Gut*, **11**, 430–7
80. Smith, D. A. and Gee, M. I. (1979). A dietary survey to determine the relationship between diet and cholelithiasis. *Am. J. Clin. Nutr.*, **32**, 1519–26
81. Williams, C. N. and Johnston, J. L. (1980). Prevalence of gallstones and risk factors in Caucasian women in a rural Canadian community. *Can. Med. Assoc. J.*, **120**, 664–8
82. Alessandrini, A., Fusco, M. A., Gatti, E. and Rossi, P. A. (1982). Dietary fibres and cholesterol gallstones: a case control study. *Ital. J. Gastroenterol.*, **14**, 156–8
83. Scragg, R. K. R., McMichael, A. J. and Baghurst, P. A. (1984). Diet, alcohol and relative weight in gallstone disease: a case–control study. *Br. Med. J.*, **228**, 1113–9
84. Reid, J. M., Fullmer, S. D., Pettigrew, K. D. *et al.* (1971). Nutrient intake of Pima Indian women: relationships to diabetes mellitus and gallbladder disease. *Am. J. Clin. Nutr.*, **24**, 1281–9
85. Friedman, G. D., Kannel, W. B. and Dawber, T. R. (1966). The epidemiology of gallbladder disease: observations in the Framingham Study. *J. Chron. Dis.*, **19**, 273–92
86. Block, G. (1982). A review of validations of dietary assessment methods. *Am. J. Epidemiol.*, **115**, 492–505
87. Attili, A. F. and the GREPCO Group (1984). Dietary habits and cholelithiasis. In Capocaccia, L., Ricci, G., Angelico, F., Angelico, M. and Attili, A. F. (eds.) *Epidemiology and Prevention of Gallstone Disease.* pp. 175–81. (Lancaster, England: MTP Press)
88. Klatsky, A. L., Friedman, G. D. and Siegelaub, A. B. (1981). Alcohol use and cardiovascular disease: the Kaiser-Permanente experience. *Circulation*, **64**, suppl. III, 32–41
89. Johnston, J. L., Williams, C. N. and Weldon, K. L. M. (1977). Nutrient intake and meal patterns of Micmac Indian and Caucasian women in Shubenacadie, NS. *Can. Med. Assoc. J.*, **116**, 1356–9
90. Pixley, F., Wilson, D., McPherson, K. and Mann, J. (1985). Effect of vegetarianism on development of gallstones in women. *Br. Med. J.*, **291**, 11–12

91. Sturdevant, R. A. L., Pearce, M. L. and Dayton, S. (1973). Increased prevalence of chole-lithiasis in men ingesting a serum-cholesterol-lowering diet. *N. Engl. J. Med.*, **228**, 24–7

92. Miettinen, M., Turpeinen, O., Karvonen, M. J., Paavilainen, E. and Elosuo, R. (1976). Prevalence of cholelithiasis in men and women ingesting a serum-cholesterol-lowering diet. *Ann. Clin. Res.*, **8**, 111–6

93. Gross, D. M. B. (1929). A statistical study of cholelithiasis. *J. Pathol. Bacteriol.*, **32**, 503–26

94. Zahor, Z. (1976). Atherosclerosis in relation to cholelithiasis and cholesterolosis. *Bull. WHO*, **53**, 531–7

95. Diehl, A. K., Stern, M. P., Ostrower, V. S. and Friedman, P. C. (1980). Prevalence of clinical gall-bladder disease in Mexican-American, Anglo and Black Women. *South. Med. J.*, **73**, 438–43

96. Tucker, L. E., Tangedahl, T. N. and Newmark, S. R. (1982). Prevalence of gallstones in obese caucasian American women. *Int. J. Obesity*, **6**, 247–51

97. Van der Linden, W. (1962). Some biological traits in female gallstone-disease patients. *Acta Chir. Scand.*, suppl. 269

98. Horn, G. (1956). Observations on the aetiology of cholelithiasis. *Br. Med. J.*, **2**, 732–7

99. Bernstein, R. A., Werner, L. H. and Rimm, A. A. (1973). Relationship of gallbladder disease to parity, obesity and age. *Health Serv. Rep.*, **88**, 925–36

100. Honore, L. H. (1980). Cholesterol cholelithiasis in adolescent females. Its connection with obesity, parity and oral contraceptive use – a retrospective study of 31 cases. *Arch. Surg.*, **115**, 62–4

101. Nestel, P. J., Whyte, H. M. and Goodman, D. S. (1969). Distribution and turnover of cholesterol in humans. *J. Clin. Invest.*, **48**, 982–91

102. Miettinen, T. A. (1971). Cholesterol production in obesity. *Circulation*, **44**, 842–50

103. Grundy, S. M., Duane, W. C., Adler, R. D., Aron, J. M. and Metzger, A. L. (1974). Biliary lipid outputs in young women with cholesterol stones. *Metabolism*, **23**, 67–73

104. Mabee, T. M., Meyer, P., DenBesten, L. and Mason, E. E. (1976). The mechanism of increased gallstone formation in obese human subjects. *Surgery*, **79**, 460–8

105. Angelin, B., Einarsson, K., Ewerth, S. and Leijd, B. (1981). Biliary lipid composition in obesity. *Scand. J. Gastroenterol.*, **16**, 1015–9

106. Sorensen, T. I. A., Jensen, L. I., Klein, H. C. *et al.* (1980). Risk of gallstone formation after jejunoileal bypass increases more with a 1:3 than a 3:1 jejunoileal ratio. *Scand. J. Gastroenterol.*, **15**, 979–84

107. Krag, E. and Hojgaard, L. (1981). Bile acid metabolism after intestinal bypass operation. *Int. J. Obesity*, **5**, 519–25

108. Layde, P. M., Vessey, M. P. and Yeates, D. (1982). Risk factors for gallbladder disease: a cohort study of young women attending family planning clinics. *J. Epidemiol. Commun. Health*, **36**, 274–8

109. Ahlberg, J. (1979). Serum lipid levels and hyperlipoproteinaemia in gallstone patients. *Acta Chir. Scand.*, **145**, 373–7

110. Angelico, F. and the GREPCO Group (1984). Factors associated with gallstone disease: observations in the GREPCO study. In Capocaccia, L., Ricco, G., Angelico, F., Angelico, M. and Attili, A. F. (eds.) *Epidemiology and Prevention of Gallstone Disease.* pp. 185–92. (Lancaster, England: MTP Press)

111. Scragg, R. K. R., McMichael, A. J. and Seamark, R. F. (1984). Oral contraceptives, pregnancy and endogenous oestrogen in gallstone disease – a case–control study. *Br. Med. J.*, **288**, 1795–9

112. Comess, L. J., Bennett, P. H. and Burch, T. A. (1967). Clinical gallbladder disease in Pima Indians. *N. Engl. J. Med.*, **277**, 894–8

113. Thistle, J. L., Eckhart, K. L., Nensel, R. E. *et al.* (1971). Prevalence of gallbladder disease among Chippewa Indians. *Mayo Clin. Proc.*, **46**, 603–8

114. Williams, C. N., Johnston, J. L. and Weldon, K. L. M. (1977). Prevalence of gallstones and gallbladder disease in Canadian Micmac Indian women. *Can. Med. Assoc. J.*, **117**, 758–60

115. Robertson, H. E. and Dochat, G. R. (1944). Pregnancy and gallstones: collective review. *Int. Abstr. Surg.*, **78**, 193–204

116. Everson, G. T., McKinley, C., Lawson, M., Johnson, M. and Kern, F. (1982). Gallbladder function in the human female: effect of the ovulatory cycle, pregnancy and contraceptive steroids. *Gastroenterology*, **82**, 711–9

117. Dokert, B., Jaross, W., Schentke, K., Trubsbach, A. and Sarembe, B. (1978). Schwan-

gerschaft, orale hormonale kontrazeption und gallenlipidzusammensetzung. *Dtsch. Gesundheitswesen*, **33**, 1153–5

118. Boston Collaborative Drug Surveillance Programme (1973). Oral contraceptives and venous thromboembolic disease, surgically confirmed gallbladder disease, and breast tumours. *Lancet*, **1**, 1399–404

119. Stolley, P. D., Tonascia, J. A., Tockman, M. S., Sartwell, P. E., Rutledge, A. H. and Jacobs, M. P. (1975). Thrombosis with low-estrogen oral contraceptives. *Am. J. Epidemiol.*, **102**, 197–208

120. Vessey, M., Doll, R., Peto, R., Johnson, B. and Wiggins, P. (1976). A long-term follow-up study of women using different metods of contraception – an interim report. *J. Biosoc. Sci.*, **8**, 373–427

121. Boston Collaborative Drug Surveillance Program (1974). Surgically confirmed gallbladder disease, venous thromboembolism, and breast tumors in relation to postmenopausal estrogen therapy. *N. Engl. J. Med.*, **290**, 15–9

122. Coronary Drug Project Research Group (1977). Gallbladder disease as a side effect of drugs influencing lipid metabolism. *N. Engl. J. Med.*, **296**, 1185–90

123. Pertsemlidis, D., Panveliwalla, D. and Ahrens, E. H. (1974). Effects of clofibrate and of an estrogen–progestin combination on fasting biliary lipids and cholic acid kinetics in man. *Gastroenterology*, **66**, 565–73

124. Bennion, L. J., Ginsberg, R. L., Garnick, M. B. and Bennett, P. H. (1976). Effects of oral contraceptives on the gallbladder bile of normal women. *N. Engl. J. Med.*, **294**, 189–92

125. Bennion, L. J., Mott, D. M. and Howard, B. V. (1980). Oral contraceptives raise the cholesterol saturation of bile by increasing biliary cholesterol secretion. *Metabolism*, **29**, 18–22

126. Ramcharan, S., Pellegrin, F. A., Ray, R. and Hsu, J-P. (1981). *The Walnut Creek Contraceptive Drug Study*. Vol. 3, pp. 151–2. (Bethesda: National Institutes of Health)

127. Royal College of General Practitioners' Oral Contraception Study (1982). Oral contraceptives and gallbladder disease. *Lancet*, **2**, 957–9

128. Evron, S., Frankel, M. and Diamant, Y. (1982). Biliary disease in young women and its association with pregnancy or oral contraceptives. *Int. Surg.*, **67**, 448–50

129. Scragg, R. K. R. and McMichael, A. J. (1984). Letter. *Br. Med. J.*, **289**, 252

130. Everson, R. B., Byar, D. P. and Bischoff, A. J. (1982). Estrogen predisposes to cholecystectomy but not to stones. *Gastroenterology*, **82**, 4–8

131. Olefsky, J. M., Farquhar, J. W. and Reaven, G. M. (1974). Reappraisal of the role of insulin in hypertriglyceridemia. *Am. J. Med.*, **57**, 551–60

132. Braunsteiner, H., Di Pauli, R., Sailer, S. and Sandhofer, F. (1966). Cholelithiasis und latent diabetische stoffwechsellage. *Schweiz Med. Wochenschr.*, **96**, 44–6

133. Kadziolka, R., Nilsson, S. and Schersten, T. (1977). Prevalence of hyperlipoproteinaemia in men with gallstone disease. *Scand. J. Gastroenterol.*, **12**, 353–5

134. Scragg, R. K. R., Calvert, G. D. and Oliver, J. R. (1984). Plasma lipids and insulin in gallstone disease: a case–control study. *Br. Med. J.*, **289**, 521–5

135. Einarsson, K., Hellstrom, K. and Kallner, M. (1975). Gallbladder disease in hyperlipoproteinaemia. *Lancet*, **1**, 484–7

136. Van der Linden, W. and Bergman, F. (1977). An analysis of data on human hepatic bile. Relationship between main bile components, serum cholesterol and serum triglycerides. *Scand. J. Clin. Lab. Invest.*, **37**, 741–7

137. Hassan, T. J., Maqsood, R. and Zuberi, S. J. (1979). Lipid patterns in cholelithiasis. *J. Pak. Med. Assoc.*, **29**, 93–6

138. Thornton, J. R., Heaton, K. W. and MacFarlane, D. G. (1981). A relation between high-density-lipoprotein cholesterol and bile cholesterol saturation. *Br. Med. J.*, **283**, 1352–4

139. Marks, J. W., Cleary, P. A. and Albers, J. J. (1984). Lack of correlation between serum lipoproteins and biliary cholesterol saturation in patients with gallstones. *Dig. Dis. Sci.*, **29**, 1118–22

140. Hove, E. and Geill, T. (1968). Serum cholesterol and incidence of gallstones. *Geriatrics*, **23**, 114–8

141. Albers, J. J., Grundy, S. M., Cleary, P. A., Small, D. M., Lachin, J. M. and Schoenfield, L. J. (1982). National Cooperative Gallstone Study: the effect of chenodeoxycholic acid on lipoproteins and apolipoproteins. *Gastroenterology*, **82**, 638–46

142. Sievers, M. L. (1968). Serum cholesterol levels in southwestern American Indians. *J. Chron. Dis.*, **21**, 107–15

143. Savage, P. J., Hamman, R. F., Bartha, G., Dippe, S. E., Miller, M. and Bennett, P. H. (1976). Serum cholesterol levels in American (Pima) Indian children and adolescents. *Pediatrics*, **58**, 274–82

144. Thorbjarnarson, B. J. (1969). Lipid in blood and bile from the normal and the person with cholelithiasis. *Arch. Surg.*, **98**, 372–4

145. Maqsood, R., Zuberi, S. J., Nizami, H. M. and Chaudhry, S. A. (1976). Gallstone composition and biochemical alterations in the serum of patients with cholelithiasis. *J. Pak. Med. Assoc.*, **28**, 167–8

146. Angelico, M. and the GREPCO Group (1984). Relationships between serum lipids and cholelithiasis: observations in the GREPCO study. In Capocaccia, L., Ricci, G., Angelico, F., Angelico, M. and Attili, A. F. (eds.) *Epidemiology and Prevention of Gallstone Disease.* pp. 77–84. (Lancaster, England: MTP Press)

147. Petitti, D. B., Friedman, G. D. and Klatsky, A. L. (1981). Association of a history of gallbladder disease with a reduced concentration of high density lipoprotein cholesterol. *N. Engl. J. Med.*, **304**, 1396–8

148. Carlson, L. A. and Ericsson, M. (1975). Quantitative and qualitative serum lipoprotein analysis. Part 2. Studies in male survivors of myocardial infarction. *Atherosclerosis*, **21**, 435–50

149. Stout, R.W., Balmer, J. P., Henry, R. W. and Buchanan, K. D. (1978). Plasma lipids and gastrointestinal hormones in subjects with gallstones. *Horm. Metab. Res.*, **10**, 357–8

150. Kolterman, O. G., Gray, R.S., Griffin, J. *et al.* (1981). Receptor and post-receptor defects contribute to the insulin resistance in noninsulin-dependent diabetes mellitus. *J. Clin. Invest.*, **68**, 957–69

151. Olefsky, J. M. and Kolterman, O. G. (1980). *In vivo* studies of insulin resistance in human obesity. In Bjorntop, P., Cairella, M. and Howard, A. N. (eds.) *Recent Advances in Obesity Research.* Vol. 3, pp. 254–67. (London: John Libbey)

152. Ponz de Leon, M., Ferenderes, R. and Carulli, N. (1978). Bile lipid composition and bile acid pool size in diabetes. *Am. J. Dig. Dis.*, **23**, 710–16

153. Kajiyama, G., Oyamada, K., Nakao, S. and Miyoshi, A. (1981). The effect of diabetes mellitus and its treatment on the lithogenicity of bile in man. *Hiroshima J. Med. Sci.*, **30**, 221–7

154. Haber, G. B. and Heaton, K. W. (1979). Lipid composition of bile in diabetes and obesity-matched controls. *Gut*, **20**, 518–22

155. Castelli, W. P., Doyle, J. T., Gordon, T. *et al.* (1977). Alcohol and blood lipids. The cooperative lipoprotein phenotyping study. *Lancet*, **2**, 153–5

156. Wynn, V., Adams, P. W., Godsland, I. *et al.* (1979). Comparison of effects of different combined oral-contraceptive formulations on carbohydrate and lipid metabolism. *Lancet*, **1**, 1045–9

157. Puavilai, G., Drobney, E. C., Domont, L. A. and Baumann, G. (1982). Insulin receptors and insulin resistance in human pregnancy: evidence for a postreceptor defect in insulin action. *J. Clin. Endocrinol. Metab.*, **54**, 247–53

158. Williams, P. F., Simons, L. A. and Turtle, J. R. (1976). Plasma lipoproteins in pregnancy. *Horm. Res.*, **7**, 83–90

159. Bailey, C. J. and Ahmed-Sorour, H. (1980). Role of ovarian hormones in the long-term control of glucose homeostasis: effects on insulin secretion. *Diabetologia*, **19**, 475–81

160. Kim, H. J. and Kalkhoff, R. K. (1975). Sex steroid influence in triglyceride metabolism. *J. Clin. Invest.*, **56**, 888–96

161. Sodhi, H. S. and Kudchodkar, B. J. (1973). Correlating metabolism of plasma and tissue-cholesterol with that of plasma-lipoproteins. *Lancet*, **1**, 513–9

162. Shaffer, E. A. and Small, D. M. (1977). Biliary lipid secretion in cholesterol gallstone disease: the effect of cholecystectomy and obesity. *J. Clin. Invest.*, **59**, 828–40

3
Natural History and Prevention

A. F. ATTILI

Prevention of a chronic non-infectious disease such as cholelithiasis can be divided into primary and secondary areas. Primary prevention means prevention of the occurrence of the disease while secondary prevention means prevention of the progression of the disease.

First of all, one might consider if it is necessary to prevent gallstone formation. Preventive measures are particularly warranted by the incidence, morbidity, mortality and social costs of the disease. The results of epidemiological studies[1], now based on ultrasound screening, indicate that in Caucasian adult populations the prevalence of gallstones is approximately 10%. Calculations, based on the epidemiological studies performed in Italy[2-4], show that 2.6 million (1.7 females and 0.9 males), out of the 57 million Italian inhabitants, suffer from gallstone disease (presence of gallstones in the gallbladder or previous cholecystectomy). Approximately 135 000 subjects (85 000 females and 50 000 males) form stones each year. Cholecystitis and obstructive jaundice are common clinical problems. Although only a minority of gallstone carriers will ever undergo surgery, cholecystectomy is the most common abdominal operation performed in western societies[5]. About 500 000 cholecystectomies are performed each year in the USA. The standardized rate of cholecystectomy in England is one third of that in Canada[6]. Differences in cholecystectomy rates, which are not explained by different prevalence rates of gallstones, are probably due to different clinical indications for the operation. The risks of mortality from gallbladder disease and cholecystectomy are relatively low in young and middle-aged adults, but increase greatly with advancing years. Cholecystectomy performed electively on an otherwise healthy young patient carries a mortality rate of 0.2%; however, the overall USA surgical mortality rate is 1.8% with a morbidity rate of 7%. Gallstone disease is undoubtedly costly, both in financial terms and in time lost from work.

Attempts towards primary and secondary prevention of gallstones should be made if these are feasible and practical.

Planning of primary or secondary prevention trials largely depends on our knowledge of the aetiology, epidemiology and natural history of the disease.

Very few data are available on the aetiology of pigment stones which, however, represent the minority of stones. Attention will thus be focused on primary and secondary prevention of cholesterol stones.

PRIMARY PREVENTION

Prevention of a chronic disease can be attempted through modification of the risk factors. We will report, here, the evidence obtained in the course of epidemiological studies in favour of, or against, the commonly indicated risk factors from gallstone disease. Diet will be discussed separately because of the importance it might have in the large-scale prevention of gallstones.

Risk factors from epidemiological studies

Epidemiological risk factors are those which are associated with an increased incidence of the disease, as demonstrated in longitudinal studies. With the sole exception of the Framingham study[7], no longitudinal study has been carried out on the incidence of gallstones in the general population. This study was, however, primarily devoted to cardiovascular diseases and recorded only cases of symptomatic or clinically diagnosed gallstone cases; no attempt was made to discover silent gallstones. In the Framingham study, the overall incidence of gallbladder disease was about twice as high in women as in men. Increases in weight and number of pregnancies were each associated with increased incidence. No relationship was demonstrated between serum cholesterol levels and gallbladder disease. The level of physical activity was also not related to gallbladder disease.

Risk factors may be suspected on the basis of cross-sectional epidemiological studies looking for factors which are associated with an increased prevalence of gallstones. Few of such studies have been performed, so far, on free-living samples of Caucasian populations. The first of these studies was performed by Bainton et al.[8] who investigated, by means of limited cholecystography, the prevalence of gallstones in Barry (an industrial town in South Wales). This technique has the advantage of giving information on the X-ray characteristics of stones thus allowing differentiation between subjects with radiolucent gallstones, which are mainly cholesterol stones, and those with radio-opaque stones, which are mainly pigment stones[9,10]. This would make it possible to analyse separately the associated factors for the two types of gallstones, which have different pathogenic mechanisms[11]. Cholecystography cannot, however, be applied to large scale epidemiological surveys as a result of the high costs and the hazards due to X-ray exposure. Bainton et al.[8] have not reported any results concerning the analysis of associated factors.

The advent of accurate ultrasound diagnosis of gallstones has favoured large-scale cross-sectional and longitudinal epidemiological surveys. Ultrasonography has the disadvantage that it does not directly make identification of pigment or cholesterol stones possible. Cholecystography, however, performed following gallstone identification, by means of ultrasonography, would overcome the problem of discrimination. The first studies, using ultrasonography as a diagnostic tool, were performed in Italy[2-4]. The Rome group for Epidemiology and Prevention of Cholelithiasis (GREPCO) studied two populations (each made up of about 1100 subjects) of civil servants in Rome, aged 20–69 years. Associated factors were studied by univariate and multivariate[12] statistical analysis. Subjects with gallstones present in the gallbladder and subjects who had been previously submitted to cholecystectomy were considered separately. The age-standardized results of the univariate analysis (unpublished observations of the GREPCO group) showed that, in men, HDL-cholesterol was significantly lower in subjects with gallstones than in those without them. In women, the mean number of pregnancies was significantly higher in subjects with gallstones than in those without. Women who had been previously submitted to cholecystectomy were significantly smaller in height and had significantly higher serum glucose levels than women without gallstones. In the multivariate analysis, the presence of gallstones was significantly and positively associated with age and serum triglycerides in both sexes. In men, a negative interaction between serum triglyceride levels and age was observed, demonstrating that young men with high levels of serum triglycerides are more frequently affected by gallstones than older men. In women, a positive association was also observed between the presence of gallstones and the number of pregnancies of the body mass index; a negative association was observed between the presence of gallstones and the serum HDL-cholesterol levels or the square of serum total cholesterol levels. A negative interaction was observed between age and number of pregnancies. The multivariate analysis, using previous cholecystectomy as independent variable, showed that age was positively associated in both sexes. In women, cholecystectomy was positively associated with serum triglyceride and glucose levels. No association was found between presence of gallstones in the gallbladder or cholecystectomy and the use of oral contraceptives or hypolipidaemic drugs. Similar results were obtained by the other Italian study[4,13] carried out on the general population of a small town (Sirmione) in the north of Italy. 1930 subjects participated in this study. At variance with the GREPCO studies, no association was found with total serum cholesterol levels (unpublished observations of the Sirmione study).

Factors associated to gallstone disease have also been investigated by means of case–control studies. Three basic criticisms of these studies are that all of them enrolled mostly symptomatic and clinically diagnosed cases, many studied inadequate controls and many used small sample sizes. The largest case–control studies published so far are those by Scragg and co-workers[14-16]. In these studies, the presence of gallstones was positively associated with obesity only in young women and with increased plasma triglyceride concentrations only in young subjects; after controlling for plasma insulin and triglyceride concentrations, an increased plasma total cholesterol concentration was associated with a decreased risk of gallstones. The probability of having gallstone disease increased in association with increasing parity, particularly among younger women. Use of oral contraceptives was associated with an increased prevalence of gallstones among young subjects and with a decreased prevalence among older subjects.

Petitti et al.[17] studied the prevalence and factors associated with gallstone disease in a population of 868 female twins. These authors found that the history of gallbladder disease was positively associated to age, body mass index and oestrogen use. A negative association was found with HDL-cholesterol serum levels.

Epidemiological evidence for factors associated with gallstone disease may also be derived by studying prevalence and incidence in cohorts of subjects exposed for a period of time to the supposed risk factor. These studies demonstrated that an increased frequency of gallstones occurs among users of clofibrate[18-20]. Women users of oral contraceptives[21-22] or men receiving long-term treatment with oestrogen[18].

Diet

Diet has long been suspected of playing a key role in the formation of cholesterol gallstones. High intake of calories, cholesterol, polyunsaturated fats, refined carbohydrates and a low intake of fibre have been, from time to time, indicated as putative risk factors. The Framingham study[7] demonstrated in a longitudinal survey, that dietary fat, protein and cholesterol intake are not risk factors for gallbladder disease. The diet interviews were, however, conducted in most cases after the disease had been diagnosed so that symptoms or medical advice may have modified levels of intake. This problem was overcome in the two Italian epidemiological studies[2-4], as both of these studies enrolled mostly asymptomatic and previously undiagnosed series of cases and the questionnaire interviews were conducted before ultrasonography. Both the GREPCO and Sirmione protocols were based on the use of the food frequency method which is the most reliable method for assessing food consumption in large-scale epidemiological surveys. Methods in which food is weighed and the nutritional assessment is made by expert personnel are probably more accurate than the food frequency method but are much more time-consuming and expensive. From the univariate analysis in the GREPCO study[22,23], the level of consumption for most of the food items examined, was lower in gallstone subjects than in subjects without gallstones, both in terms of daily mean quantitative consumption and in terms of frequency of consumption. A reduced frequency of consumption in gallstone subjects was evidently mostly for fatty foods. Women with gallstones were less likely to have a snack between meals than women without gallstones. After controlling in the multivariate analysis for possible confounding variables such as age, body mass index, presence of symptoms, awareness of having gallstones and levels of physical activity, a weak negative association was observed between the presence of gallstones and the mean daily consumption of pasta in men, and of sugar in women, and with frequency of consumption of vegetables in men. This latter finding could fit into the low fibre intake theory. The former results do not corroborate the hypothesis that a high calorie intake is a risk factor for gallstones. Similar results have been obtained by the Sirmione study (unpublished observations of the Sirmione Group) in which a low fibre intake, in particular, was demonstrated in gallstone subjects. At variance with the GREPCO study, a weak negative association was noted with alcohol consumption.

The results of case–control studies investigating the association of diet with gallstone disease have not been consistent. Some studies showed, for instance, a higher energy intake[14,24,25], some others a lower[26] and others no difference[27-29] between subjects with and those without gallstones. Only the daily intake of fibre was uniformly reported as 'reduced' in subjects with gallstones[14,30]. In accordance with the same theory, prevalence of gallstones was found to be lower in vegetarian women than in women who ate meat[31].

As far as the type of dietary fat is concerned, the GREPCO group reported that, in women, the percentage composition of erythrocyte fatty acids[22,32], which is an objective index of the long-term changes of dietary lipids[33], was not different in subjects with or without gallstones. Substituting polyunsaturated fat for saturated fat, in the American diet, has been reported to increase the incidence of gallstones[34]. This finding was not confirmed by another study performed in Scandinavian countries[35].

In brief, only a low fibre intake was invariably (although in some cases, weakly) associated with gallbladder disease. The other putative dietary risk factors do not seem to be firmly linked to the pathogenesis of gallstones. These conclusions should, however, be considered with great caution as they are mainly based on cross-sectional studies and could greatly be modified by the results of prospective longitudinal studies. Dietary factors could, for instance, be important in conditioning obesity and when this has been established, gallstones could form without any further involvement of dietary factors. Little attention has been paid so far in epidemiological studies to frequency of meals and duration of overnight fast. Both these factors could cause a decreased gallbladder contraction and bile stasis.

In conclusion, factors associated to gallstone disease which have received almost invariable confirmation through epidemiological studies are age, female sex, parity (especially in young women), serum triglycerides and obesity. These factors are the most likely to become true risk factors after confirmation of an association with an increased incidence of gallstones in longitudinal studies. Factors which have received substantial epidemiological evidence are the low serum total or HDL-cholesterol levels and low dietary fibre. Factors which have received little epidemiological evidence but that are known[36] pathogenic mechanisms responsible for conditions predisposing to gallstone formation (supersaturated bile, nucleation defects or impaired gallbladder motor function) are gastrointestinal disorders involving major malabsorption of bile acids[37], total parenteral nutrition, rapid weight loss during slimming diets, use of oral contraceptives or hypolipidaemic drugs. Some of these factors, on the other hand, might never be confirmed by epidemiological studies in free-living population samples on account of their too low prevalence rates.

Preventive measures

What measures can we take to prevent gallstone disease? From the foregoing, it is reasonable to expect that prevention or correction of obesity and reduction of serum triglycerides should reduce the incidence of gallstone disease in the general population. These objectives could be reached through modification of diet, such as reduction of energy intake and increase of dietary fibre. The reduction of the period of overnight fast could be another practical preventive measure but other changes in the diet such as reduction of dietary fat or modification of the fatty acid composition, could have unpredictable results. The above-outlined preventive measures overlap, at least in part, with those currently believed of importance in the prevention of cardiovascular diseases. Some points, however, deserve consideration. Firstly, it has been demonstrated that during caloric restriction and weight-loss the secretion of all biliary lipids decrease and the bile acid pool shrinks[36]. In some subjects, the secretion of bile acids decreases more than that of cholesterol, with a resulting rise in bile saturation. The lack of a proportional fall in cholesterol secretion may be due to biliary excretion of the cholesterol mobilized from adipose tissue. A new more favourable equilibrium between biliary lipids is reached only when weight maintenance is obtained. Patients who embark cyclically on 'crash diets', but regain weight between each therapeutic attempt, may achieve nothing or be worse in terms of susceptibility to gallstones. Secondly, reduction of serum triglycerides should not be achieved with the use of clofibrate and possibly also not with other hypolipidaemic drugs. Thirdly, reduction of obesity is, in most cases, followed by a reduction of total serum cholesterol levels. According to some epidemiological studies, this situation is associated with a relatively high prevalence of gallstones. This hypothetical negative effect, in my opinion, would not, however, completely counteract the benefits obtained from the weight and serum triglycerides reduction.

A pharmacological approach with chenodeoxycholic or ursodeoxycholic acids should be reserved only to populations at particularly high risk of developing gallstones, such as subjects whose gallstones were dissolved by means of medical treatment. Frequent recurrence has been reported in these subjects[38] and there is no doubt that these subjects must be monitored for early detection of recurrent stones and possibly protected against gallstone recurrence. Low dose (375 mg/day) continuous CDCA was no more effective than a placebo in preventing recurrence[39]. A large prospective random allocation post dissolution trial is now in progress in Great Britain and Belgium[38]. This study, which has a yet unbroken code, compares the effects of low dose (3 mg/kg per day) ursodeoxycholic acid, placebo and a diet, high in fibre and low in refined carbohydrate, in preventing gallstone recurrence. Another group of subjects at particularly high risk of developing gallstones is that of obese subjects undergoing rapid weight reduction. A trial which compares placebo and ursodeoxycholic acid (1200 mg/day) or aspirin (1300 mg/day) for a 16-week period is now in progress in California (J. Marks: personal communication). The long-term prevention of gallstone disease with exogeneous bile acids should be considered with extreme caution since administration of chenodeoxycholic acid has been demonstrated to induce a low, but epidemiologically important, increase in total serum cholesterol levels[40]. A similar side-effect has not been reported for ursodeoxycholic acid, but trials, as large and as well-planned as that published by the National Co-operative Gallstone Study for chenodeoxycholic acid[41], have not been performed so far.

SECONDARY PREVENTION

Natural history after gallstone formation

Once gallstones are formed they are, at least for a short period, silent (Figure 3.1). The natural fate of silent stones is (a) to remain in the gallbladder for

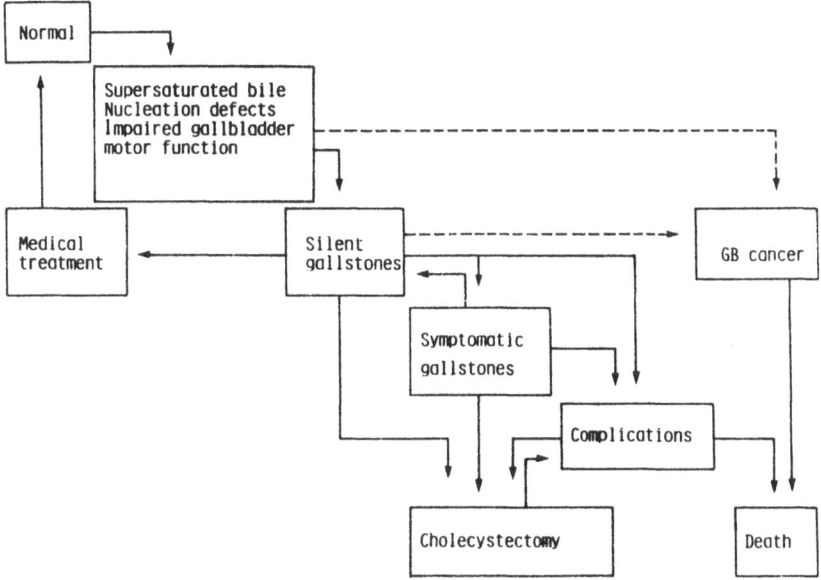

Figure 3.1   Natural history of gallstone disease

the rest of the subject's life without inducing symptoms or complications; (b) to become symptomatic; (c) to induce complications (cholecystitis, extrahepatic jaundice, pancreatitis, etc.). Stage (c) is preceded in most cases by stage (b). The natural fate may be modified by prophylactic surgery or by medical treatment. The rate at which silent gallstones become symptomatic largely depends on the definition of silent gallstones which, in turn, is derived from the definition of symptoms related to gallstones. In the past it was believed that gallstones caused many dyspeptic symptoms such as belching, flatulence, intolerance to fatty foods, abdominal discomfort after meals, variations in bowel habits, etc. Several studies[2,8,42], however, have clearly shown that dyspeptic symptoms are no more frequent in subjects with gallstones than in those without them. In two epidemiological studies[2,43] subjects submitted to cholecystectomy presented dyspeptic symptoms more often than subjects who had not previously been operated upon. Two possibilities may explain this finding: the dyspeptic symptoms were induced by cholecystectomy or cholecystectomy was performed on subjects who presented dyspeptic symptoms which favoured diagnosis, but the cholecystectomy did not relieve symptoms which were related to causes other than gallstones. What seems clear is that patients with 'non-specific' symptoms should not be considered symptomatic. As far as pain is concerned, it has recently been shown by GREPCO[3] that in the 5 years before examination, an unspecified abdominal pain was equally frequent among 66 women with gallstones and in 979 without gallstones (66.6% and 59.4% respectively). When location and duration of pain were analysed, a first discrimination was obtained between subjects with or without gallstones. Women with gallstones had in fact suffered at least one episode of abdominal pain in the right hypocondrium or epigastrium lasting more than 30 min more frequently (34.8%) than women without gallstones (20.7%). The difference was statistically significant ($p < 0.05$). On the basis of this observation, the following definition of symptomatic gallstone subjects can be offered: symptomatic gallstone subjects are those who complained of at least one episode of abdominal pain in the right hypocondrium or in the epigastrium which lasted more than 30 min during the 5-year period prior to examination. Further specifications of biliary pain (radiation, use of antispasmodics or bed rest, accompanying fever or mild jaundice) would increase the specificity of the symptom but necessarily decrease the sensitivity.

Although the definition of symptomatic gallstone subjects, given above, might be criticized from a clinical point of view, it represents the first clear-cut epidemiological approach to the problem to which future reports might refer for comparison. Previous studies either gave an ambiguous definition, or none at all, of symptomatic gallstones. Gracie and Ransohoff[44] defined biliary pain as an episode of upper abdominal pain that was not clearly due to another cause. Comfort et al.[45] included symptoms of indigestion (gaseous indigestion, intolerance to certain foods and heartburn) in the definition of symptomatic subjects. It is clear that it is difficult to make a comparison between different studies with different definitions. Nevertheless, the incidence rates of biliary pain and of complications, observed by the various authors, are shown in Table 3.1. The annual incidence rates of biliary colic in both

Table 3.1 Studies of the natural history of silent gallstones

Authors	No. of asymtomatic gallstone subjects	Years of follow-up	Yearly incidence rates (%)	
			Biliary pain	Complications
Lund[46]	34	5–20	4.24*	1.64*
Comfort et al.[45]	112	10–20	1.25*	0.3*
Newman et al.[47]	191	2–22	2.2	NA
Gracie and Ransohoff[44]	123	11–24	2 in 0–4 years 1 in 5–9 years 0.5 in 10–14 years 0 thereafter	0.15*
McSherry et al.[48]	135	3.8**	2.6*	0.6*
GREPCO†	67	2–4	4.5	0
Sirmione‡	101	2	5.5	0.5

NA: not available
* Calculated from the authors' overall incidence rate figures and assuming a mean follow-up between the minimum and maximum
† Unpublished observations of GREPCO
‡ Unpublished observations of the Sirmione study
** Median

the GREPCO and Sirmione studies are very high. This fact may be, on one hand, explained by differences in the definition of biliary colic and, on the other, as both the GREPCO and Sirmione studies included mostly previously undiagnosed cases who were probably more alert to abdominal symptoms after they had been informed of the presence of gallstones.

The natural fate of symptomatic gallstones is (a) to remain symptomatic; (b) to revert to an asymptomatic situation; (c) to give rise to complications. In many cases the natural history of symptomatic gallstones is modified by cholecystectomy. On the basis of the definition of symptomatic gallstones given above, symptomatic gallstones may revert to an asymptomatic stage when a 5-year free-of-pain period interrupts the pain sequence. The fate of patients with untreated but diagnosed and symptomatic gallstones is even less defined than that of the asymptomatic patients. In most cases, symptomatic gallstone patients are advised to undergo cholecystectomy presuming that symptoms would continue and that complications would continue and that complications would appear. However, data to support these assumptions are more deductive than factual. McSherry et al.[48] reported that 44% of 556 symptomatic gallstones, followed up for a mean of 82.9 ± 63.2 months, underwent biliary tract operations, most often because of persistent symptoms. The calculated annual incidence rate of cholecystectomy is 6.4%. The incidence rate of surgery for persistent symptoms during the 2–4 years of follow-up of 54 symptomatic gallstone subjects in the GREPCO and Sirmione studies considered together was 12.6%. During the same follow-up 46% of initially symptomatic gallstone subjects did not experience new episodes of biliary pain.

The possibility of a causal link between cholelithiasis and gallbladder cancer has been noted since 1924[49]. The following evidence suggests an association between gallbladder cancer and cholelithiasis: gallstones are present in more than 80% of subjects with gallbladder cancer[51–53]; risk factors for cholelithiasis overlap, to a certain extent, with those for gallbladder cancer[54,55]. These factors include age, female sex, parity, dietary habits, exogenous oestrogens, clofibrate and gastrointestinal disorders. However, differences in the geographical distribution of gallbladder cancer may not be explained only by differences in the prevalence of gallbladder disease, thus suggesting that at least some other risk factors are active, one of which could be a chronic carrier state in the gallbladder of Salmonella typhi[54,56]. The incidence of gallbladder cancer in gallstone patients is not easy to establish in prospective studies, nor can it be derived from official statistics on the causes of death because, until recently, the International Classification of Diseases has classified cancers of the gallbladder and of the extrahepatic bile ducts under the same heading (cancer of the biliary tract) instead of separately. Calculations, based on the supposed prevalence of gallstones in Italy and on mortality from cancer of the biliary tract, indicate that the annual incidence rate of cancer of the biliary tract among subjects with gallstones should be around 0.05%. According to Donaldson[57] the overall occurrence of gallbladder cancer is 0.5% in patients with gallstones. One case–control study[58] conducted by a retrospective chart review even noted an association between the size of gallstones and the risk of gallbladder cancer. However, other researchers have disagreed[59,60], as they felt that there is no aetiological relationship between the two. In any case, incidence of gallbladder cancer is very low.

In conclusion, subjects with gallstones cannot be classified as symptomatic if they only complained of dyspeptic symptoms. Silent gallstones become symptomatic when an abdominal pain appears in the right hypocondrium or in the epigastrium lasting more than 30 min and remain symptomatic (by definition) until a 5-year pain-free period interrupts the pain sequence. Both symptomatic and asymptomatic gallstone subjects can become complicated whenever a major complication (acute cholecystitis, jaundice, etc.) occurs. Gallbladder cancer is associated with gallstones and factors predisposing to gallstones. In few cases, death may be due to complications linked to gallstone disease and to gallbladder cancer.

Early diagnosis

Early detection of gallstones might facilitate secondary prevention, also because recently formed stones are more likely to be pure cholesterol stones which can be dissolved by medical treatment. With regard to this, ultra-sonographic screening of high-risk populations is advisable. Attempts at defining those conditions which can identify groups of subjects with a high probability of having gallstones are in progress, mostly derived from the data base of cross-sectional epidemiological studies[3]. Among 35 variables which could easily be recorded with a questionnaire without expensive or invasive techniques, only five were found associated to the presence of gallstones by the GREPCO group: age, number of pregnancies, body mass index, presence of at least one episode of biliary colic and biliary colic restricting the patient to bed rest. The sum of the predictive scores attributed to each variable would enable us to calculate the probability of having stones of each interviewed subject. It was calculated that, if this finding was available before the beginning of the first female GREPCO study, the ultrasound examination of only one fifth of the population would have permitted detection of three fifths of the women with gallstones. Prospective evaluation of this procedure in further population samples is needed.

Preventive measures

Prevention of symptoms or complications in asymptomatic gallstone patients is obviously achieved by medical dissolution or surgical removal of gallstones. According to the epidemiological observations of GREPCO and of the Sirmione studies[61,62], only 25–35% of gallstones are suitable for medical dissolution (i.e. the gallstones are radiolucent, less than 15 mm in diameter, in a visualized gallbladder). Only one half of these subjects will have their stones dissolved under an appropriate therapeutic regimen and about 50% of those dissolved will re-form within a few years. Thus only 5–8%, a figure not far from a surgical approach to the problem[63], of asymptomatic gallstone subjects will receive a definite prevention of symptoms or complications by means of medical treatment. Is it necessary for all, or part of, the remaining 92–95% of asymptomatic gallstone subjects to undergo surgical removal of gallstones?

This subject is presently being widely discussed and the great perplexities have been condensed in a humorous editorial in the *New England Journal of Medicine*[57]. Doubts mostly arise from the vague information about the natural history of silent gallstones and could be cleared up only by large, time-consuming and expensive clinical trials comparing expectant management or prophylactic cholecystectomy. A decision analysis approach (a hypothetical clinical trial which uses data on probabilities from medical literature) has been attempted in three different papers[62,64,65]. Such studies are obviously influenced by an optimistic or pessimistic view of the natural history of gallstone disease. The conclusion was, however, in any case, that expectant management is the treatment of choice for silent gallstones. A similar conclusion was also drawn in a recent 'surgical' paper[48] describing the natural history of symptomatic and asymptomatic gallstones in which, however, a decision analysis approach was not attempted. We believe that data larger than those presently available are necessary, particularly those deriving from epidemiological unselected series of cases. Such studies could also answer some potentially important questions regarding risk factors for biliary pain or for complications. Are there any differences between the sexes in the natural history? In the cross-sectional studies of GREPCO[3], women with gallstones were more frequently symptomatic than men. This result was not, however, confirmed by the Sirmione study. Do silent gallstones behave differently according to the characteristics of the gallbladder or of the gall-stones? With regard to this, patients in the National Cooperative Gallstone Study[66], with multiple stones, were more likely than those with solitary stones to have had biliary pain during the 12 months before entry into the study and to develop symptoms during the prospective follow-up. In the cross-sectional studies performed by GREPCO[66], no association was found between presence of biliary colic in the 5 years prior to the study and the X-ray characteristics of the gallbladder or gallstones (e.g. visualization of gallbladder, number, transparency or diameter of stones). Are there other risk factors for biliary pain or complications which could be prevented during expectant management? The internationally accepted medical advice given to patients to avoid intake of cholecystokinetic foods (eggs, fat, etc.) is based on the concept that increased pressure within the biliary tree, due to the gallbladder contraction against an impacted stone or an unrelaxed sphincter of Oddi, is the cause of biliary pain. The efficacy of this medical counsel has, however, never been scientifically tested. The era of primary and secondary prevention of gallstones has begun and during the next 10–20 years these problems should be solved.

References

1. Ingelfinger, F. J. (1968). Digestive disease as a national problem. V. Gallstones. *Gastroenterology*, 55, 102–4
2. Rome Group for the Epidemiology and Prevention of Cholelithiasis (GREPCO) (1984). Prevalence of gallstone disease in an Italian adult female population. *Am. J. Epidemiol.*, 119, 796–805
3. Capocaccia, L. and Ricci, G. (1985). Epidemiology of gallstone disease. In Barbara, L.,

Dowling, R. H., Hofmann, A. F. and Roda, E. (eds.) *Recent Advances in Bile Acid Research.* pp. 231–8. (New York: Raven Press)

4. Barbara, L. and the 'Progetto Sirmione' (1984). Epidemiology of gallstone disease: the 'Sirmione study'. In Capocaccia, L., Ricci, G., Angelico, F., Angelico, M. and Attili, A. F. (eds.) *Epidemiology and Prevention of Gallstone Disease.* pp. 23–5. (Lancaster: MTP Press)

5. Fisher, M. M. (1979). Perspectives in gallstones. In Fisher, M. M., Goreski, C. A., Shaffer, E. A. and Strasberg, S. M. (eds.) *Gallstones.* pp. 1–17. (New York: Plenum Press)

6. Holland, C. and Heaton, K. W. (1972) Increasing frequency of gallbladder operations in the Bristol clinical area. *Br. Med. J.,* **3**, 672–5

7. Friedman, G. D., Kannel, W. B. and Dawber, T. R. (1966). The epidemiology of gallbladder disease: observations in the Framingham study. *J. Chron. Dis.,* **19**, 273–92

8. Bainton, D. B., Davies, G. T., Evans, K. T. and Gravelle, I. H. (1976). Gallbladder disease. Prevalence in a South Wales industrial town. *N. Engl. J. Med.,* **294**, 1147–9

9. Trotman, B. W., Ostrow, J. D., Soloway, R. D., Cheong, E. B. and Longyear, R. B. (1974). Pigment vs. cholesterol cholelithiasis: comparison of stone and bile composition. *Am. J. Dig. Dis.,* **19**, 585–90

10. Dolgin, S. M., Sanford Schwartz, J., Kressel, H. Y., Soloway, R. D., Miller, W. T., Trotman, B. W., Soloway, A. S. and Good, L. I. (1981). Identification of patients with cholesterol or pigment gallstones by discriminant analysis of radiographic features. *N. Engl. J. Med.,* **304**, 808–11

11. Bennion, L. J. and Grundy, S. M. (1978). Risk factors for the development of cholelithiasis in man. (First of two parts.) *N. Engl. J. Med.,* **299**, 1161–7

12. Capocaccia, R. and the GREPCO Group (1984). Appendix, Logistic regression analysis in epidemiological research. In Capocaccia, L., Ricci, G., Angelico, F., Angelico, M., and Attili, A. F. (eds.) *Epidemiology and Prevention of Gallstone Disease.* pp. 223–31. (Lancaster: MTP Press)

13. Roda, E. and the 'Progetto Sirmione' (1984). Factors associated with gallstone disease: observations in the 'Sirmione study'. In Capocaccia, L., Ricci, G., Angelico, F., Angelico, M. and Attili, A. F. (eds.) *Epidemiology and Prevention of Gallstone Disease.* pp. 207–9. (Lancaster: MTP Press)

14. Scragg, R. K. R., McMichael, A. J. and Baghurst, P. A. (1984). Diet, alcohol, and relative weight in gallstone disease: a case–control study. *Br. Med. J.,* **288**, 1113–9

15. Scragg, R. K. R., Calvert, G. D. and Oliver, J. R. (1984). Plasma lipids and insulin in gallstone disease: a case–control study. *Br. Med. J.,* **289**, 521–5

16. Scragg, R. K. R., McMichael, A. J. and Seamark, R. F. (1984). Oral contraceptives, pregnancy and endogenous oestrogen in gallstone disease. A case–control study. *Br. Med. J.,* **288**,1795–1799

17. Petitti, D. B., Friedman, G. D. and Katsky, A. L. (1981). Association of a history of gallbladder disease with a reduced concentration of high density lipoprotein cholesterol. *N. Engl. J. Med.,* **304**, 1396–1398

18. The Coronary Drug Project Research Group, (1977). Gallbladder disease as a side effect of drugs influencing lipid metabolism. *N. Engl. J. Med.,* **296**, 1185–90

19. Bateson, M. C., Maclean, D., Ross, P. E. and Bouchier, I. A. D. (1978). Clofibrate therapy and gallstone induction. *Dig. Dis.,* **23**, 623–8

20. Cooper, J., Geizerova, H. and Oliver, M. F. (1975). Clofibrate and gallstones. *Lancet,* **1**, 1083

21. Heaton, K. W. (1973). The epidemiology of gallstones and suggested aetiology. *Clin. Gastroenterol.,* **2**, 67–83

22. Attili, A. F. and the GREPCO Group (1984). Dietary habits and cholelithiasis. In Capocaccia, L., Ricci, G., Angelico, F., Angelico, M. and Attili, A. F. (eds.) *Epidemiology and Prevention of Gallstone Disease.* pp. 175–81. (Lancaster: MTP Press)

23. Attili, A. F. and the GREPCO group (1986). Diet and gallstones: results of an epidemiological study performed in male civil servants. In Barbara, L., Cheli, R., Bianchi Porro, G. and Libkin, M. (eds.) *Nutrition and Digestive Diseases.* (New York: Raven Press) (In press)

24. Sarles, H., Chalvet, H., Ambrosi, L., Gazeix, N. and D'Ortoli, G. (1957). Etude statistique des facteurs diététiques dans la patologie de la lithiase biliaire humaine. *Sem. Hop. Paris,* **33**, 3424–38

25. Sarles, H., Chabert, C., Pommeau, Y., Save, E., Mouret, H. and Gerolami, A. (1969). Diet and cholesterol gallstones. A study of 101 patients with cholelithiasis compared to 101 matched controls. *Am. J. Dig. Dis.,* **14**, 531–4

26. Burnett, W. (1971). The epidemiology of gallstones. *Tijdsch. Gastroenterol.* **14**, 79–89

27. Sarles, H., Gerolami, A. and Cros, R. C. (1978). Diet and cholesterol gallstones. *Digestion*, **17**, 121–7

28. Wheeler, M., Hills, L. L. and Laby, B. (1970). Cholelithiasis, a clinical and dietary survey. *Gut*, **11**, 430–7

29. Coste, T., Karsenti, P., Berta, J. L., Cubeau, J. and Guilloud-Bataille, M. (1979). Facteurs dietetiques de la lithiase biliaire: comparaison de l'alimentation d'un groupe de lithiasiques a l'alimentation d'un groupe témoin. *Gastroenterol. Clin. Biol*, **3**, 417–24

30. Alessandrini, A., Fusco, M. A., Gatti, E. and Rossi, P. A. (1982). Dietary fibres and cholesterol gallstones: a case control study. *Ital. J. Gastroenterol.*, **14**, 156–8

31. Pixley, F., Wilson, D., McPherson, K. and Mann, J. I. M. (1985). Effect of vegetarianism on development of gallstones in women. *Br. Med. J.*, **291**, 11–12

32. The Rome Group for Epidemiology and Prevention of Cholelithiasis (1986). Erythrocyte fatty acid composition and gallstone disease: results of an epidemiological survey. *Am. J. Clin. Nutr.* (In press)

33. Farquhar, J. W. and Ahrens, E. H. Jr. (1963). Effects of dietary fats on human erythrocyte fatty acid pattern. *J. Clin. Invest.*, **42**, 657–86

34. Sturdevant, R. A., Pearce, M. L. and Dayton, S. (1973). Increased prevalence of cholelithiasis in men ingesting a serum-cholesterol-lowering diet. *N. Engl. J. Med.*, **288**, 24–7

35. Miettinen, M., Turpeinen, O., Karvonen, M. J., Paavilainen, E. and Elosuo, R. (1976). Prevalence of cholelithiasis in men and women ingesting a serum-cholesterol-lowering diet. *Ann. Clin. Res.*, **8**, 111–16

36. Bennion, L. J. and Grundy, S. M. (1978). Risk factors for the development of cholelithiasis in man. (Second of two parts.) *N. Engl. J. Med.*, **299**, 1221–7

37. Heaton, K. W. and Read, A. E. (1969). Gallstones in patients with disorders of the terminal ileum and distributed bile salt metabolism. *Br. Med. J.*, **3**, 494–6

38. Dowling, R. H., Gleeson, D., Ruppin, D. C., Murphy, G. M. and the British/Belgian Gallstone Study Group (1984). Gallstone recurrence and post-dissolution management. In Paumgartner, G., Stiehl, A. and Gerok, W. (eds.) *Enterohepatic Circulation of Bile Acids and Sterol Metabolism.* pp. 361–9. (Lancaster: MTP Press)

39. Marks, J. W. and the National Co-operative Gallstone Study Group (1984). Low dose chenodiol to prevent gallstone recurrence after dissolution therapy. *Ann. Intern. Med.*, **100**, 376, 381

40. Albers, J. J., Grundy, S. H., Cleary, P. A., Small, D. H., Lachin, J. M., Shoenfield, L. J. and The National Cooperative Gallstone Study Group (1982). The effect of chenodeoxycholic acid on lipoproteins and apolipoproteins. *Gastroenterology*, **82**, 638–46

41. The Steering Committee and The National Co-operative Gallstone Study Group (1981). Chenodiol (chenodeoxycholic acid) for dissolution of gallstones: The National Cooperative Gallstone Study. A controlled trial of efficacy and safety. *Ann. Intern. Med.*, **95**, 257–82

42. Price, W. H. (1963). Gallbladder dyspepsia. *Br. Med. J.*, **2**, 138–41

43. Janzon, L., Aspelin, P., Eriksson, S., Hildell, J., Trell, E. and Ostberg, H. (1985). Ultrasonographic screening for gallstone disease in middle-aged women. Detection rate, symptoms, and biochemical features. *Scand. J. Gastroenterol.*, **20**, 706–10

44. Gracie, W. A. and Ransohoff, D. F. (1982). The natural history of silent gallstones. The innocent gallstone is not a myth. *N. Engl. J. Med.*, **307**, 798–800

45. Comfort, M. W., Gray, H. K. and Wilson, J. M. (1948). The silent gallstone: a ten to twenty year follow-up study of 112 cases. *Ann. Surg.*, **128**, 931–7

46. Lund, J. (1960). Surgical indications in cholelithiasis: prophylactic cholecystectomy elucidated on the basis of long-term follow-up on 526 non-operated cases. *Ann. Surg.*, **151**, 153–62

47. Newman, H. F., Northup, J. D., Rosenblum, M. and Abrams, H. (1968). Complications of cholelithiasis. *Am. J. Gastroenterol.*, **50**, 476–96

48. McSherry, C. K., Ferstenberg, H., Ford Calhoun, W., Lahman, E. and Virshup, M. (1985). The natural history of diagnosed gallstone disease in symptomatic and asymptomatic patients. *Ann. Surg.*, **202**, 59–63

49. Leitch, A. (1924). Gallstones and cancer of the gallbladder: an experimental study. *Br. Med. J.*, **2**, 451–4

50. Strauch, G. O. (1960). Primary carcinoma of the gallbladder. *Surgery*, **47**, 368–81
51. Klein, R. H. and DeWeese, M. S. (1973). Primary carcinoma of the gallbladder. *Arch. Surg.*, **104**, 769–72
52. Andrews, E. C., Bennett, D. E. and Arhelger, R. B. (1969). Carcinoma of the gallbladder. *South. Med. J.*, **62**, 573–8
53. Hart, J., Shani, M. and Modan, B. (1972). Epidemiological aspects of gallbladder and biliary tract neoplasms. *Am. J. Publ. Health*, **62**, 36–9
54. Strom, B. L. (1984). Epidemiological and biochemical aspects of an important sequel to cholelithiasis: gallbladder cancer. In Capocaccia, L., Ricci, G., Angelico, F., Angelico, M. and Attili, A. F. (eds.) *Epidemiology and Prevention of Gallstone Disease*. pp. 64–76. (Lancaster: MTP.)
55. Bismuth, H. and Malt, R. A. (1979). Current concepts in cancer. Carcinoma of the biliary tract. *N. Engl. J. Med.*, **301**, 704–6
56. Nervi, F., Paz, B. and Montiel, F. (1984). Pathogenic and clinical relationships between endemic salmonellosis and gallbladder disease. In Capocaccia, L., Ricci, G., Angelico, F., Angelico, M. and Attili, A. F. (eds.) *Epidemiology and Prevention of Gallstone Disease*. pp. 144–52. (Lancaster: MTP Press)
57. Donaldson, R. M. (1982). Advice for the patient with 'silent' gallstones. *N. Engl. J. Med.*, **307**, 815–17
58. Diehl, A. K. (1983). Gallstone size and the risk of gallbladder cancer. *J. Am. Med. Assoc.*, **250**, 2323–6
59. Deyman, H., Gerbarg, D. S., Kelly, J. H., Parker, S. and Singer, J. (1961). Are gallstones and gallbladder carcinoma related? *J. Am. Med. Assoc.*, **176**, 450–1
60. Parkash, O. (1975). On the relationship of cholelithiasis to carcinoma of the gallbladder and on the sex dependency of the carcinoma of the bile ducts. *Digestion*, **12**, 129–33
61. The Rome Group for Epidemiology and Prevention of Cholelithiasis (GREPCO) (1986). Radiologic appearance of gallstones and its relationship with biliary symptoms and awareness of having gallstones: observations during epidemiological studies. *Dig. Dis.* (In press)
62. Roda, E., Sama, C., Morselli, A. M., Taroni, F. and Rusticali, A. G. (1985). Silent stones. In Barbara, L., Dowling, R. H., Hofmann, A. F. and Roda, E. (eds.) *Recent Advances in Bile Acid Research*. pp. 239–42. (New York: Raven Press)
63. Shersten, T. (1978). Medical treatment of gallstones. *Scand. J. Gastroenterol.*, **13**, 129–31
64. Ransohoff, D. F., Gracie, W. A., Wolfenson, L. B. and Neuhauser, D. (1983). Prophylactic cholecystectomy or expectant management for silent gallstones. A decision analysis to assess survival. *Ann. Int. Med.*, **99**, 199–204
65. Fitzpatrick, G., Neutra, R. and Gilbert, J. P. (1977). Cost-effectiveness of cholecystectomy for silent gallstones. In Bunker, J. P., Barnes, B. A. and Monsteller, F. (eds.) *Costs, Risks and Benefits of Surgery*. pp. 246–61. (New York: Oxford University Press)
66. Thistle, J. L., Cleary, P. A., Lachin, J. M., Tyor, M. P., Hersh, T., the Steering Committee and The National Co-operative Gallstone Study Group (1984). The natural history of cholelithiasis: the National Cooperative Gallstone Study. *Ann. Int. Med.*, **101**, 171–5

4
Diagnosis

D. L. CARR-LOCKE

INTRODUCTION

A diagnosis of gallstones may be made in a variety of clinical settings, some specifically related to gallstone disease or its consequences, some commonly considered to be related but on analysis found to be non-specific and others where gallstones are discovered incidentally. The logical application of diagnostic tools for the documentation of gallstone disease naturally depends upon the correct recognition of clinical presentations. Single or recurrent attacks of classical biliary pain, often mistakenly referred to as 'colic', acute cholecystitis, empyema and mucocoele of the gallbladder, extrahepatic biliary obstruction causing cholestasis, bacterial cholangitis, and single or recurrent attacks of acute pancreatitis may all be specific effects of gallstones within the gallbladder or bile ducts and are the clinical problems discussed later. The non-specific complaints of dyspepsia, dietary fat intolerance, flatulence, upper abdominal bloating, postprandial fullness, heartburn, nausea, vomiting and vague abdominal pains or discomfort are common to a wide variety of upper and lower gastrointestinal conditions and the finding of gallstones in patients with these symptoms may be coincidental. The differential diagnosis for this group of symptoms with or without abdominal signs is well known[1] but it is increasingly apparent from experience of investigating many mainly young and middle-aged females with 'biliary' symptoms that the 'right upper quadrant' or 'hepatic flexure syndrome' variant of irritable bowel syndrome accounts for many more cases of right hypochondrial pain than do gallstones. Thus it cannot be overemphasized that a carefully taken history is essential before embarking on what should be a thorough assessment of the biliary tract when this is indicated. Technology should complement not substitute for good clinical practice. Indeed, interpretation of the investigative findings, their accuracy and limitations will only be possible in the light of pre-existing knowledge of the patient's problems and condition. Unnecessary overuse of imaging techniques can be avoided in an individual patient by suitable discussion between clinician and investigator, whether this be radiologist, ultrasonographer, gastroenterologist or medical physicist, in order to arrive at a diagnosis of gallstone disease with accuracy and safety.

DIAGNOSTIC MODALITIES

A full clinical examination will be an integral part of the initial assessment of any patient presenting with symptoms suggestive of gallstone disease. Apart from the findings in the acute problems of cholecystitis, jaundice, cholangitis and pancreatitis or their complications, clinical signs are unlikely to be helpful to indicate that gallstones are present since right hypochondrial tenderness alone is not specific. The history is therefore all-important.

The many imaging techniques available for the potential diagnosis of gallstones are considered here in terms of their disadvantages, such as patient preparation, degree of acceptability and risk, set against their diagnostic accuracy for gallbladder and bile duct stones. Details of standard techniques are not given unless germane to the discussion. All methods described in this chapter will not be available together in any but the most well-endowed institution, but the vast majority of patients will be successfully investigated by the 'simpler' modalities currently present in most district general hospitals with a minority requiring further assessment at a local or distant referral centre where additional expertise is offered.

Plain abdominal radiography

A plain abdominal radiograph will detect between 10% and 30% of gallstones within the gallbladder[2,3], with the lower figure more likely in the UK due to the low incidence of calcium-containing stones (Figure 4.1). The majority of gallstones, composed of more than 70% cholesterol, are radiolucent and are not seen on plain films. Bile duct stones are more rarely calcified still, in about 2% or less[2,3] (Figure 4.2) even when calcified stones are present in the gallbladder and thus, in situations where choledocholithiasis is suspected, a plain radiograph is not worthwhile. This is a simple procedure, is acceptable to the patient, requires no special preparation, carries no particular risk, has a very low sensitivity but high specificity, making this an initial investigation with limited benefit. Detection of calcification in gallstones will have implications for medical dissolution therapy but calcified gallstones must be distinguished from other causes of right upper quadrant calcification[2,3].

Occasionally a plain radiograph will show a complication of gallstone disease which may be diagnostic[2,3], e.g. the opaque mass of a mucocoele or empyema of the gallbladder, calcification in the wall of the gallbladder resulting from chronic cholecystitis (Figure 4.3), acute emphysematous cholecystitis showing gas in the gallbladder wall, or air in the biliary tree which, in the absence of a previous biliodigestive anastomosis or any endoscopic or surgical operation on the biliary sphincter, represents a bilioenteric fistula (Figure 4.4).

Oral cholecystography (OCG)

Oral cholecystography has been in use for 60 years[4] with little change in radiographic technique other than the development of improved contrast agents[5]. Until the advent of ultrasound it was the most commonly performed examination for suspected gallbladder stones but now takes second place to

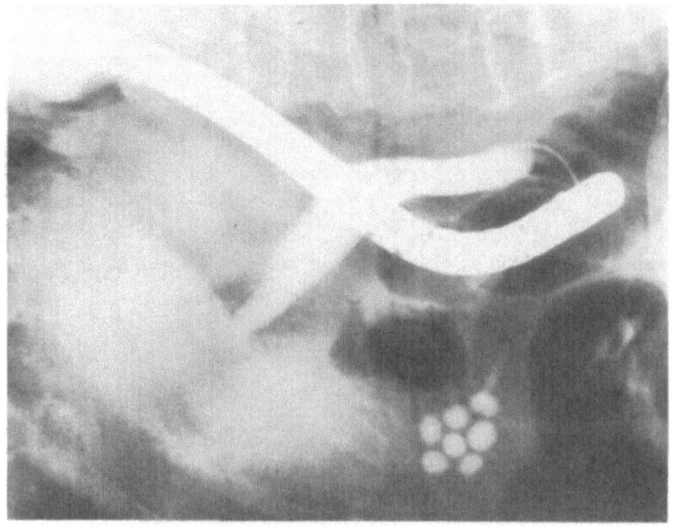

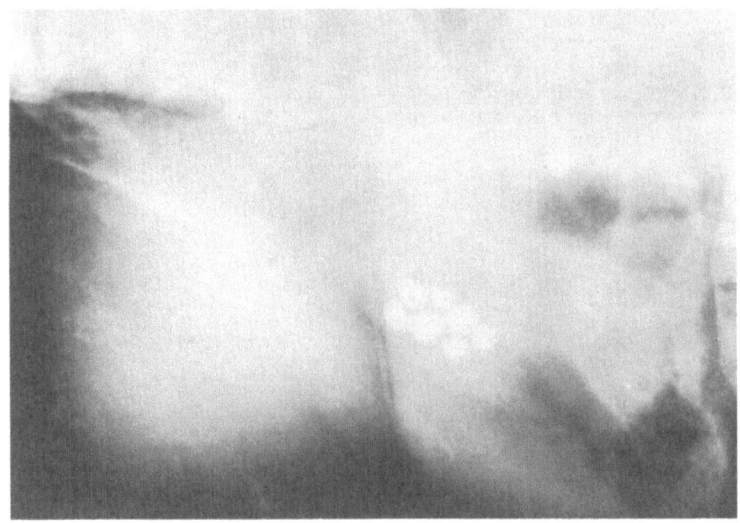

Figure 4.1 Plain abdominal radiograph showing (a) a collection of calcified gallbladder stones and a separate stone near the spine confirmed at ERCP (b)

73

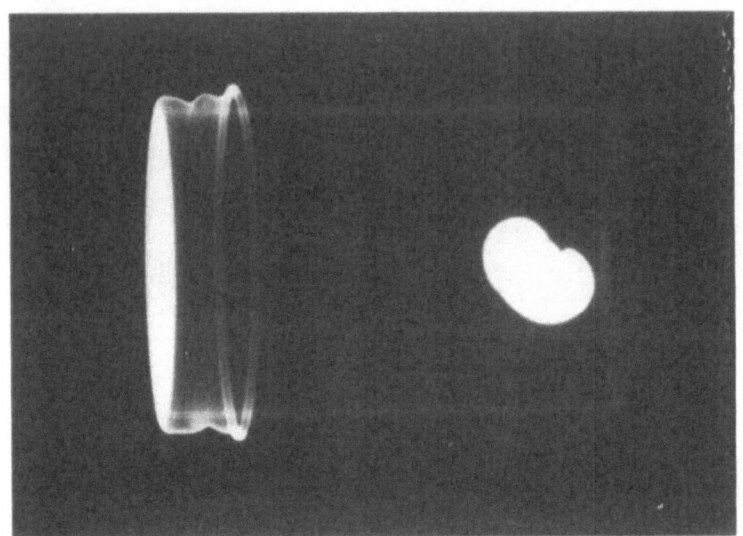

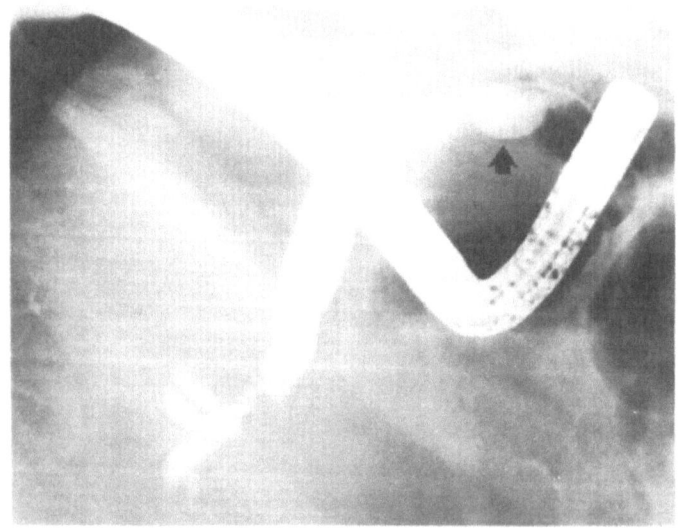

Figure 4.2 ERCP showing (a) a single calcified bile duct stone (arrow) and (b) its radiographic appearance after endoscopic removal

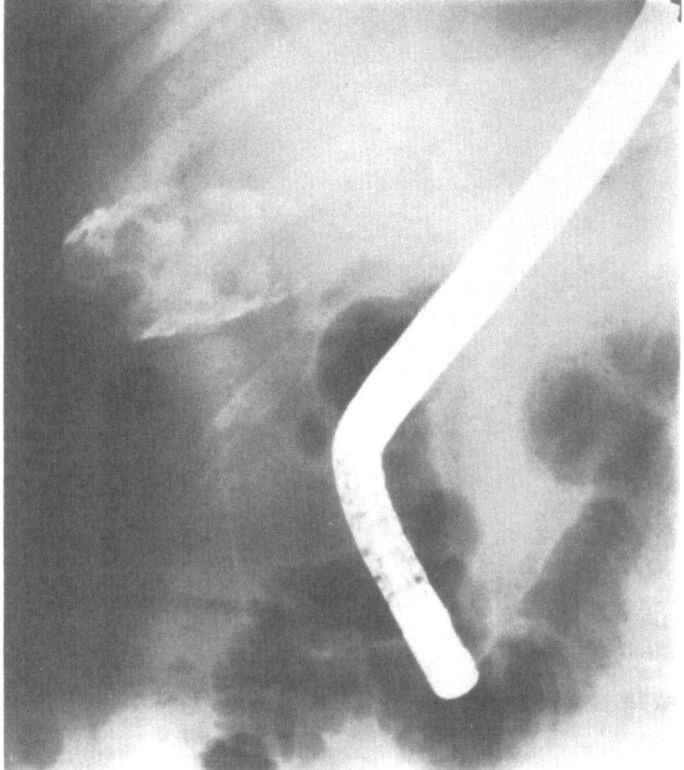

Figure 4.3 Abdominal radiograph prior to contrast injection at ERCP showing calcification in the wall of the gallbladder

ultrasound in most radiology departments. The patient is asked to attend for a plain radiograph to detect any radio-opaque gallbladder stones which, if present, may prevent obscuration by contrast and may obviate the need for a contrast study. The low incidence of calcified stones and logistic considerations may make this initial visit impracticable. In the absence of calcification the subject is given an oral contrast agent such as sodium iopodate (Biloptin or Solu-Biloptin, Schering) or iopanoic acid (Telepaque, Sterling Research), which is lipid-soluble and is absorbed principally from the small bowel and, to a lesser extent, from the colon. After transport via the bloodstream bound to albumin, it is taken up by hepatocytes, conjugated with glucuronide and excreted into bile where it concentrates in the gallbladder as water is reabsorbed. Radiographic imaging of the gallbladder area is obtained 12–15 hours after contrast ingestion with supine and supine oblique projections. If adequate views of the gallbladder are obtained and do not demonstrate stones many radiologists would consider this a normal examination and proceed no further. There is variation between centres in the use of measures to induce gallbladder contraction in order to identify stones in

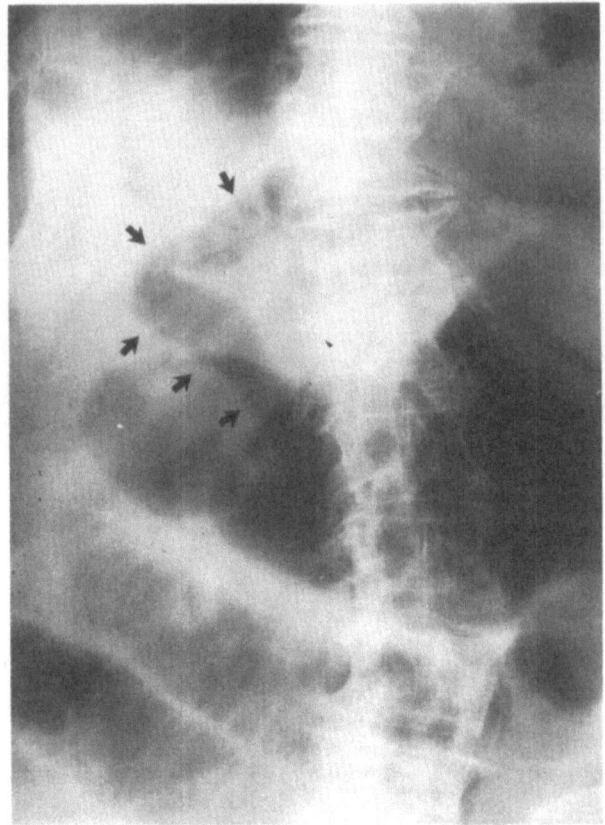

Figure 4.4 Plain abdominal radiograph showing an air-filled biliary tree (arrows)

the cystic duct or extrahepatic bile ducts[6,7]. This can be achieved physiologically by the ingestion of a fat stimulus[6,7] such as Calogen LCT emulsion (Scientific Hospital Supplies), or more rapidly pharmacologically by the intravenous injection of cholecystokinin[8] or its octapeptide, sincalide (Kinevac, Squibb)[9] or caeruletide[7,10]. Failure of the gallbladder to contract after a fatty meal is probably without significance[7]. The expected success rate of visualization of the bile ducts during OCG is only 10% with standard techniques, 20% after a fatty meal, but over 80% after a cholecystokinetic peptide[7]. Other aspects of technique have been well described[11].

This is a simple non-invasive radiographic method and thus acceptable to most patients but there are side-effects from the contrast material, some of which may be serious, and the fat stimulus or peptide injection may induce intense nausea and vomiting. Serious morbidity from orally administered biliary contrast agents is rare but minor symptoms of nausea, vomiting and diarrhoea occur in up to 50%[5] and are probably dose-related. Renal toxicity is the most significant side-effect but is confined to those patients receiving large doses or a simultaneous intravenous agent and this combined exam-

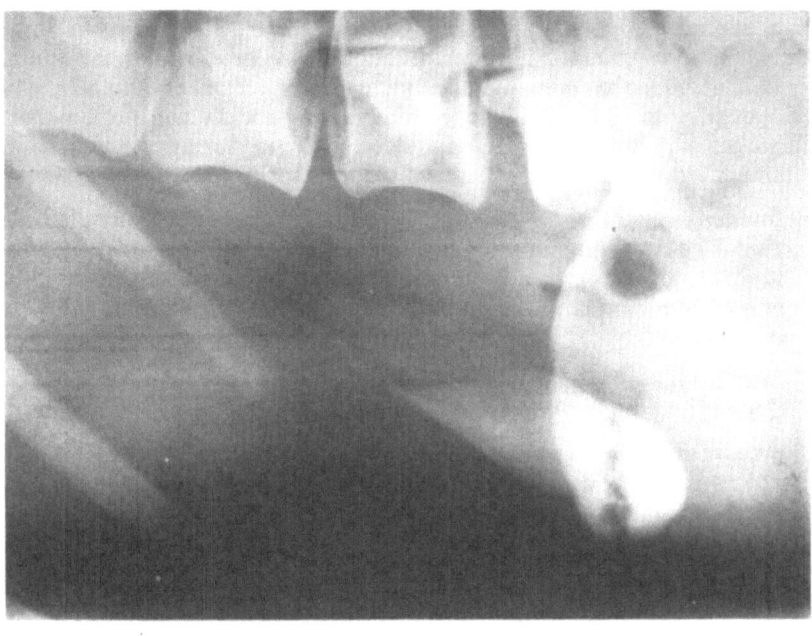

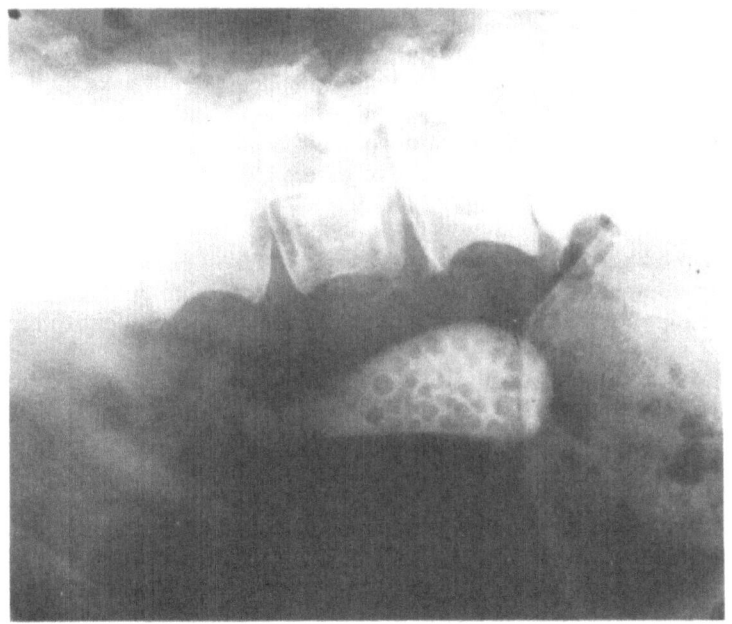

Figure 4.5 Oral cholecystography showing (a) multiple gallbladder stones and (b) layering on an erect view (donated by Dr D. C. James)

ination is therefore not recommended. A technically satisfactory chole-cystogram will diagnose radiolucent gallstones (Figure 4.5) with a sensitivity of more than 90%[12-15]. Technical success, however, may only be achieved after a second examination with or without tomography using a single increased dose of contrast medium, fractionated dose or other technique[6] since at least 10% of patients with complete non-opacification and 60% with poor opacification of the gallbladder after a single OCG will have normal gallbladders[16]. A non-opacified gallbladder, often mistakenly termed 'non-functioning', may result from a number of factors.

(1) Interference with contrast absorption, e.g. failure by the patient to take the tablets, vomiting occasionally induced by the contrast agent, delayed gastric emptying for any reason, small bowel disease causing obstruction or malabsorption, and the presence of diarrhoea or its induction by the contrast itself.

(2) Interference with contrast liver uptake, e.g. acute or chronic liver disease, and drugs competing for the same hepatic pathway.

(3) Interference with contrast excretion or entry into the gallbladder, e.g. any cause of cholestasis or mechanical obstruction to the extrahepatic bile ducts and cystic duct.

In the absence of interfering factors a non-opacified gallbladder has a high probability of indicating disease (over 90%[12-15]) of which gallstones will be the most likely cause of the presumed cystic duct obstruction. The specificity of oral cholecystography is not precisely known as this will depend on how assiduously the patients have been further investigated following an apparently normal examination. The false negative rate has been estimated to be between 2% and 10%[17]. When endoscopic retrograde chol-angiopancreatography (ERCP) was used in this context in two studies involving 84[18] and 206[19] patients in whom normal ultrasound examinations had also been obtained, 14% and 16% respectively were found to have gallbladder stones (Figure 4.6), suggesting a specificity for cholecystography of about 80%. When considering patients for medical dissolution therapy to gallbladder stones, oral cholecystography is the investigation of choice to assess gallbladder function and the suitability of stones for this treatment. Detection of recurrence after treament may also best be studied by cholecystography[20]. This method is most appropriately used for patients with recurrent biliary pain as an interval investigation rather than in acute conditions and it has no place in cholestasis nor the detection of bile duct stones.

Ultrasound

Ultrasonography of the gallbladder and surrounding structures had rapidly developed technologically and in its clinical application such that it now represents the first line investigation in suspected biliary and pancreatic disease in most hospitals. Techniques of ultrasound imaging in its static grey-scale[21] and real-time[22] modes have been well documented in their application to the biliary tract[21-25]. The principle depends on the application of a trans-

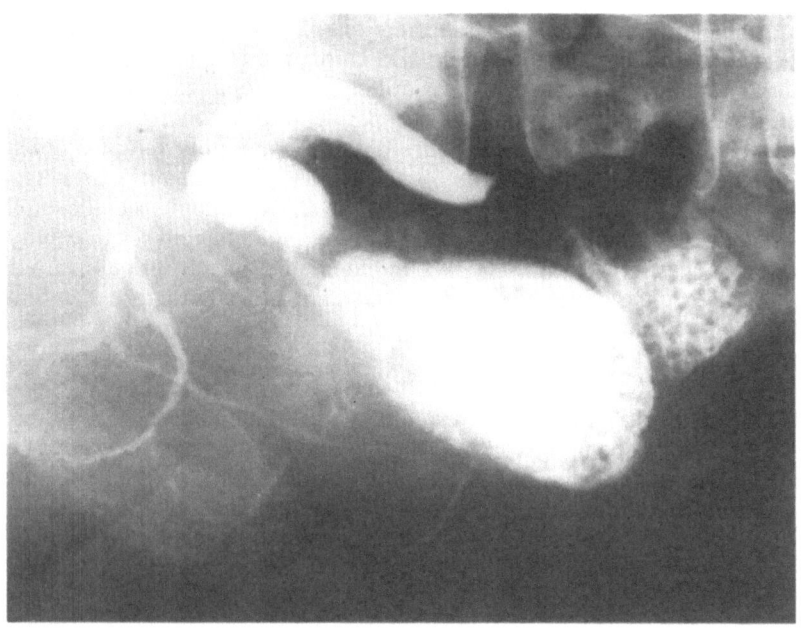

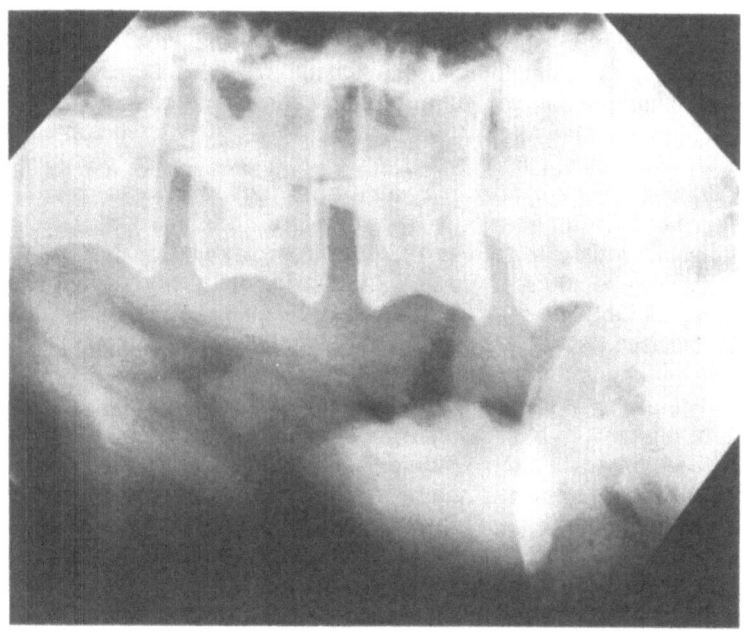

Figure 4.6 (a) False negative oral cholecystogram and (b) ERCP from the same patient showing multiple gallbladder stones (ultrasound also negative)

ducer emitting high frequency sound of 3.5–5 MHz to the skin and the transmission of these sound waves through the abdomen until their reflection by intra-abdominal organs. The reflected sound is collected by a receiver carried within the transducer module and converted to a static or dynamic display which may be permanently recorded on appropriate film. Each generation of instruments reduces operator dependence but, as with many other investigative techniques, best results are obtained by highly skilled enthusiasts. Recognition of normal and abnormal biliary structures has been well defined[23-26] and gallbladder stones have characteristic image of high amplitude intraluminal reflections that cast an acoustic shadow and show gravity-dependent movement (Figure 4.7). Technical factors play an important part in achieving a good gallbladder image and care must be taken with skin contact using a suitable sonic coupling fluid, such as mineral oil, correct positioning of the patient to minimize the transducer–gallbladder distance and avoid overlying bowel gas if possible, and repetition on another occasion if conditions are not optimal. Patient preparation is minimal with an 8-hour fast preferable if not being performed as an acute examination. Acceptability is excellent with little disturbance to the patient even if acutely ill or if repeated examinations are required, and there are no known risks to the patient or staff.

Allowing for technical failures, real-time ultrasound can detect gallbladder stones with a sensitivity and specificity of more than 95%[7,14,15,22,25,27]. This compares very favourably with OCG[14,15] and in many situations achieves more accurate results or images when the former technique has failed, is equivocal or inappropriate. Ultrasound has the advantages of allowing rapid assessment of the gallbladder when OCG has failed to produce opacification, accurate imaging of the gallbladder wall, measurement of the calibre of the bile ducts and simultaneous hepatic and pancreatic imaging. As there is a known small false negative rate further biliary investigation is warranted in those patients with typical biliary symptoms but negative scans. Identifiable artefacts causing stone-like appearances on ultrasound are acoustic shadows from bowel gas or barium, from bowel positioned 'behind' the gall bladder, from the gallbladder neck, from reverberation from gas or ribs, respiratory movement and compound scanning in the static mode. Non-imaging of the gallbladder may be due to it being packed with stones with very little surrounding bile (see Figures 4.6 and 4.19), a small contracted gallbladder, lack of fasting, obesity or an atypical gallbladder position.

Ultrasound detection of bile duct stones (Figure 4.8) has not attained the same levels of sensitivity as in the gallbladder and figures of 10–81% are reported[28,29] and the advent of real-time scanners for routine use has not improved success[28]. Reasons for failure in choledocholithiasis may be the relative inaccessibility of the bile duct to sound waves owing to surrounding structures and bowel gas, refraction of the ultrasound beam by duct walls, lack of surrounding bile and less common production of an acoustic shadow. recent introduction of endoscopic ultrasound may improve detection of bile duct stones[40] but this becomes an invasive procedure. Ultrasound demonstration of dilated intrahepatic and extrahepatic bile ducts in obstructive

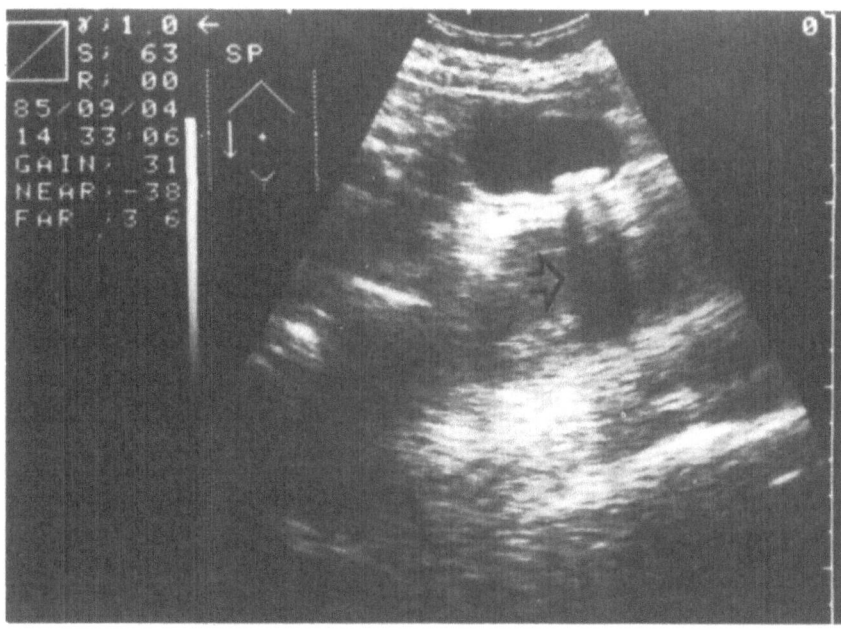

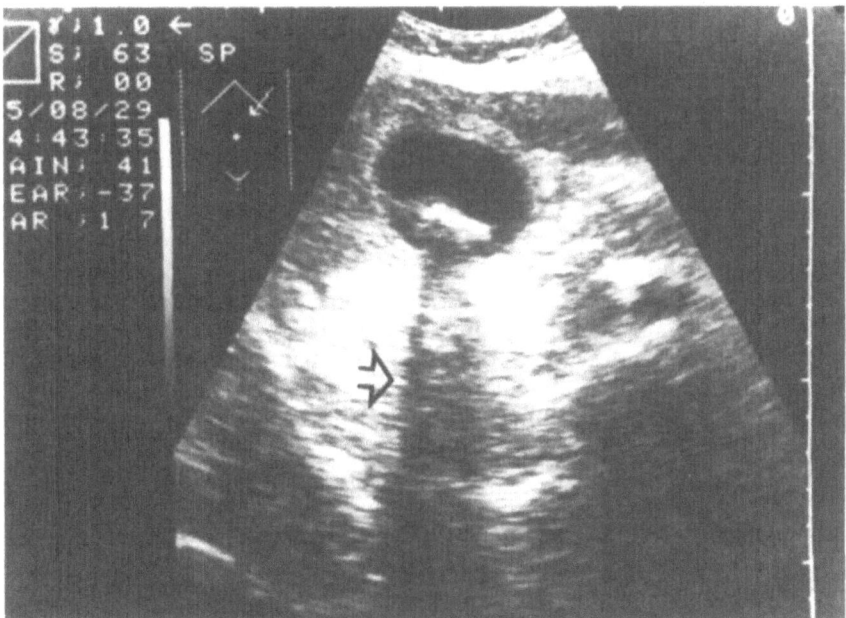

Figure 4.7 Ultrasonic imaging of gallbladder stones with characteristic sonic shadow (arrow) shown (a) longitudinally and (b) in cross-section (donated by Dr A. E. Crozier)

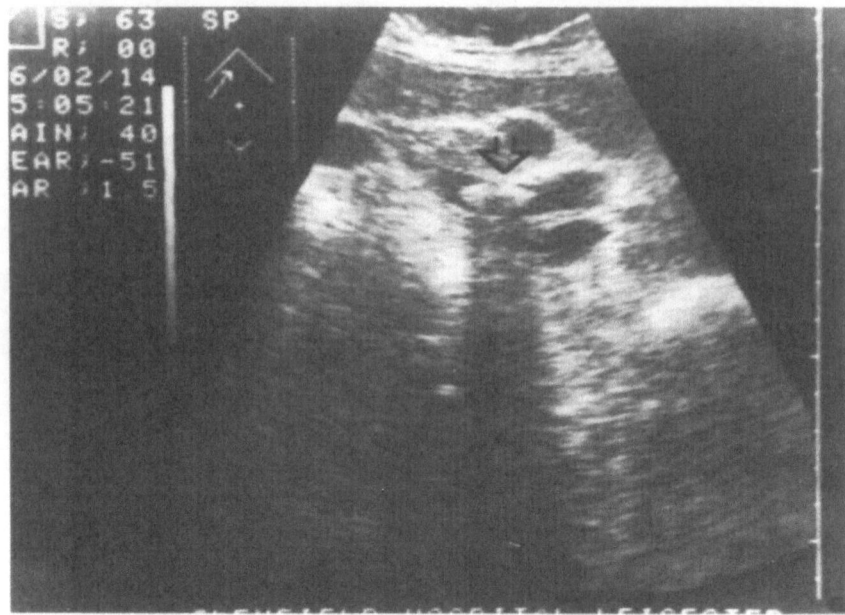

Figure 4.8 Ultrasonic image of large bile duct stone (arrow) with sonic shadow (donated by Dr A. E. Crozier)

jaundice carries a high sensitivity of more than 90%[24,25,41] but exact definition of the cause is less accurate.

Radionuclide scanning

Early hepatobiliary radiopharmaceuticals, like [^{131}I]Rose Bengal[42] were designed to be excreted in bile in order to provide a potential for static and dynamic imaging of the bile pathway by radiation emission detection but were soon abandoned for practical and safety reasons, although they paved the way for their modern equivalents now in widespread use. Radionuclide imaging has the advantages of being non-invasive, low radiation and allowing prolonged biliary observation, but has the disadvantage of low morphological resolution. Departments of radionuclide imaging currently offer a facility for emergency biliary scanning with one of the ^{99m}Tc-labelled derivatives of iminodiacetic acid (IDA), of which HIDA has become the most popular, all of which have a short halflife and are good gamma-ray emitters[7,43,44]. Normally 3–5 mCi of the radionuclide is injected intravenously as a sterile solution and after an interval of 20–60 min will have been taken up by the liver and excreted into bile where it will readily produce a representation of the biliary tract on gamma camera imaging (Figure 4.9). Uptake, liver handling and bile excretion behaviour vary with different side-chain substitutions of the IDA molecule and some will enhance biliary imaging in the presence of cholestasis better than others[7,43,44]. The information is stored on magnetic tape or

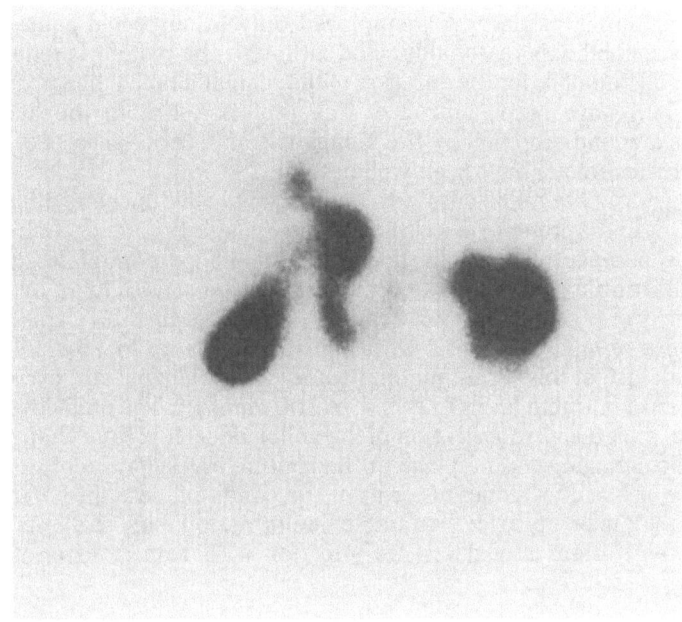

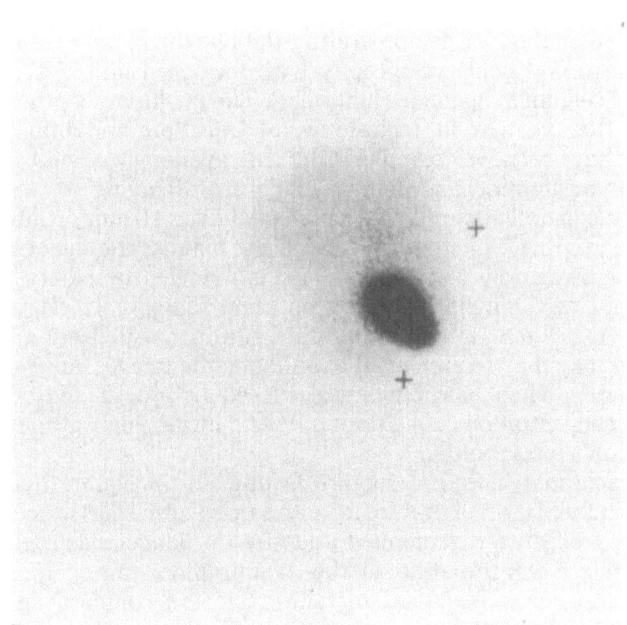

Figure 4.9 Normal HIDA radionuclide image showing (a) gallbladder, bile ducts and small bowel on anterior projection and (b) liver and gallbladder on right lateral projection (donated by Dr J. M. Berry)

computer disc for later replay and enhancement if necessary. Patient preparation is minimal, as the test is employed only in suspected acute cholecystitis. Acceptability is reasonably good although the patient is required to be supine and immobile for the duration of the scan at a time when abdominal pain may not have been controlled. The radiation risk to the liver and intestine is low and excretion by the kidney is small. Other aspects of biliary scintigraphy technique have been well described[44].

Non-imaging of the gallbladder with imaging of the bile duct and duodenum (Figure 4.10) in the presence of a clinical picture suggesting acute cholecystitis and in the absence of alcoholic liver disease and parenteral feeding[45] is virtually diagnostic of cystic duct obstruction with a sensitivity of over 95% and specificity of nearly 100%[7,43,45–49] and is more accurate than ultrasound[50]. The presence of mild cholestasis with bilirubin levels up to 75 μmol/l does not preclude use of this technique and some IDA analogues are excreted in the presence of bilirubin levels in excess of 200 μmol/l[44]. The predictive value of a normal scan (i.e. demonstration of the gallbladder) is greater than 98%[43]. Radionuclide imaging has no place in the routine investigation of suspected gallbladder or bile duct stones other than the condition described above and although it may provide valuable information in patients with cholestasis[7,43,44] other modalities are superior with respect to anatomical definition.

Intravenous cholangiography (IVC)

A non-invasive method for demonstrating the bile ducts radiographically as a companion to oral cholecystography was developed in 1953[51] with the availability of sodium iodipamide (Biligrafin). The evolution of other contrast agents and the changes in techniques of injection and infusion cholangiography have been well reviewed[5,51,52]. Intravenously administered contrast such as meglumine ioglycamate (Biligram, Schering) or meglumine iotroxate (Biliscopin, Schering) may be injected over 10 min or infused over 40–60 min and provides between 5 and 8.5 g iodine. The agent is cleared from the bloodstream by liver uptake and is followed by biliary excretion sufficient to image the main bile ducts on plain radiographs (Figure 4.11). Spot films are taken at 30 min intervals until bile duct visualization is optimal when tomography may be employed to enhance the image. Imaging success falls significantly when bilirubin levels exceed 68 μmol/l and/or alkaline phosphatase concentrations are elevated[7,52] and increasing the contrast dose does not improve resolution[51].

Patient preparation does not require fasting and adequate hydration is important to minimize any renal toxicity and uricosuric effects. Acceptability is low as the procedure is prolonged and often produces side-effects which may necessitate discontinuation of the examination. Minor symptoms of nausea, vomiting, skin rash and metallic taste are common and resolve rapidly on withdrawal of the agent. Severe life-threatening reactions are more frequent than with oral contrast media but the incidence is probably exaggerated. Intravenous cholangiography is contraindicated in patients with renal disease, significant cardiovascular disease, known hypersensitivity

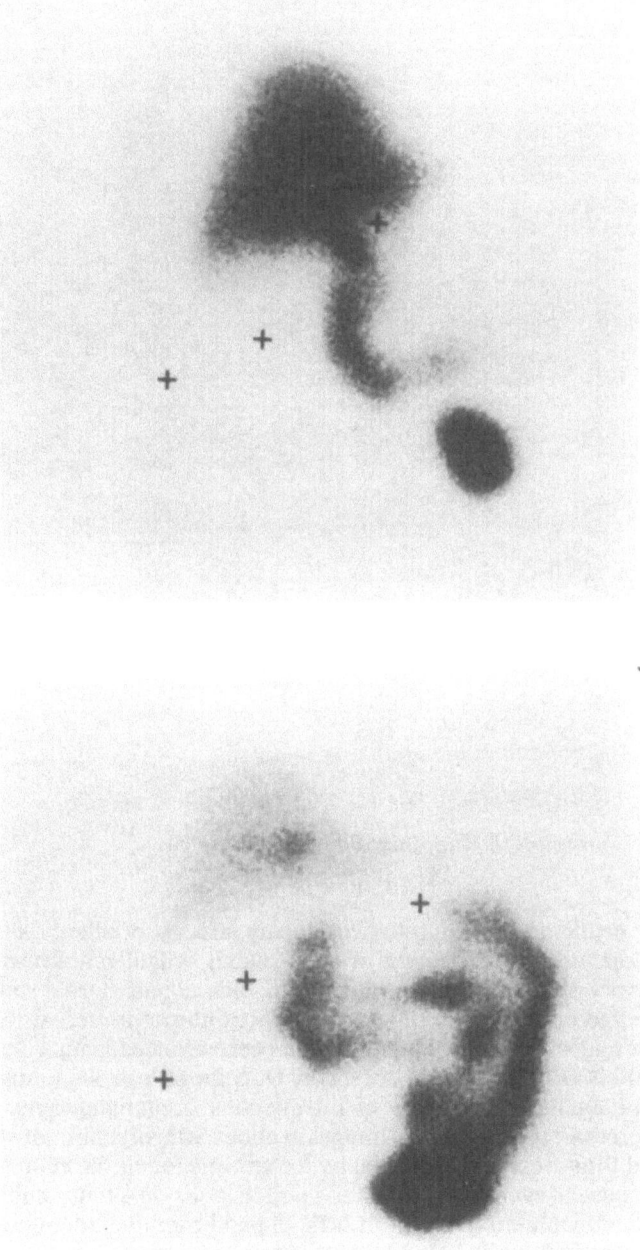

Figure 4.10 HIDA scan in acute cholecystitis showing (a) isotope in the liver, bile ducts and duodenum and (b) in liver and intestine, but no gallbladder image on either scan

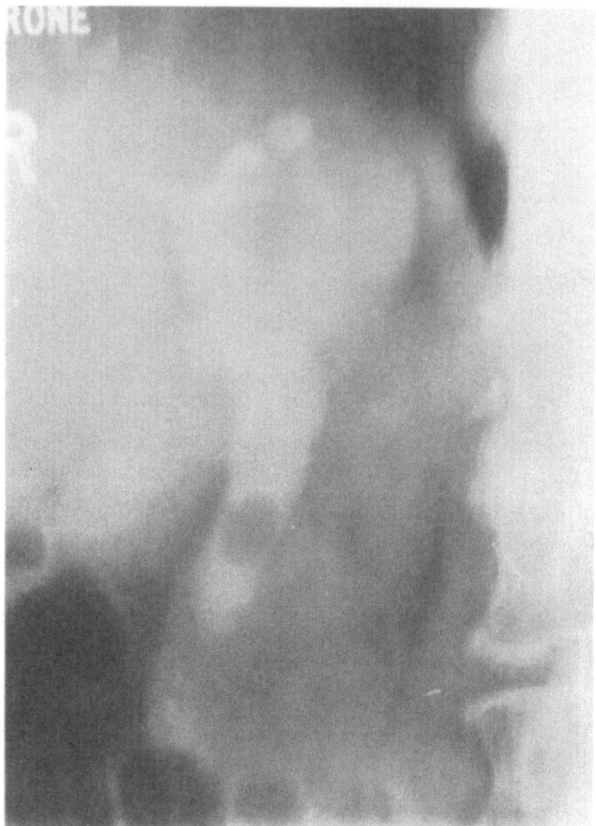

Figure 4.11 Intravenous cholangiogram showing bile duct stone

to iodine, myeloma and thyrotoxicosis. Any history of allergy should alert the radiologist to the possibility of anaphylaxis, vagal bradycardia or cardiopulmonary arrest. Prior administration of a corticosteroid and/or antihistamine and a test dose of the contrast agent do not protect the individual from such major incidents. Mortality has been reported from 1 in 5000[5] to 22 in 6 200 000[51]. IVC should not follow OCG for at least 48 hours[51].

The fundamental limitations of intravenous cholangiography lie in its failure to produce optimal biliary images in about 50% of examinations (Figure 4.12), and thus requiring tomography for enhancement, its complete failure in the presence of even mild cholestasis and its poor sensitivity and specificity which are probably no better than 60% of good quality cholangiograms. Its use in suspected acute cholecystitis to demonstrate non-filling of the gallbladder has been supplanted by radionuclide scanning and safer and more accurate radiographic methods for imaging the bile ducts are available although these are invasive. IVC may be the only method for bile duct imaging available to some clinicians at present but with wider use of alternative

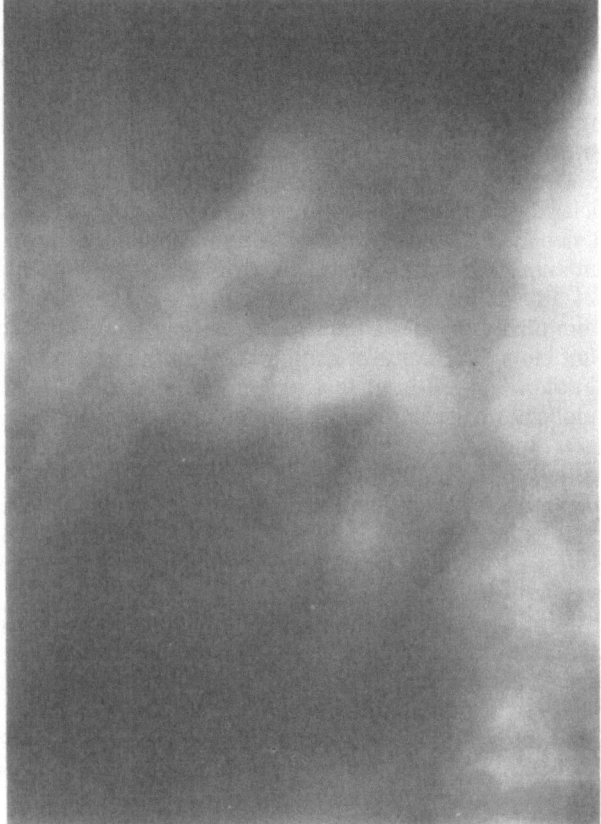

Figure 4.12   Intravenous cholangiogram not allowing adequate interpretation

techniques this method of imaging should almost certainly disappear from our radiology departments before the end of this decade.

Percutaneous transhepatic cholangiography (PTC)

Accurate anatomical imaging of the biliary tract in the presence of jaundice in order to attempt definition of the presence and nature of an obstructing lesion is not possible with any of the techniques described above. Recent improvements in ultrasound have allowed a more precise anatomical and pathological diagnosis but there is often still a need to outline the biliary tree prior to any interventional therapy whether this be surgical, endoscopic, radiological or pharmacological. A method for instilling radiographic contrast material directly into the biliary system by a percutaneous, transhepatic route was first introduced in 1921[53] for opacifying the gallbladder and in 1937[54] for direct puncture of intrahepatic bile ducts. The technique gained initial popularity but increasing complications from the use of large bore needles (of 18 or 20 gauge) and catheters led to the decline of this mode of investigation, only to be rekindled in the 1970s by the development of a fine needle technique[55-57]. Following Okuda's documentation of this 'skinny' or 'Chiba' needle method[58] using a new 22 gauge steel needle of outer diameter 0.7 mm, the technique has now become the most commonly practised invasive method for achieving anterograde cholangiography in the jaundiced patient[59] and is probably performed in most radiology departments where such patients are investigated. The needle carries a fine inner stilatte, measures 18 cm in length, and is sufficiently flexible to allow respiration to continue during needle withdrawal deeply inserted into liver tissue. Preparation of the patient involves admission to hospital, a mandatory check of coagulation status and correction of any abnormality with vitamin K or fresh frozen plasma as indicated, administration of an appropriate prophylactic antibiotic or combination of antibiotics such as ampicillin and gentamicin, or cefotaxime alone or pipericillin alone[60], an 8-hour fast, and informed consent with the risks of possible complications explained. Untreated cholangitis, severe dyspnoea, marked ascites and an inability of the patient to co-operate are relative contraindications to the procedure.

Intravenous sedation, such as diazepam or midazolam, is commonly used and the skin site for puncture prepared as for liver biopsy. The standard approach is via an intercostal space, usually the 7th or 8th, in the right mid-axillary line after infiltration with local anaesthesia with the patient in suspended expiration and with the needle perpendicular to the skin surface, parallel to the tabletop and being directed toward the estimated site of hepatic duct bifurcation. A number of different aids to defining this position have been described but a point midway between the dome of the right hemi-diaphragm and the apex of the duodenal loop or a point 5 cm above the liver edge on fluoroscopy and 2 cm to the right of the right lateral border of the spine are commonly used. On withdrawal of the needle an intrahepatic bile duct is opacified close to the hilum of the liver and contrast injected under fluoroscopic control, adjusting the needle position to give optimal filling of the biliary tree (Figure 4.13). Many standard contrast media are suitable for PTC, e.g. diatrizoate with an iodine content of 292 mg/ml (Urografin 290, Schering) or 270 mg/ml (Hypaque 45%, Sterling Research), iothalamate with 280 mg/ml (Conray 280, May and Baker), or the newer non-ionic media such as lopamidol 200 or 300 mg/ml (Niopam, Merck). In the case of an obstructed biliary system it must be remembered that increasing intraductal pressure may not only induce pain but may lead to many of the recognized complications following this procedure. It is possible to exchange the diagnostic needle for a plastic catheter to provide temporary external bile drainage either before or after contrast injection to obviate this problem. When the intrahepatic ducts are grossly dilated PTC is often achieved at the first needle pass, but with lesser degrees of dilatation or normal sized ducts several passes may be required with failure determined by the enthusiasm and experience of the radiologist and the resilience of the patient! In the presence of dilated intrahepatic ducts, PTC will be obtained after one to four passes in 90% and all patients with a bile duct diameter of more than 10 mm should be entered with ten passes or less[59], whereas in non-dilated intrahepatic ducts one to ten passes includes 85% of patients and up to 16 needle passes have been

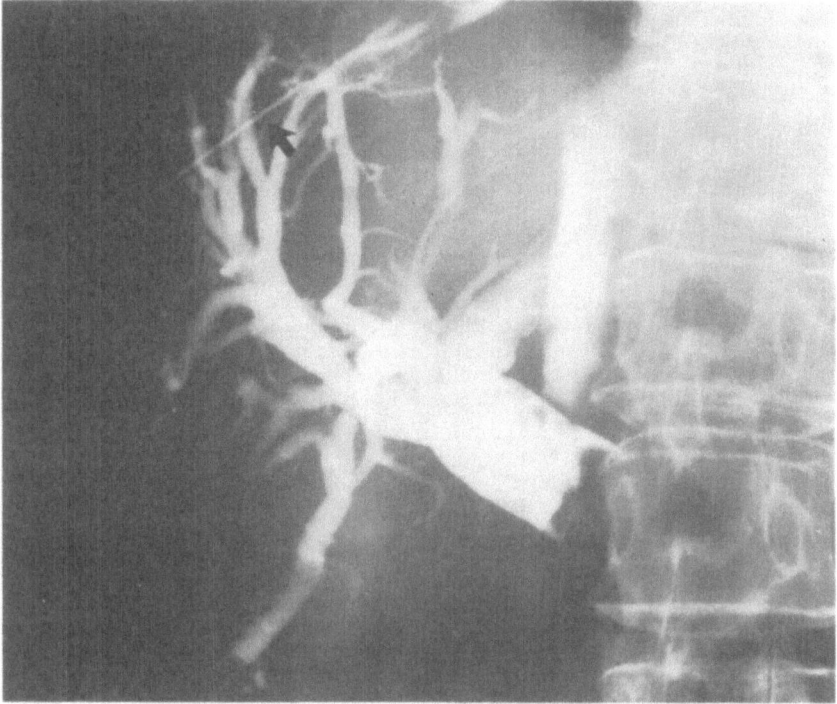

Figure 4.13 PTC showing needle in peripheral intrahepatic duct (arrow) and multiple small stones in a dilated bile duct above a large obstructing stone (donated by Mr C. I. Massey)

described in non-dilated ducts without an increase in complication rate[59,61,62]. Spot radiographs are taken as indicated by the appearances on fluoroscopy and delayed films may be required after an interval of minutes or hours if insufficient filling of the distal bile duct has been obtained during PTC. Care with patient positioning, correct timing of films and insistence on high quality radiographs are essential to achieve a high diagnostic accuracy. With the equipment and radiological expertise available in most hospitals in the UK an incorrect diagnosis on PTC should never be the result of inadequate technique. Other aspects of technique are well documented[59,61-66].

PTC should therefore be technically successful in nearly 100% of attempts in the presence of a dilated biliary system (Figure 4.14) and over 70% when not dilated[59,63,66] (Figure 4.15). The reported accuracy to be expected from PTC for the detection of the level of biliary obstruction is over 95% and 90% for defining the cause[62,65] but interpretation of intraluminal filling defects may be difficult and a false diagnosis of calculous obstruction reported (Figure 4.16).

In general, patients find PTC tolerable when sedation is employed but distension of an obstructed biliary tree by contrast can induce pain, nausea and vomiting and occasionally requires termination of the investigation. A review of all major and minor complications[67] indicates an incidence of

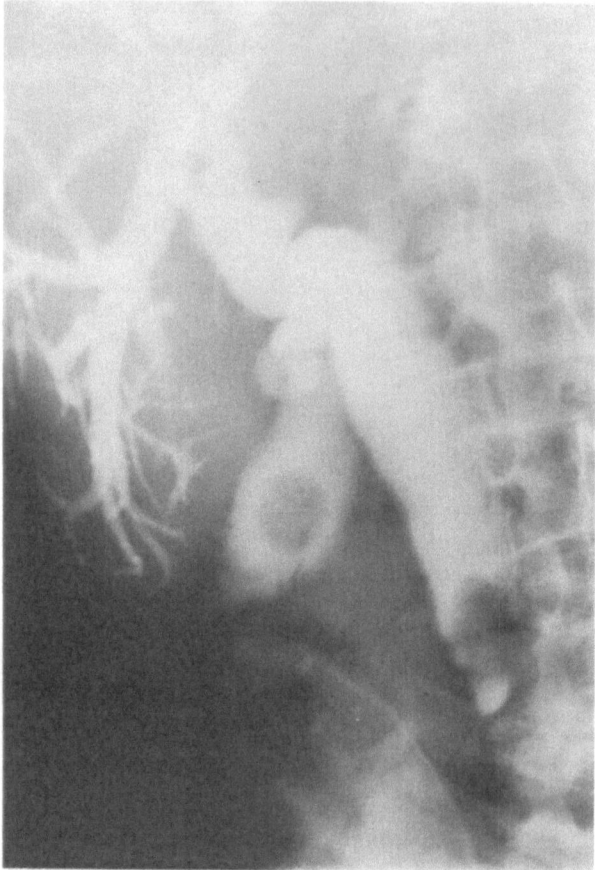

Figure 4.14 PTC showing stones in a dilated bile duct and gallbladder stone (needle not shown)

31.7% but serious complications occur in 3–10%[59,66]. Despite the variation in reported complications the distribution of sepsis (53%), bile leakage (27%), haemorrhage (7%) and other events (13%), including pneumothorax, bile embolization and adverse reactions to contrast, are fairly uniform[59] with a mortality rate of 0.1%[59] to 0.3%[66]. Avoidance of overdistension of the biliary tree with contrast, pre-, intra- or post procedure bile drainage and judicious use of prophylactic antibiotics should reduce complications. Thus PTC is an accurate modality for defining biliary anatomy and pathology but requires a degree of patient selection using other non-invasive tests in order to optimize the risk–benefit ratio.

Endoscopic retrograde cholangiopancreatography (ERCP)

The advent of the side-viewing fibre-optic duodenoscope in the 1970s allowed direct access to the duodenal papilla and its cannulation permitting retrograde

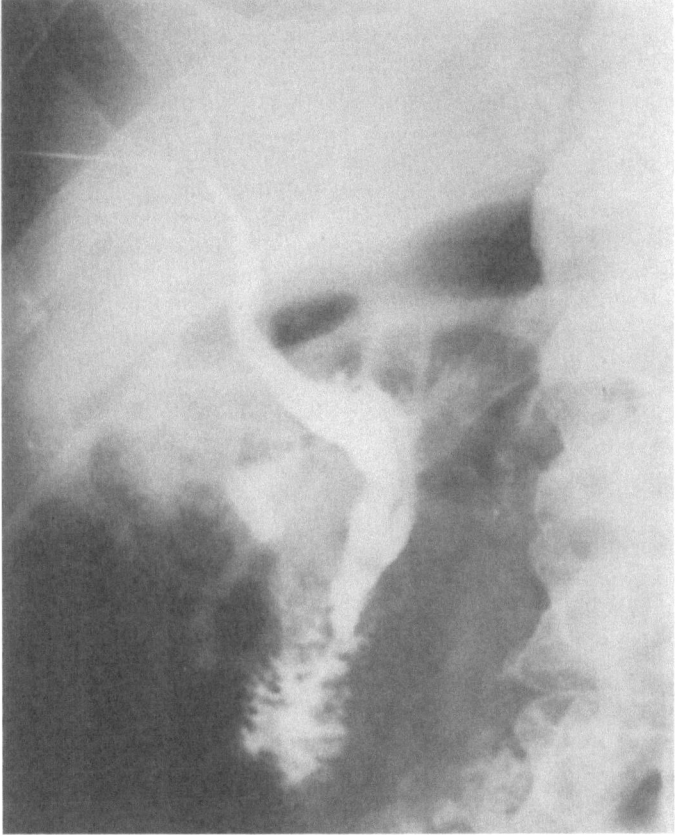

Figure 4.15 PTC showing stone in a non-dilated bile duct

injection of radiographic contrast into the pancreatic and bile ducts[68]. The general proliferation of gastrointestinal endoscopy at that time encouraged the technique of ERCP to grow rapidly in its application to the investigation of suspected biliary disease and, with its therapeutic development, endoscopic sphincterotomy[69,70], there was a further impetus to investigate and consider treatment of bile duct stone disease by endoscopic approaches (see Chapter 7). Although equally applicable to patients with obstructive jaundice suitable for PTC (Figure 4.17) and probably with similar accuracy in the demonstration of biliary disease[63], ERCP has a number of potential advantages. The additional information gained from the endoscopic examination of the upper gastrointestinal tract with the facility to biopsy lesions and a concomitant pancreatogram, as well as the ability to treat biliary disorders at the same examination, increases the value of ERCP over PTC but it is undoubtedly a more difficult technique to learn and its availability nationally is far more limited, being concentrated in specialized centres. ERCP is also able to provide cholangiography in patients with suspected bile duct stones in whom

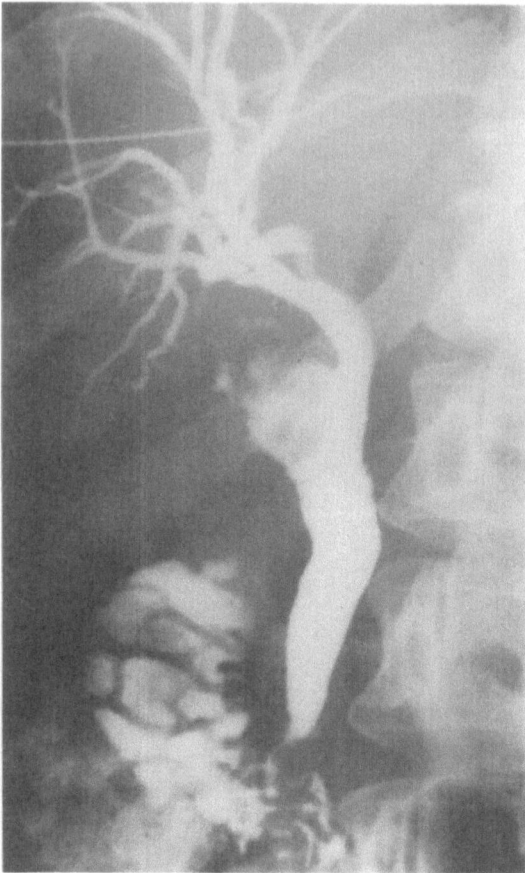

Figure 4.16 PTC showing filling defect in mid bile duct misinterpreted as tumour but found to be a large gallbladder stone causing the Mirizzi syndrome

no dilatation is apparent on ultrasound (Figure 4.18) and when all other methods have failed to provide a biliary image or a confident diagnosis (Figure 4.19).

Preparation for ERCP requires an 8-hour fast, understanding by the patient of the manoeuvres to be undertaken and the provision of informed consent, prophylactic antibiotics for patients with cholestasis or heart valve lesions, a check of coagulation status if there is any likelihood of proceeding to endoscopic sphincterotomy and facilities for observation following the procedure, if being carried out as a day case examination, or admission to hospital if a therapeutic procedure is undertaken or planned. A fully equipped radiology room is essential providing high quality image intensification and permanent radiographs with sufficient physical space to accommodate the endoscopy personnel and equipment. Adequately trained medical, nursing, radiographic and portering staff are needed to accomplish safe, accurate and efficient ERCP, allow management decisions to be made during ERCP and cope with any

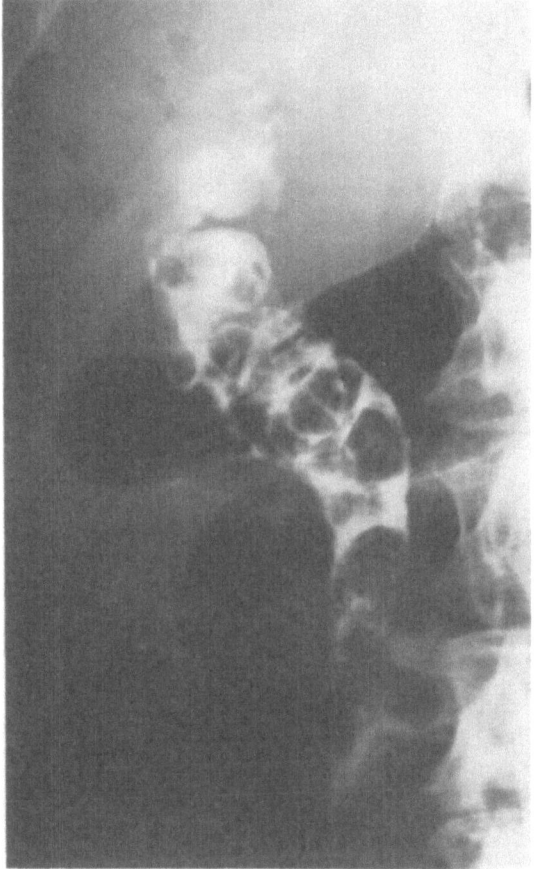

Figure 4.17   ERCP showing a dilated bile duct packed with stones

complications which might arise. Following local pharyngeal anaesthesia, intravenous sedation with diazepam or midazolam and passage of the duod-enoscope to the second part of the duodenum, temporary duodenal paralysis is induced with hyoscine-N-butyl bromide (Buscopan, Boeringer) or glucagon (Nova) and the major papilla cannulated with a catheter preflushed with radiographic contrast. This should be one containing an equivalent iodine concentration of 200–300 mg/ml and may be ionic, e.g. diatrizoate (Urografin 290, Schering; Hypaque 45%, Sterling Research) and iothalamate (Conray 280, May and Baker), or non-ionic, e.g. Iopamidol (Niopam 200 or 300, Merck). Use of less concentrated contrast in a dilated biliary tree is an ideal to be attained but changing syringes after cannulation of a duct may allow entry of air bubbles and hamper interpretation of cholangiography. There may be a slight advantage in using non-ionic media to reduce or avoid the complication of acute pancreatitis but in general these are considerably more expensive and the risk of pancreatitis is small in most centres performing ERCP

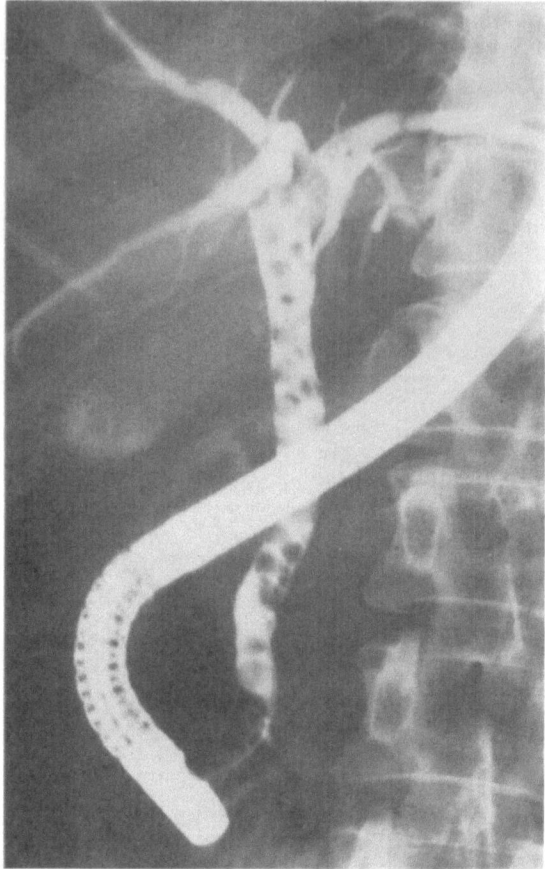

Figure 4.18 ERCP showing multiple stones in a normal-sized bile duct

regularly. Continuous fluoroscopy during contrast injection is mandatory in order to identify ductal opacification and recognize stones as they are demonstrated. Over opacification of the bile ducts induces pain and may obscure small stones but adequate filling of the intrahepatic and extrahepatic ducts is required to complete cholangiography and ensure gallbladder filling if the cystic duct is patent. Spot films are taken during contrast injection and after its completion with further views obtained after withdrawal of the endoscope and repositioning of the patient in a supine or supine oblique projection as the left hepatic duct system fills preferentially in the prone position owing to its more anterior anatomy. Occasionally delayed radiographs will be needed if the gallbladder has failed to outline or if drainage of contrast from the biliary tree is being observed. Attention to detail and obsessional demand for high quality radiographs make for improved accuracy in the diagnosis of calculi (Figure 4.20). No barium studies should have been undertaken within 3 days of ERCP as residual barium in the colon interferes

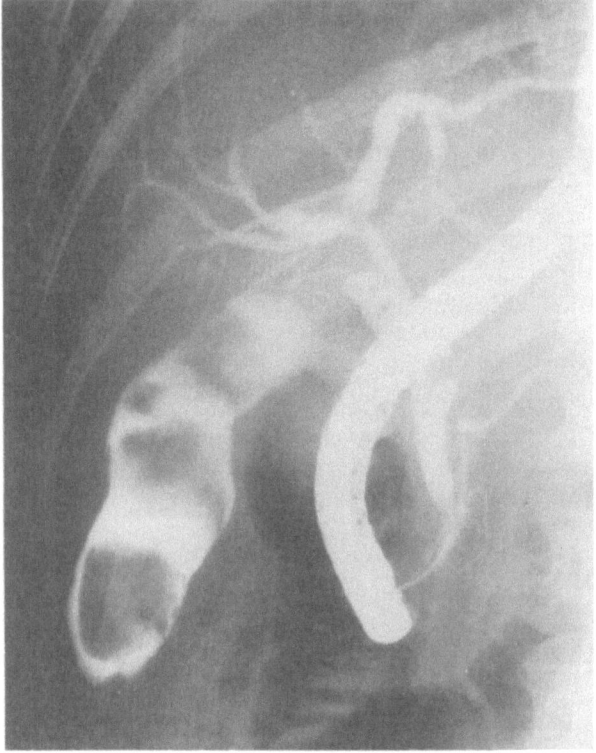

Figure 4.19 ERCP showing large gallbladder stones and stone in cystic duct not identified by ultrasound

with adequate visualization of the lower bile duct area. Initial endoscopic examination of the upper gastrointestinal tract, especially the area around the papilla, will sometimes reveal additional diagnostic information relevant to gallstone disease. Spontaneous and iatrogenic choledochoduodenal fistulae, a dilated intramural common bile duct and stone impaction at the papilla itself are such features. Other aspects of ERCP methodology have been reviewed[68,71].

Successful cholangiography should be achieved in well over 90% of cases in a centre performing ERCP regularly, irrespective of bile duct diameter and is a highly accurate method for identifying gallstones in the bile ducts and gallbladder (Figures 4.17–4.19). Sensitivity and specificity for bile duct stones are over 90% in all clinical settings where ERCP is applicable, which in all cases involves some selection of patients and in many involves further selection after other preliminary investigations. ERCP may be the only appropriate method of identifying bile duct stones in some patients (see Clinical Problems) but in others is an adjunct to ultrasound and an alternative to IVC or PTC with which it compares very favourably. ERCP detection of gallbladder calculi as a specific aim is usually reserved for patients in whom other investigative

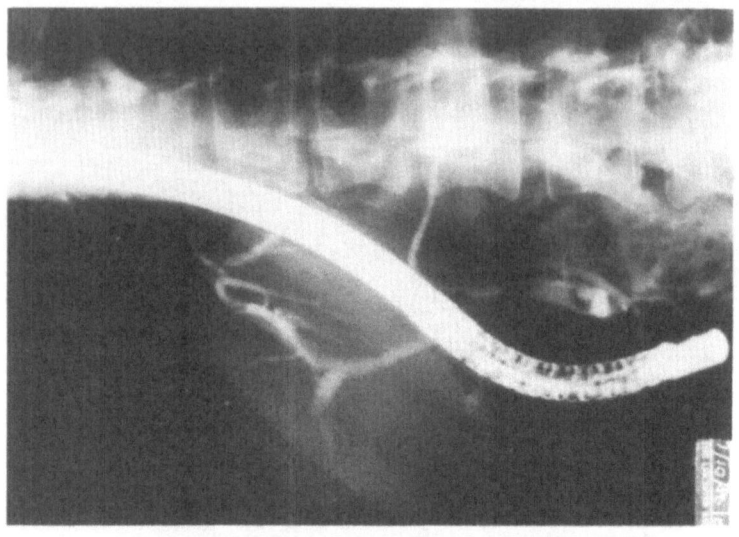

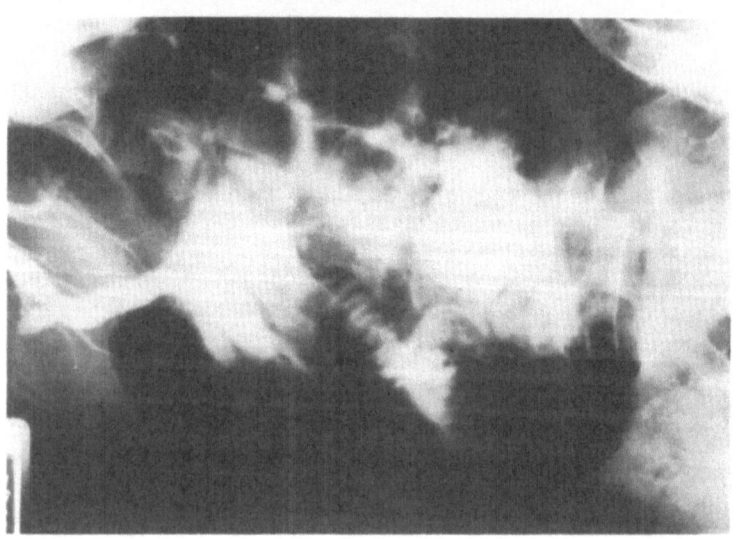

Figure 4.20 Two ERCPs in same post cholecystectomy patient showing (a) an inadequate examination with obscuring of the lower bile duct by spilled intraduodenal contrast and (b) repeat with demonstration of a small bile duct stone

modalities have been normal or equivocal in the presence of continuing symptoms suggesting biliary disease. Two studies have shown gallstone diagnosis rates of 14%[18] and 16%[19] in patients with negative ultrasonography and oral cholecystography. ERCP will fail in a small number of attempts because of inaccessibility of the duodenal papilla in patients with pyloric or duodenal stenosis, some patients with duodenal diverticulum or Billroth 2 partial gastrectomy, and in others patient co-operation or technical difficulty in achieving good cannulation will be responsible. A number of different designs of ERCP catheter with a variety of shaped tips are now available to assist the endoscopist in difficult situations and have undoubtedly reduced the technical failure rate. Where indicated a second attempt locally or at a more experienced centre may be justified.

In experienced centres ERCP for most patients is a rapid and well-tolerated procedure. With the standards of care expected in a modern endoscopy unit the risks from the endoscopic component of ERCP and the drugs employed are negligible. In the first few years after the technique was first introduced complications occurred in up to 3% of patients undergoing diagnostic ERCP and deaths in 0.2%[68] but this has steadily fallen to less than 1% for morbidity and less than 0.1% for mortality in recent years[71]. In a personal experience of over 3615 diagnostic examinations over 10 years a complication rate of 0.7% has been observed with acute pancreatitis representing the majority. Those events now recognized as being secondary to continuing biliary obstruction are few as therapeutic intervention is commonly undertaken at the same examination as the diagnostic ERCP and the stone(s) removed or a nasobiliary catheter inserted (see Chapter 7). Acute pancreatitis is usually confined to those patients with previous spontaneous attacks and although most following ERCP are mild, some are severe on standard criteria and require the same intensive therapy. There is now no question that where ERCP is available therapeutic considerations influence its use as a diagnostic imaging tool.

Peroperative cholangiography (POC)

This is an integral part of the surgical management of gallstone disease and is now accepted as routine during cholecystectomy whether or not there are clinical pointers to the presence of bile duct calculi[72,73]. Unfortunately, the standard of radiographic equipment and thus the quality of films produced in operating theatres is, in general, poor in comparison with most radiology departments as portable radiographic units are used and screening facilities are a rarity. This is compounded by the problems of unavoidable supine projection when the lower bile duct often overlies the spine, estimated intervals for radiographic exposures, frequent use of too dense contrast material, and combined with the variable level of experience of the surgeon in interpreting cholangiograms, all lead to potential inaccuracies. A well-performed POC (Figure 4.21), however, should carry a sensitivity and specificity of greater than 90%[72] for the diagnosis of bile duct stones. The addition of choledochoscopy has improved the detection rate but retained stones are still reported in up to 6–8% of some series[74,75].

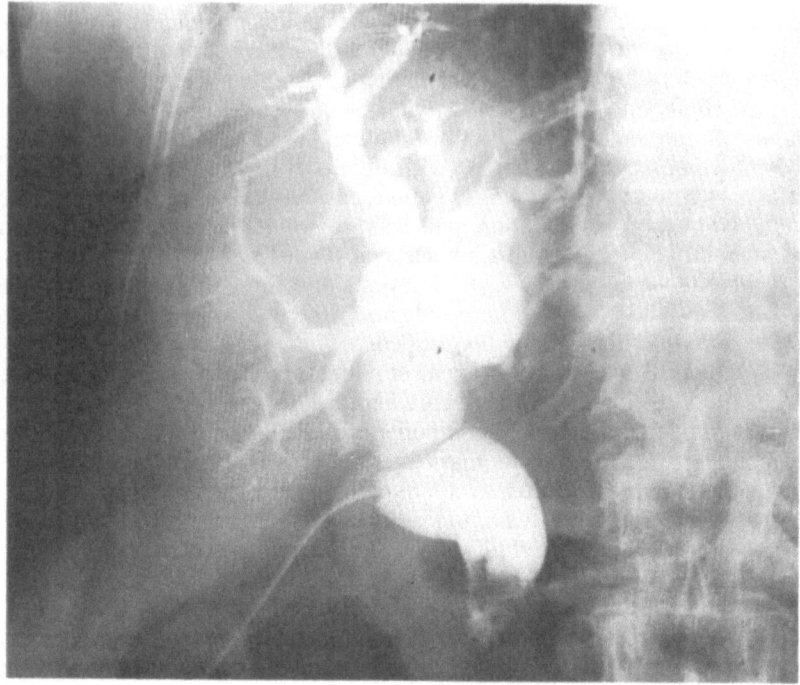

Figure 4.21 Peroperative cholangiogram of good quality showing impacted stone in lower bile duct

Despite the laudable desire to improve the intraoperative detection of bile duct stones and so avoid postoperative complications there may be an increasing attitude amongst surgeons (against traditional teaching) that, as endoscopic and T-tube extraction therapy are now so successful and safe compared with surgical bile duct exploration or re-exploration, difficult residual calculi shown on a postexploration POC may be amenable to these forms of therapy and the risks of further surgical bile duct manipulation should perhaps be avoided.

T-tube cholangiography (TTC)

The insertion of a T-tube is standard practice following surgical bile duct exploration when primary duct closure has not been performed. Cholangiography is obtained by injection of contrast via the T-tube usually between the seventh and tenth postoperative day when any retained stones will be revealed[72,73] (Figure 4.22). The procedure is carried out in the radiology department under fluoroscopy and careful observation of the biliary system during injection is essential if small stones are not to be overlooked or confusion arise with air bubbles. In cases of doubt TTC can be easily repeated. No special patient preparation is needed except an explanation of the procedure and the small risk of inducing bacteraemia or, rarely, septicaemia.

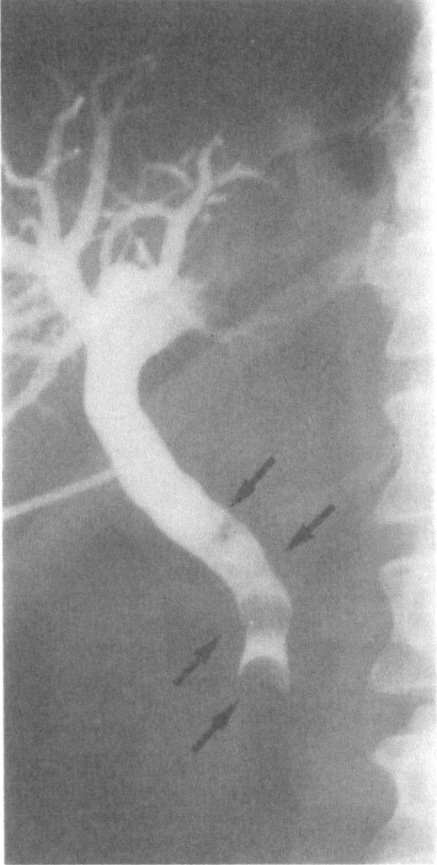

Figure 4.22 T-tube cholangiogram showing retained stones (arrows)

Discomfort may be caused during too rapid injection of contrast but sedation is not usually required. Although a false positive diagnosis of calculi is soon resolved by repeat or further investigation, the specificity of TTC is not precisely known as stones undetected may not cause symptoms for many weeks, months or years and it is often impossible to document whether or not these stones are retained or recurrent (Figure 4.23).

Computerized axial tomography (CT)

The biliary tree and gallstones are well demonstrated by CT scanning[7,76] but the cost, radiation exposure and limited availability makes this very much a third line investigation after ultrasound and invasive studies and is reserved for difficult problems which cannot be resolved by other means (Figure 4.24). Stones in the gallbladder and bile ducts not visible on plain radiographs may be visible on CT owing to the presence of small but sufficient quantities of

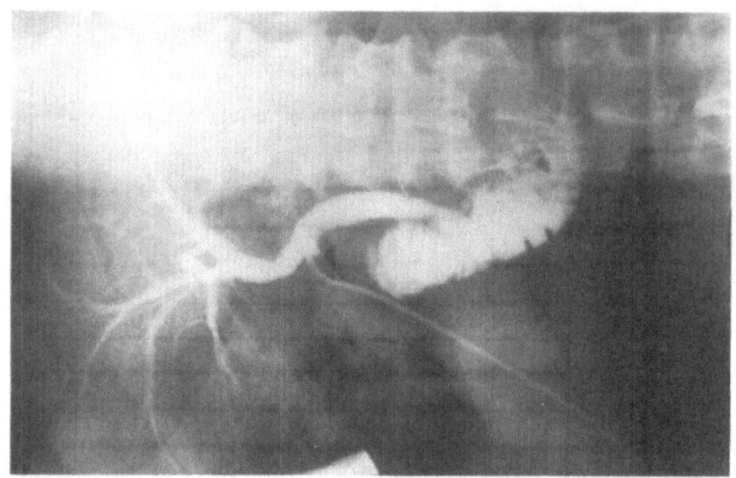

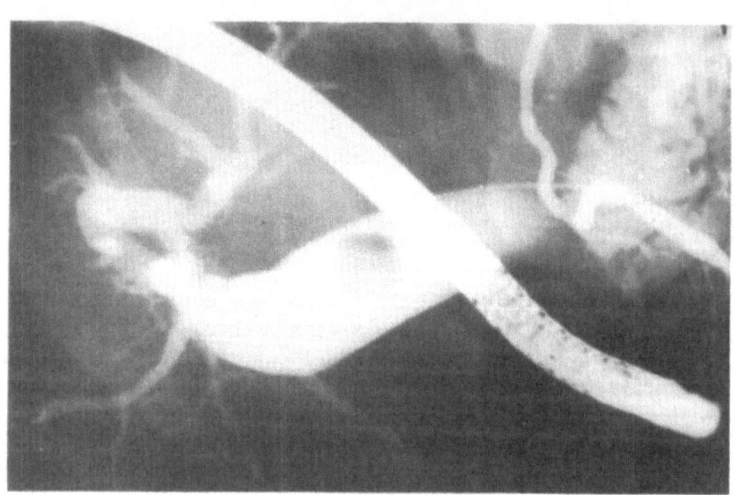

Figure 4.23 Cholangiograms in same patient performed (a) peroperatively after bile duct exploration with no abnormality apparent and (b) 4 years later by ERCP showing a large bile duct stone

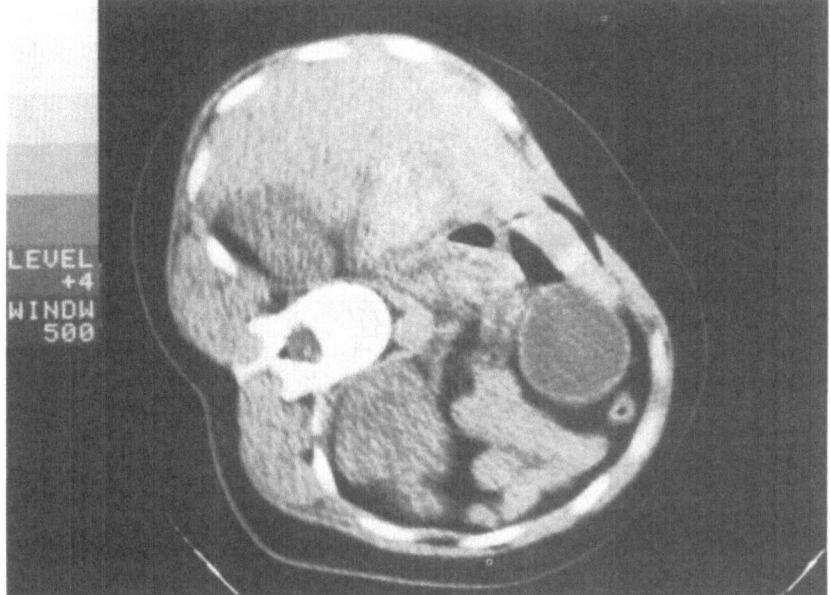

Figure 4.24 CT of patient presenting with acutely tender gallbladder mass, initially diagnosed as cholecystitis/empyema, but here shown to be intraluminal gallbladder haemorrhage with subsequent finding of haemophilia

calcium[76] when stones of 1 mm size can be imaged[7]. Pure cholesterol stones may not be distinguishable by CT from surrounding bile[7]. Diagnosis of gallbladder disease in general is likely to be 80% accurate[76] but ultrasound and OCG are more practicable first line investigations. Mucocele (hydrops) and empyema of the gallbladder are readily distinguished by measurement of gallbladder wall thickness[7] although this is also possible with real-time ultrasonography. In jaundice the distinction between dilated and non-dilated ductal systems by CT with and without vascular and biliary enhancement[77] is possible with a sensitivity of 84–88%, a specificity of 94–97% and an overall accuracy of 91%[76]. Identification of the cause of obstruction compares with ultrasound but when the lower bile duct is inaccessible to the latter, CT may provide the diagnosis (Figure 4.25).

A recent indication for CT has arisen from the development of endoscopic lithotripsy where it is advantageous to know the likelihood of success on attempted stone fragmentation of very large stones. A method for calculating a 'stone index' to predict this outcome has been described[78].

Biliary drainage and microscopy

In patients with suspected gallbladder calculi but negative findings on oral cholecystography further investigation may involve ultrasonography, repeated cholecystography, ERCP or CT. An additional indirect method was

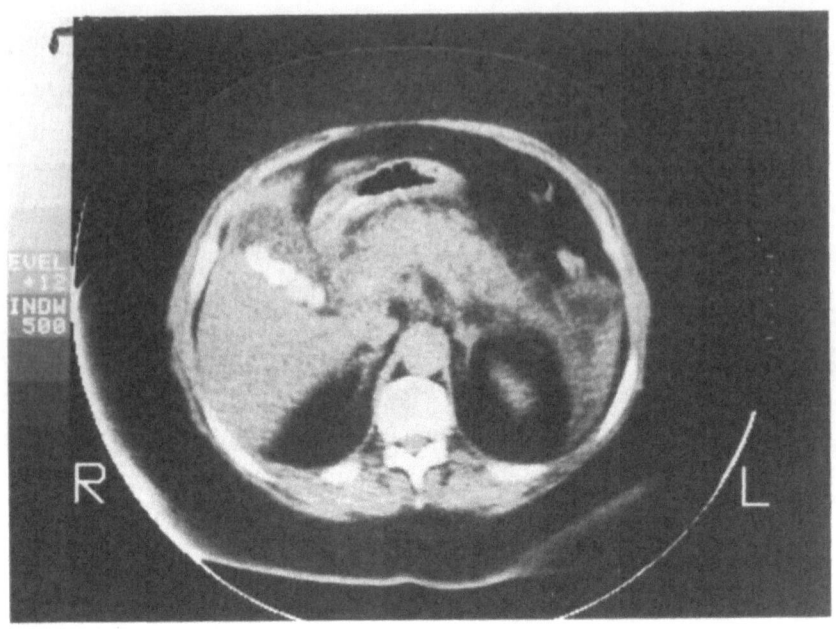

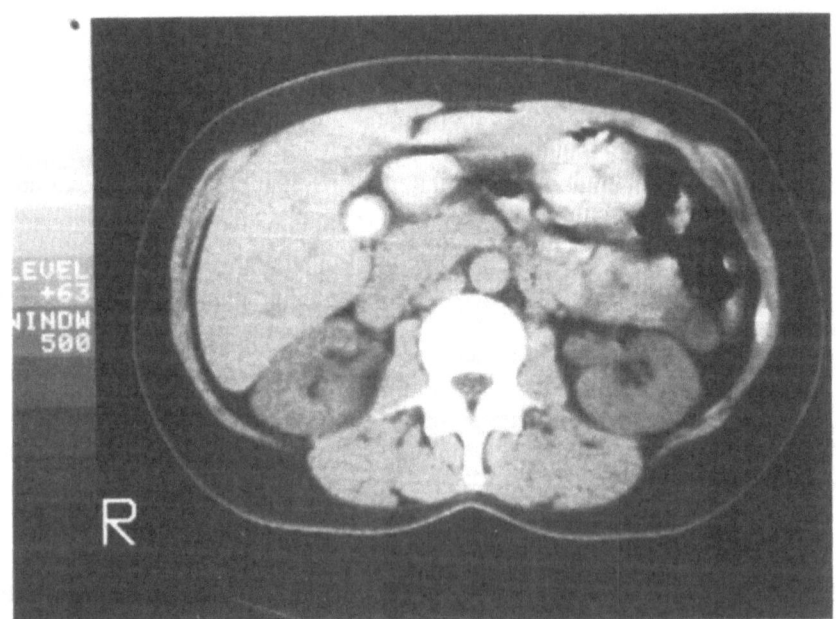

Figure 4.25   CT of jaundiced patient showing stones (a) in gallbladder and (b) in low CBD

described in 1919[79] and came to be called the Meltzer–Lyon test but has gained little popularity. The principle of the test depends on the aspiration of bile from the duodenum after a cholecystokinetic stimulus, such as intravenous CCK, and the immediate search for cholesterol crystals and calcium bilirubinate granules in the sediment of centrifuged viscous (gallbladder) bile by microscopy. Failure to obtain the viscous fraction on two attempts suggests gallbladder disease but this should manifest as a failure to opacify on cholecystography or contract after a fat stimulus during ultrasonography. Clinical results[80–82] have been variable and reflect differences in selection of patients and interpretations of the test findings. Sensitivity values of 62–100% and specificity values of 68–75%[80–82] can be deduced from the trial results. One might expect endoscopic aspiration of bile to improve detection of these constituents as there may be a small place for this type of examination in patients with recurrent biliary pain or relapsing pancreatitis but no supportive data is available. Rigorous conditions for examination of bile, such as immediate microscopy in a room maintained at 37°C, will produce best results[81].

Biochemical predictors of gallstone disease

It is well recognized that abnormal serum liver enzyme and bilirubin concentrations may lead the clinician to suspect gallstone disease as the cause of the clinical problem under investigation but there are no specific patterns peculiar to gallstones compared with other causes of extrahepatic biliary disease. The exception to this, however, may exist in acute gallstone-associated pancreatitis where study of biochemical factors early in an attack may allow a probability classification into a biliary or non-biliary cause.

CLINICAL PROBLEMS

The previous section dealt with the wide range of currently available diagnostic tests for gallstone disease with details of patient preparation, acceptability, accuracy and complications for each modality and should be referred to when statements are made in this section concerning a particular modality. In order to make sense of these sophisticated techniques and select the most appropriate and logical test or sequence of tests for an individual with suspected gallstones this section suggests a possible approach to each of four sets of clinical circumstances in an attempt to represent the most common settings in which investigative decisions require to be made.

Recurrent abdominal pain – is it gallstones?

For the patient with a history of recurrent biliary pain without jaundice in whom gallstones are at the top of the differential diagnostic list, ultrasonography is highly likely to provide the confirmatory diagnosis with little chance of a false positive result when considering gallbladder disease. If this is not available, oral cholecystography will give similar but slightly less accurate results and care must be taken in the interpretation of the non-opacifying gallbladder. A positive finding on either test will have implications

103

for therapy and for the majority this will mean surgical cholecystectomy. Consideration for medical dissolution treatment may need additional information from the complementary test to ascertain suitability.

Cholecystography may demonstrate the bile ducts after a cholecystokinetic stimulus but rarely is this sufficient to show stones or be used routinely for this purpose. Ultrasound, on the other hand, may well indicate unexpected bile duct dilatation or a luminal stone without an antecedent history or jaundice or cholangitis. When this history is present, however, or abnormal liver enzymes or bilirubin are found, an ultrasound demonstration of gallbladder stones and a dilated common bile duct gives circumstantial evidence for suspecting choledocholithiasis. Local surgical views will dictate the next step in the sequence but increasingly irrespective of history, a preoperative ERCP is requested to exclude or confirm stones within the bile ducts. This might be combined with precholecystectomy endoscopic sphincterotomy where indicated, sphincterotomy without subsequent cholecystectomy in the high risk elderly patient, or merely provide preoperative information to direct the surgeon to explore the bile duct as would be the case in the absence of an ERCP service. Intravenous cholangiography has been traditionally used in this context but is too inaccurate to provide clinically useful information.

If both oral cholecystography and ultrasonography are normal or one is equivocal, and repeat of either or both fails to solve the dilemma, ERCP would be the next investigation of choice as a significant number of such patients will be found to have gallstones. Radionuclide scanning and PTC are not indicated here but CT may be needed occasionally if the problem remains unresolved after this series of tests is completed.

Acute abdomen – is it cholecystitis?

A diagnosis of acute cholecystitis is usually made on clinical grounds based on the presenting history, physical findings and simple laboratory investigations. There is a need, however, to confirm this as soon as possible after admission to enable early surgery to be undertaken if indicated and to rule out other causes of an acute abdomen if the symptoms or signs are not characteristic. Urgent ultrasound may fail for technical reasons due to intervening bowel gas or impairment by abdominal tenderness but when successful should be capable of showing not only gallbladder stones but the local inflammatory effects on gallbladder wall and the surrounding tissues if a real-time scanner is used (Figure 4.26). Mere documentation of gallstones does not prove the diagnosis of acute cholecystitis. Urgent radionuclide scanning with HIDA or a similar agent has a high success rate for biliary imaging in this context and a highly accurate correlation with cholecystitis when the gallbladder fails to image. Plain abdominal radiography, oral cholecystography, intravenous cholangiography, and PTC are not applicable investigations but there may be a case for urgent ERCP to identify concomitant choledocholithiasis if jaundice is present. If jaundice develops subsequently it is investigated as described below.

The associated conditions of empyema and mucocele of the gallbladder may be sequels to acute cholecystitis or mimic it in presentation. The diagnosis

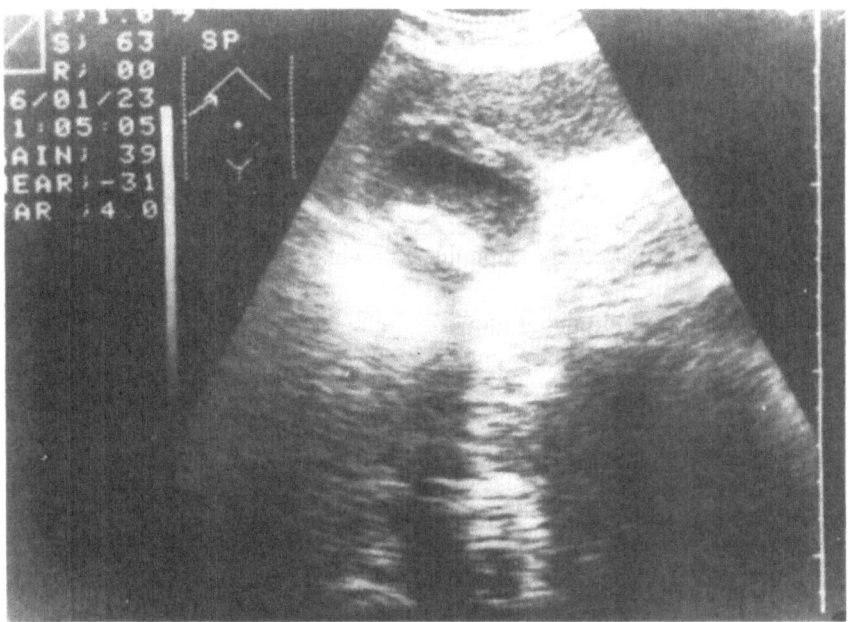

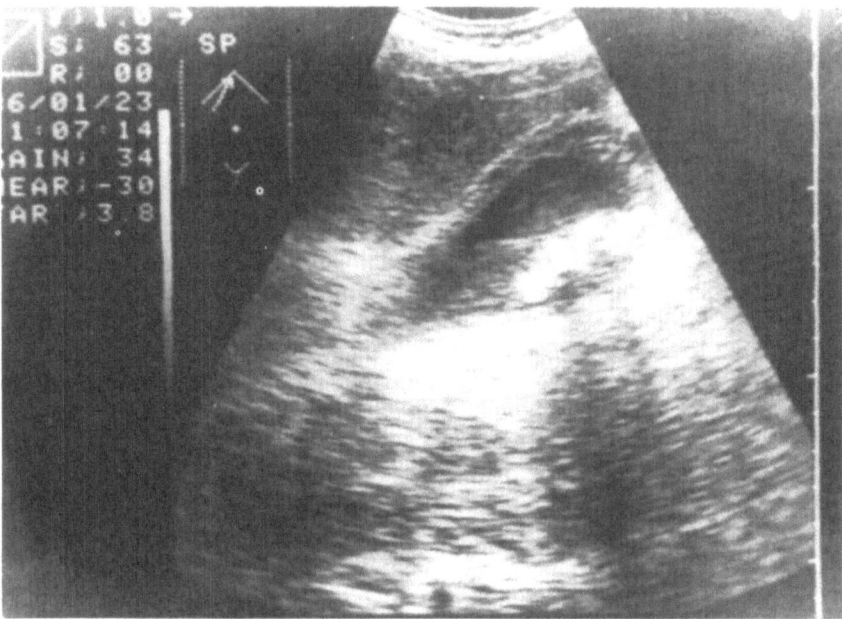

Figure 4.26 Ultrasound in acute cholecystitis showing (a) cross-sectional and (b) longitudinal appearances of gallbladder with thickened echogenic walls and containing stones (donated by Dr A. E. Crozier)

of empyema is a matter of urgency if a fatal outcome is to be avoided, especially in the elderly in whom this is particularly more common. If HIDA scanning alone is used without assiduous clinical surveillance or subsequent ultrasonography this condition will be overlooked. The same consideration is given to mucocele but requires less urgent intervention. It should also be emphasized that empyema is invariably associated with bile duct stones. If cholecystostomy has been the only treatment for these conditions, ERCP with a view to sphincterotomy may be required. CT scanning may occasionally be helpful in further definition of a gallbladder mass.

Cholestasis – is it choledocholithiasis?

Characterization of jaundice as cholestasis is mandatory before embarking on imaging investigations as this will be inappropriate for other causes of jaundice. There may be clinical indicators from the history or physical examination which may favour a diagnosis of benign (calculous or non-calculous) or malignant extrahepatic biliary obstruction or intrahepatic cholestasis but frequently these are absent or misleading. The aims of imaging tests in cholestasis are to define the anatomical abnormality and, by inference from the appearances or from additional associated methods, the pathological cause of this. Biochemical tests are unable to provide either of these facets of diagnosis with any accuracy. Ultrasonography is, in practice, the first imaging investigation in most centres and will provide a certain level of diagnosis depending on local equipment and expertise. At the least it should enable a differentiation between those patients with dilated and non-dilated ductal systems but at best can demonstrate obstructing lesions or their effects with considerable probability. Stones and other causes of low common bile duct obstruction, however, are often difficult to distinguish when a periductal mass is also present. The presence of gallstones in the gallbladder either on plain abdominal radiography or ultrasound does not necessarily imply choledocholithiasis.

Further definition of an obstructing biliary lesion can be provided by PTC or ERCP and choice will nearly always be determined by local availability and enthusiasm. The majority will probably undergo PTC as this is more likely to be available but, in those centres where access to ERCP is routine, this will be the investigation of choice. PTC will still be required for ERCP failures and occasionally when both modalities are required to solve a difficult biliary problem but this is uncommon in gallstone disease. If initial ultrasound suggests a non-dilated system this does not exclude choledocholithiasis and ERCP is the best method for elucidating this. Many patients are now seen early in their disease evolution when gross changes in the biliary tract may not have had time to develop or, alternatively, a bile duct stone may have passed spontaneously and not given rise to significant duct dilatation. Oral cholecystography, radionuclide scanning and intravenous cholangiography are worthless in the patient with cholestasis. CT may occasionally be of value when other techniques have failed to define the problem fully but this is extremely unusual in gallstone disease.

Acute pancreatitis – is it gallstone-associated?

Prompt diagnosis of a biliary cause for acute pancreatitis may influence management and it is hoped that trials will show that early endoscopic or surgical intervention in some patients will ultimately influence outcome. Selection of patients with a biliary aetiology soon after admission is incomplete if urgent ultrasound alone is used to detect gallbladder stones as the technical success and accuracy rates are poor[83]. Radionuclide scanning is also disappointing[83]. Biochemical tests are necessary in acute pancreatitis to stage severity within the first 24 hours of the attack and these can be used to predict the probability of a biliary cause. A number of different mathematical models have been employed to determine the best combination of values of bilirubin, alkaline phosphatase, gamma glutamyl transferase and alanine transferase[84]. ERCP is not now considered to be contraindicated in active pancreatitis provided that precautions are taken by an experienced operator[84]. This is undertaken only to diagnose the presence of persistent bile duct stones which may impair recovery from the current attack, produce concomitant cholangitis or give rise to a further attack and may be removed by sphincterotomy. Interim results of a trial[84] suggest that this strategy may have a part to play in the early management of acute pancreatitis and affect morbidity and mortality. Plain abdominal radiography to detect gallstones, oral cholecystography, intravenous cholangiography and PTC are of no use in the immediate investigation of this condition although some may be considered as interval investigations if there is still doubt about aetiology or if the aforementioned techniques are not available during the acute attack.

CONCLUSIONS

The common occurrence of gallstone disease in its many presentations in widely differing age groups should entreat all clinicians to understand and utilize diagnostic investigations for cholelithiasis or choledocholithiasis in an appropriate manner and sequence. The limitations of commonly used tests are often overlooked and many patients are left without a diagnosis for their continuing 'biliary' symptoms. Once the possibility of gallstone disease has been questioned in the light of a consistent clinical setting, assiduous investigation should lead to a confident diagnosis of biliary disease due to gallstones or not and this may require invasive tests in a small proportion. Increasing availability and accuracy of ultrasonography with each generation of machine and perhaps new techniques, such as endoscopic ultrasound, will undoubtedly render other long-established tests obsolete in the decades to come. Endoscopic techniques for diagnosis have been and will continue to be linked with therapy for gallstones and the possibility of rapid dissolution of bile duct and gallbladder calculi by direct luminal infusion of new cholesterol solvents is likely to influence this further. Future improvements in the diagnosis of gallstones and their treatment will only come about by continued interaction and discussion between clinicians and imaging investigators together with critical evaluation of new techniques against old.

References

1. Bell, G. D. (1984). Clinical features and medical treatment of gallstones. In Bouchier, I. A. D. Allan, R. N., Hodgson, H. J. F. and Keighley, M. R. B. (eds.) *Textbook of Gastroenterology.* pp. 1404–5. (London: Balliere Tindall)

2. McCort, J. J. (1981). Abdominal calcifications. Gallbladder and biliary tree. In McCort, J. J., Mindelzum, R. E., Filpi, R. G. and Rennell, C. (eds.) *Abdominal Radiology.* pp. 60–4. (Baltimore: Williams and Wilkins)

3. Berk, R. N. (1977). The plain abdominal radiograph. In Berk, R. N. and Clemett, A. R. (eds.) *Radiology of the Gallbladder and Bile Ducts.* pp. 1–40. (London: W. B. Saunders)

4. Graham, E. A., Cole, W. H. and Copher, G. H. (1924). Visualisation of the gallbladder by the sodium salt of tetrabromophthalein. *J. Am. Med. Assoc.*, **82**, 1777–8

5. Loeb, P. M. and Berk, R. N. (1977). Biliary contrast materials. In Berk, R. N. and Clemett, A. R. (eds.) *Radiology of the Gallbladder and Bile Ducts.* pp. 71–100. (London: W. B. Saunders)

6. Berk, R. N. (1983). Oral cholecystography. In Margulis, A. R. and Burhenne, H. J. (eds.) *Alimentary Tract Radiology.* pp. 1441–2. (St Louis: C. V. Mosby)

7. Frommhold, W. and Wolf, F. (1983). Radiological and radionuclide methods for the diagnosis of biliary disorders. *Clin. Gastroenterol.*, **12**, 65–100

8. Hopman, W. P. M., Jansen, J. B. M., Rosenbusch, G. and Lamers, C. B. H. W. (1986). Gallbladder contraction induced by cholecystokinin: bolus injection or infusion? *Br. Med. J.*, **292**, 375–6

9. Sargent, E. N., Meyers, H. I. and Hubsher, J. (1976). Cholecystokinetic cholecystography: efficacy and tolerance study of sincalide. *Am. J. Roentgenol.*, **127**, 267–71

10. Sargent, E. N., Wieler, M. and Halls, J. (1979). Cholecystokinetic cholecystography: comparison of the effect of intramuscular ceruletide to a fatty meal. *Am. J. Roentgenol.*, **133**, 489–92

11. Berk, R. N. (1983). Radiology of the gallbladder. In Margulis, A. R. and Burhenne, H. J. (eds.) *Alimentary Tract Radiology.* pp. 1434–60. (St Louis: C. V. Mosby)

12. Berk, R. N. (1977). Oral cholecystography. In Berk, R. N. and Clemett, A. R. (eds.) *Radiology of the Gallbladder and Bile Ducts.* pp. 101–99. (London: W. B. Saunders)

13. Cooley, R. N. and Donner, M. W. (1963). The diagnostic accuracy of radiologic studies of the biliary tract, small intestine and colon. *Am. J. Med. Sci.*, **246**, 610–38

14. Krook, P. M., Allen, F. H., Bush, W. H., Ginger Malmer, R. T. and MacLean, M. D. (1980). Comparison of real-time cholecystosonography and oral cholecystography. *Radiology*, **135**, 145–8

15. De Lacey, G., Gajjar, B., Twomey, B., Levi, J. and Cox, A. G. (1984). Should cholecystography or ultrasound be the primary investigation for gallbladder disease? *Lancet*, **1**, 205–7

16. Watts, J. McK. and Toouli, J. (1984). Cholecystitis and choledocholithiasis. In Bouchier, I. A. D., Allan, R. N., Hodgson, H. J. F. and Keighley, M. R. B. (eds.) *Textbook of Gastroenterology.* p. 1419. (London: Balliere Tindall)

17. Gough, M. H. (1977). 'The cholecystogram is normal' ... but ... *Br. Med. J.*, **1**, 960–2

18. Neoptolemos, J. P., Lloyd, D. M. and Carr-Locke, D. L. (1984). Diagnosing gallbladder disease (letter). *Br. Med. J.*, **289**, 108

19. Venu, R. P., Geenen, J. E., Toouli, J., Stewart, E. and Hogan, W. J. (1983). Endoscopic retrograde cholangioancreatography. Diagnosis of cholelithiasis in patients with normal gallbladder X-ray and ultrasound studies. *J. Am. Med. Assoc.*, **249**, 758–61

20. Gleeson, D., Ruppin, D. C. and Dowling, R. H. (1983). British Gall Stone Study Group postdissolution trial: interim report on overall recurrence rates and discrepancies between ultrasonography and oral cholecystography. *Gut*, **24**, A1006

21. Bartrum, R. J., Crow, H. C. and Foote, S. R. (1977). Ultrasonic and radiographic cholecystography. *N. Engl. J. Med.*, **296**, 538–43

22. Cooperberg, P. L. and Burhenne, H. J. (1980). Real-time ultrasonography. *N. Engl. J. Med.*, **302**, 1277–9

23. Cosgrove, D. O. and McCready, V. R. (1983). Biliary system. In *Ultrasound Imaging: Liver, Spleen and Pancreas.* pp. 225–72. (London: John Wiley and Sons)

24. Sanders, R. C. and Conrad, M. R. (1977). Ultrasonic examination of the gallbladder. In Berk, R. N. and Clemett, A. R. (eds.) *Radiology of the Gallbladder and Bile Ducts.* pp. 331–51. (London: W. B. Saunders)

25. Filly, R. A., Laing, F. C., Callen, P. W. and Gooding, G. A. W. (1983). Ultrasonography. In Margulis, A. R. and Burhenne, H. J. (eds.) *Alimentary Tract Radiology*. pp. 1479–1510. (St Louis: C. V. Mosby)
26. Okuda, K. and Tsuchiya, Y. (1983). Ultrasonic anatomy of the biliary system. *Clin. Gastroenterol.*, 12, 49–63
27. Ferucci, J. T. (1979). Body ultrasonography. *N. Engl. J. Med.*, 300, 590–602
28. Einstein, D. M., Lapin, S. A., Ralls, P. W. and Halls, J. M. (1984). The insensitivity of sonography in the detection of choledocholithiasis. *Am. J. Roentgenol.*, 142, 725–8
29. Behan, M. and Kazam, E. (1978). Sonography of the common bile duct: value of the right anterior oblique view. *Am. J. Roentgenol.*, 130, 701–9
30. Roenigsberg, M., Wiener, S. N. and Walzer, A. (1979). The accuracy of sonography in the differential diagnosis of obstructive jaundice: a comparison with cholangiography. *Radiology*, 133, 157–65
31. Dewbury, K. C., Joseph, A. E. A., Hayes, S. and Murray, C. (1979). Ultrasound in the evaluation and diagnosis of jaundice. *Br. J. Radiol.*, 52, 276–80
32. Vallon, A. G., Lees, W. R. and Cotton, P. B. (1979). Grey-scale ultrasonography in obstructive jaundice. *Gut*, 20, 51–4
33. Malini, S. and Sabel, J. (1977). Ultrasonography in obstructive jaundice. *Radiology*, 123, 429–33
34. Weinstein, B. J. and Weinstein, D. P. (1980). Biliary tract dilatation in the non-jaundiced patient. *Am. J. Roentgenol.*, 134, 899–906
35. Wild, S. R., Cruickshank, J. G., Fraser, G. M., Coupland, W. A. and Grieve, D. C. (1980). Grey-scale ultrasonography and percutaneous transhepatic cholangiography in biliary tract disease. *Br. Med. J.*, 281, 1524–6
36. Taylor, J. K. W. and Rosenfield, A. T. (1977). Grey-scale ultrasonography in the differential diagnosis of jaundice. *Arch. Surg.*, 112, 820–5
37. Cronan, J. J., Mueller, P. R. and Simeone, J. F. (1983). Prospective diagnosis of choledocholithiasis. *Radiology*, 146, 467–9
38. Gross, B. H., Harter, L. P. and Gore, R. M. (1983). Ultrasonic evaluation of common bile duct stones. *Radiology*, 146, 471–4
39. Laing, F. C. and Jeffrey, R. B. (1983). Choledocholithiasis and cystic duct obstruction: difficult ultrasonographic diagnosis. *Radiology*, 146, 475–9
40. Strohm, W. D., Kurtz, W. and Classen, M. (1984). Detection of biliary stones by means of endosonography. *Scand. J. Gastroenterol.*, 19, (suppl. 94), 60–4
41. Meire, H. B. (1984). Ultrasound in gastroenterology. *Clin. Gastroenterol.*, 13, 191–4
42. Verow, P. W. and Wisbey, M. (1975). Sequential liver and biliary tract scanning with ^{131}I labelled Rose Bengal. *Clin. Radiol.*, 26, 499–504
43. Rhys Davies, E. (1984). Radionuclide investigations. *Clin. Gastroenterol.*, 13, 210–16
44. Rosenthall, K. (1983). Nuclear medicine of the biliary tract. In Margulis, A. R. and Burhenne, H. J. (eds.) *Alimentary Tract Radiology*. pp. 1554–64. (St Louis: C. V. Mosby)
45. Shuman, W. P., Gibbs, P., Rudd, T. G. and Malk, L. A. (1982). PIPIDA scintigraphy for cholecystitis: false positives in alcoholism and total parenteral nutrition. *Am. J. Roentgenol.*, 138, 1–5
46. Bouchier, I. A. D. (1984). Imaging procedures to diagnose gallbladder disease. *Br. Med. J.*, 288, 1632–3
47. Down, R. H. L., Goldin, A., Arnold, J., Watts, J. McK. and Benness, G. (1979). Comparison of accuracy of ^{99m}Tc-pyridoxylidene glutamate scanning with oral cholecystography and ultrasonography in diagnosis of aute cholecystitis. *Lancet*, 2, 1094–7
48. Weissmann, H. S., Frank, M. S., Bernstein, L. H. and Freeman, L. M. (1979). Rapid and accurate diagnosis of acute cholecystitis with ^{99m}Tc-HIDA cholescintigraphy. *Am. J. Roentgenol.*, 132, 523–8
49. Nicholson, R. W., Hastings, D. L., Testa, H. J. and Torrance, B. (1980). HIDA scanning in gallbladder disease. *Br. J. Radiol.*, 53, 878–82
50. Freitas, J. E. (1982). Cholescintigraphy in acute and chronic cholecystitis. *Sem. Nucl. Med.*, 12, 18–28
51. Burhenne, H. J. and Murray, J. B. (1983). Intravenous cholangiography. In Margulis, A. R. and Burhenne, H. J. (eds.) *Alimentary Tract Radiology*. pp. 1461–78. (St Louis: C. V. Mosby)

52. Berk, R. N. (1977). Intravenous cholangiography. In Berk, R. N. and Clemett, A. R. (eds.) *Radiology of the Gallbladder and Bile Ducts.* pp. 200–40. (London: W. B. Saunders)
53. Burchhardt, H. and Muller, W. (1921). Versuche uber die punktion der Gallenblase und ihre Rontgendarstellung. *Dtsch. Med. Wochschr.,* **161,** 168
54. Huard, P. and Do-Xuan-Hop. (1937). La ponction transhepatique des canaux biliaires. *Bull. Soc. Med. Chir. Indoch.,* **15,** 1090
55. Ariyama, J. (1971). Percutaneous transhepatic cholangiography. In Saitoh, T. (ed.) *Clinical X-ray Diagnosis.* (Tokyo: Igaku-Shoin)
56. Kubota, H., Wagai, K. and Hasegawa, M. (1969). The gallbladder and bile ducts. In Shirakabe, H. and Ichikawa, H. (eds.) *Gastrointestinal Radiology.* (Tokyo: Kanehara and Co.)
57. Ohto, M. (1973). *Percutaneous Transhepatic Cholangiography.* (Tokyo: Igaku-Shoin)
58. Okuda, K., Tanikawa, K., Emura, T., Kuratomi, S., Jinnuochi, S., Urabe, K., Sumikoshi, T., Kanda, Y., Fukuyama, Y., Musha, H., Mari, H., Shimokawa, Y., Yakushiji, F. and Matsuura, Y. (1974). Non-surgical percutaneous trans-hepatic cholangiography – diagnostic significance in medical problems of the liver. *Am. J. Dig. Dis.,* **19,** 21–36
59. Ariyama, J. (1983). Percutaneous transhepatic cholangiography. In Margulis, A. R. and Burhenne, H. J. (eds.) *Alimentary Tract Radiology.* pp. 2229–41. (St Louis: C. V. Mosby)
60. Dooley, J. S., Hamilton-Miller, J. M. T., Brumfitt, W. and Sherlock, S. (1984). Progress report: antibiotics in the treatment of biliary infection. *Gut,* **25,** 988–98
61. Ariyama, J., Shirakabe, H. and Ohashi, K. (1978). Experience with percutaneous transhepatic cholangiography using the Japanese needle. *Gastrointest. Radiol.,* **2,** 359–65
62. Harbin, W. P., Mueller, P. R. and Ferrucci, J. T. (1980). Transhepatic cholangiography: complications and use patterns of fine needle transhepatic cholangiography: a multiinstitutional study. *Radiology,* **135,** 15–22
63. Cotton, P. B. (1983). Direct choledochography and related diagnostic methods. *Clin. Gastroenterol.,* **12,** 101–7
64. Ferrucci, J. T. and Wittenberg, J. (1977). Refinements in Chiba needle transhepatic cholangiography. *Am. J. Roentgenol.,* **129,** 11–23
65. Gold, R. P., Casarella, W. J., Stern, G. and Seaman, W. B. (1979). Transhepatic cholangiography: the radiological method of choice in suspected obstructive jaundice. *Radiology,* **133,** 39–44
66. Mueller, P. R., Van Sonnenberg, E. and Simeone, J. F. (1982). Fine-needle transhepatic cholangiography: indications and usefulness. *Ann. Int. Med.,* **97,** 567–72
67. Kreek, M. J. and Balint, J. A. (1980). 'Skinny needle' cholangiography – results of a pilot study of a voluntary prospective method for gathering risk data on new procedures. *Gastroenterology,* **78,** 598–604
68. Cotton, P. B. (1977). Progress report. ERCP. *Gut,* **18,** 316–41
69. Classen, M. and Demling, L. (1974). Endoscopische Sphinkterotomie der papilla Vater. *Dtsch. Med. Wochschr.,* **99,** 496–7
70. Kawai, K., Akasaka, Y., Murakami, K., Tada, M., Kohli, Y. and Nakajima, M. (1974). Endoscopic sphincterotomy of the ampulla of Vater. *Gastrointest. Endosc.,* **20,** 148–51
71. Stewart, E. T. and Vennes, J. A. (1983). Endoscopic retrograde cholangiopancreatography. In Margulis, A. R. and Burhenne, H. J. (eds.) *Alimentary Tract Radiology.* pp. 2263–80. (St Louis: C. V. Mosby)
72. Burhenne, H. J. (1983). Postoperative radiology: intestinal and biliary tract. In Margulis, A. R. and Burhenne, H. J. *Alimentary Tract Radiology.* (eds.) pp. 1783–91. (St Louis: C. V. Mosby)
73. Clemett, A. R. (1977). Operative and postoperative cholangiography. In Berk, R. N. and Clemett, A. R. (eds.) *Radiology of the Gallbladder and Bile Ducts.* pp. 272–84. (London: W. B. Saunders)
74. Rattner, D. W. and Warshaw, A. L. (1981). Impact of choledochoscopy in the management of choledocholithiasis. *Ann. Surg.,* **194,** 76–9
75. Feliciano, D. W., Mattox, K. L. and Jordan, G. L. (1980). The value of choledochoscopy in exploration of the common bile duct. *Ann. Surg.,* **191,** 649–53
76. Stanley, R. J. and Sagel, S. S. (1983). Computed tomography. In Margulis, A. R. and Burhenne, H. J. (eds.) *Alimentary Tract Radiology.* pp. 1511–34. (St Louis: C. V. Mosby)
77. Pedrosa, C. S., Casanova, R., Lezana, A. H. and Fernandez, M. C. (1981). CT in obstructive jaundice part II. The cause of obstruction. *Radiology,* **139,** 635–46

78. Staritz, M., Ewe, K., Meyer zum Buschenfelde,, K.-H., Schreyer, T. and Dahnert, W. (1984). Computed tomography to predict hardness of bile duct stones before endoscopic lithotripsy. *Lancet*, 1, 460
79. Lyon, B. B. V. (1919). Diagnosis and treatment of diseases of the gallbladder and biliary ducts; preliminary report on a new method. *J. Am. Med. Assoc.*, 73, 980
80. Freeman, J. B. and Cohen, W. N. (1975). Cholecystokinin cholangiography and analysis of duodenal bile in the investigation of pain in the right upper quadrant of the abdomen without gallstones. *Surg. Gynecol. Obstet.*, 140, 371–6
81. Delchier, J.-C., Benfred, P., Preaux, A.-M., Metreau, J.-M. and Dhumeaux, D. (1986). The usefulness of microscopic bile examination in patients with suspected microlithiasis. *Hepatology*, 6, 118–22
82. Foss, D. C. and Laing, R. R. (1977). Detection of gallbladder disease in patients with normal oral cholecystograms. Results using a simplified biliary drainage technique. *Dig. Dis.*, 22, 685–9
83. Neoptolemos, J. P., Hall, A. W., Finlay, D. F., Berry, J. M., Carr-Locke, D. L. and Fossard, D. P. (1984). The urgent diagnosis of gallstones in acute pancreatitis: a prospective study of three methods. *Br. J. Surg.*, 71, 230–3
84. Neoptolemos, J. P., London, N., Slater, N. D., Carr-Locke, D. L., Fossard, D. P. and Moossa, A. R. (1986). A prospective study of ERCP and endoscopic sphincterotomy in the diagnosis of gallstones acute pancreatitis. *Arch. Surg.* (In press)

5
Surgical Management

S. A. SADEK and A. CUSCHIERI

INTRODUCTION

There is a high prevalence of gallstones in Britain, Europe, Australia and North America[1-5]. In Britain 9 out of 10 subjects with gallstones do not have a cholecystectomy, and females are three times more likely to have their gallstones removed than males[6]. There are major differences in the cholecystectomy rates between different countries. Thus in the UK, the cholecystectomy rate is 70–79/100 000 whereas in North America and Canada, the figure is 3–4 times higher[7,8]. As these different rates cannot be explained by differences in disease prevalence, it appears likely that the indications for cholecystectomy vary from country to country in accordance with the type of health care system which predominates. Within the UK, the cholecystectomy rate has risen during the past two decades. This rise has not been accompanied by a reduction in the overall mortality rate from gallstone disease and has been attributed to changes in the diagnostic and surgical resources[9]. Chronic administration of thiazide diuretics does not predispose to the development of gallstones but two studies have implicated this treatment with the subsequent development of acute cholecystitis[10,11] in patients known to harbour stones. The widespread use of diuretic therapy in the treatment of hypertension may well have been a factor in the rising cholecystectomy rate for gallstone disease in the UK.

SPECTRUM OF GALLSTONE-RELATED DISORDERS

An important differentiation is between silent and symptomatic gallstones since this affects management in the individual case.

Silent (asymptomatic) gallstones

Most surveys indicate that silent gallstones outnumber symptomatic ones. The arguments for cholecystectomy in this group have included the risk of gallbladder cancer and the eventual development of symptoms/acute life-threatening disease. This viewpoint emanated from early retrospective and poorly controlled reports[12,13], and is not supported by more recent prospective studies which have shown that the vast majority of silent gallstones will not cause symptoms or complications during life[14,15]. Comparative evaluation of the relative risks of expectant versus surgical management of silent gallstones employing *decision analysis* techniques, which incorporate the probabilities of all the risk factors of both conservative and surgical treatment, has demonstrated that surgical intervention reduces marginally the life expectancy in addition to being substantially more costly[15]. A case could be made for the periodic review of patients with silent gallstones since approximately 1 in 5 will develop symptoms or complications and there are currently no reliable predictor criteria that can identify these patients.

As gallstones are present in the majority of patients who develop carcinoma of the gallbladder, cholecystectomy has been advocated as a prophylactic measure in patients with silent gallstones. However, carcinoma of the gallbladder is rare and its reported necropsy incidence[6,9] is 0.3–0.4%. The operative mortality of cholecystectomy varies with age but overall it certainly exceeds that resulting from gallbladder cancer by a significant margin[16]. The evidence linking cholecystectomy with the development of colon cancer remains conflicting[17] and cannot be used as a further argument against cholecystectomy for silent gallstones. The majority of surgeons in the West are convinced by the available data quoted above that surgical intervention is not warranted for symptomless gallstones, and those few who are not, ought to be.

Symptomatic gallstone disease

The management of these patients is best discussed in terms of the clinical presentation which may be vague and ill-defined or acute with established physical signs signs Table 5.1).

Table 5.1   Spectrum of symptomatic gallstone disease

Chronic cholecystitis
Acute biliary colic/acute cholecystitis
Jaundice due to large bile duct obstruction
Cholangitis/septicaemia
Acute gallstone pancreatitis
Biliary fistulous disease
Gallstone ileus

Chronic cholecystitis

Chronic right hypochondrial pain when of biliary tract origin is usually due to chronic calculous cholecystitis. The presence of chronic symptoms attributed to gallstones is currently the commonest indication for routine cholecystectomy. There is little doubt that these patients should have their gallbladder removed as approximately one third of them will develop complications if surgical treatment is delayed[18]. Furthermore, the morbidity and certainly following surgical intervention are considerably enhanced in those patients who develop complications necessitating urgent surgical intervention[19]. In practice, the problem concerns the careful selection of patients for cholecystectomy since the symptoms are by no means specific and can be caused by other common gastrointestinal disorders. A large cohort of patients who continue to experience symptoms after cholecystectomy (post-cholecystectomy syndrome) are subsequently found to have disease outside the biliary tract.

Acute biliary colic and acute cholecystitis

The condition of acute biliary colic is usually ascribed to those patients who are restless from the pain especially when this is of short duration (30 min to 3 h). However, the clinical differentiation between acute biliary colic and acute cholecystitis is often impossible, and absence of fever, leukocytosis and minimal physical signs do not exclude gallbladder inflammation, particularly in the elderly. Both conditions emanate from the same underlying pathology (acute cystic duct obstruction) and require the same treatment – cholecystectomy.

In over 95% of cases, acute cholecystitis is obstructive in nature and results from impaction of a stone in Hartmann's pouch/cystic duct[20]. Much less commonly acute cholecystitis is acalculous. The relative incidence of acute calculous, acute acalculous and acute emphysematous cholecystitis in a consecutive series of 510 patients undergoing early surgery is shown in Figure 5.1.

Acute calculous (obstructive) cholecystitis

In this condition, the gallbladder becomes acutely inflamed with transmural oedema. The initial inflammation is chemically induced and is not of bacterial origin although sepsis is an important feature of the complications of the disease. The release of mucosal phospholipase which converts the lecithin in the bile to lysolecithin is currently held responsible for the initiation of the inflammatory response although bacterial lysosomal enzymes have also been implicated. Prostaglandins have also been implicated in the inflammation of the gallbladder[21]. At the time of surgery carried out during the same admission, approximately 50% of cultures of gallbladder contents are sterile. Aerobic enteric organisms account for 94% of positive cultures and anaerobes for the remainder[22].

Physical signs include pyrexia, tenderness with rebound in the right hypochondrium, positive Murphy's sign (inspiratory arrest), ileus and mild abdominal distention. A tender palpable mass in the right hypochondrium is observed in 25% of patients and may signify empyema of the gallbladder, abscess due to localized perforation or carcinoma of the gallbladder. Jaundice is encountered in 20–25% of patients with acute calculous cholecystitis, but common duct stones are found in only 12% of cases[23,24]. In the absence of ductal calculi, jaundice has been ascribed to reactive hepatitis or oedema

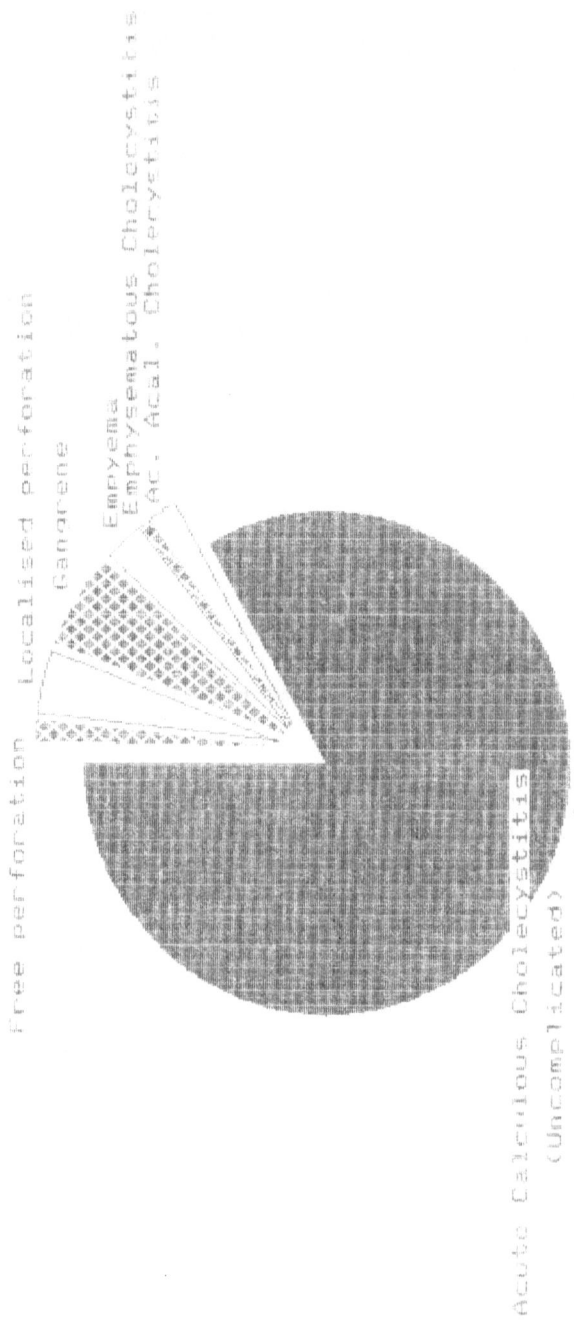

Figure 5.1 Operative findings in 501 patients undergoing urgent or early cholecystectomy at Ninewells hospital

of the common bile duct. A raised serum amylase (>1200 IU) is used to differentiate acute cholecystitis from acute gallstone pancreatitis. However, in a preliminary report on the operative findings in patients with 'acute pancreatitis' randomized to early surgery, acute or acute on chronic cholecystitis without any obvious pancreatic inflammation was found in 50% of cases[25].

The important imaging tests aside from plain radiology of the abdomen, include ultrasound scanning, gallbladder scintigraphy ([99mTc]HIDA, IDA, Iprofenin) and intravenous cholangiography. Ultrasound examination has been advocated as the initial diagnostic procedure for acute cholecystitis since it enables the determination of tenderness over the sonographically identified gallbladder and is able to detect stones, sludge and gallbladder wall thickening[26]. However, the sensitivity and specificity of ultrasound examination for the diagnosis of acute cholecystitis, as opposed to gallstone disease, is low[27,28]. Moreover, this investigative modality is highly observer dependent, and its diagnostic yield will therefore vary from centre to centre depending on local expertise. Gallbladder scintiscanning is the most accurate test of acute cholecystitis[28,32]. It has a sensitivity of 91–97% and a specificity of 87%. False positives are due to chronic cholecystitis and are also encountered in patients with gallstone pancreatitis[33]. A normal gallbladder scintiscan is virtually 100% accurate in excluding acute cholecystitis. Intravenous cholangiography is less accurate than biliary scintigraphy for the diagnosis of acute cholecystitis[29], and cannot be employed when the serum bilirubin exceeds 50μmol/l. Oral cholecystography is unpredictable in the ill patient who is nauseous and may vomit. The technique is, however, useful after the acute episode has subsided and in patients with mild attacks.

Acute acalculous cholecystitis

This accounts for between 2 and 8% of cases and is usually encountered in critically ill elderly patients[34], but the condition has been reported in children[35]. The disease usually develops on a background of prolonged illness, e.g. multiple trauma, major surgery, extensive burns, severe sepsis and drug overdosage. The risk factors which have been associated with the development of gallbladder inflammation include blood volume depletion, prolonged ileus, morphine administration exceeding 6 days, intravenous hyperalimentation, multiple blood transfusions, infected wounds and starvation[36,37]. The presumed pathophysiology involves prolonged distention of the gallbladder, bile stasis and inspissation together with a mucosal injury and thrombosis of the blood vessels of the seromuscular layer consequent on a postulated activation of factor XII[38]. Macroscopically, the gallbladder shows marked oedema of the seromuscular coat with focal necrotic areas. Emergency cholecystectomy is necessary to prevent the onset of free perforation of the inflamed gallbladder.

Acute emphysematous cholecystitis

This is a severe and fulminant form of acute cholecystitis which is caused by a mixed infection including gas-forming organisms (*E. coli, Cl. welchii*, aerobic and anaerobic streptococci). It is usually but not always acalculous. Thrombosis of the cystic artery has been implicated in the development of the condition. Acute emphysematous cholecystitis has a predilection for males (70% of reported cases) and diabetic individuals[39,40].

Complications of acute cholecystitis

The important complications of acute cholecystitis are empyema (suppurative cholecystitis), perforation and gangrene. They all contribute significantly to the morbidity and mortality from the disease and all require urgent surgical intervention.

Empyema – This is an uncommon complication with a reported incidence of 2–3% of all patients with gallstone disease. It usually affects elderly patients[41]. The gallbladder contents are positive in 80%.

Gangrene – Patchy gangrene of the gallbladder wall was encountered in 7.3% in the Ninewells series of 510 patients undergoing early surgery for acute cholecystitis. It usually affects the fundus and may lead to localized or free perforation. The risk factors for the development of gangrene are old age, diabetes, empyema, acalculous cholecystitis and especially, emphysematous cholecystitis.

Perforation – Free perforation into the general peritoneal cavity results in generalized peritonitis and carries a high mortality variously reported as 30–50%. Perforation into the duodenum results in a cholecystoduodenal fistula with resolution of the cholecystitis but the condition may then progress to gallstone ileus.

Jaundice due to ductal calculi

The majority of ductal calculi are found in the common bile duct, and in the Western hemisphere only an estimated 5% are intrahepatic (usually in the left ductal system) although a much higher incidence is encountered in Eastern countries in association with bacterial infection (*E. coli, Bacteroides fragilis*), parastic infestations and oriental cholangitis[42-44]. Most instances of multiple intrahepatic calculi arise proximal to strictures in the intrahepatic biliary tree.

Ductal calculi are classified as primary, originating *de novo* within the bile ducts; or secondary, which are stones that have migrated from the gallbladder. Primary ductal calculi consist of amorphous soft concretions of cholesterol and bilirubinate with a low calcium content[45]. The important factors concerned with their formation include stasis due to obstructing lesions and congenital cystic disease of the biliary tract; and infection with beta-glucuronidase producing bacteria[46].

Ductal calculi may present with episodic upper abdominal pain and dyspepsia, recurrent bouts of biliary colic accompanied by jaundice, painless jaundice, and acutely, with cholangitis and septicaemia or gallstone pancreatitis. However, 15–20% of patients with ductal calculi have no symptoms[47]. The management depends on the age, presence of intercurrent disease and the clinical picture but there is an increasing tendency towards the utilization of endoscopic papillotomy particularly in the elderly and the poor risk patient.

Gallstone pancreatitis

The association between acute pancreatitis and the passage of ductal calculi through the sphincter of Oddi is now well established[48] and gallstone pancreatitis remains the commonest form of acute pancreatitis in Britain. Clinical reports of emergency surgery, carried out within 3 days of onset of the illness, have shown an incidence of ductal impaction varying from 6% in one prospective clinical trial[49] to 62–72% in two retrospective reports[50,51]. These findings have been widely interpreted as evidence for the role of calculous obstruction in the aetiology of acute gallstone pancreatitis as originally reported by Opie[52]. The findings when surgery is undertaken early during the same hospital admission but beyond 3 days of onset of acute pancreatitis cast serious doubt on this hypothesis. In two retrospective reports[53,54] and one prospective clinical trial[25] of early surgery, ampullary calculous obstruction was absent. Urgent surgical or endoscopic decompression by papillotomy[55] is therefore unwarranted. The opposite view to the obstructive theory postulates that the passage of ductal calculi through the sphincter indicates an open channel, perhaps due to a functionally incompetent sphincter permitting duodenobiliary/pancreatic reflux. Direct evidence for a hypotonic sphincter in patients with previous gallstone pancreatitis was obtained by ceruletide biliary manometry in a recent study[56].

Surgical management of gallstone disease

The current status of biliary tract surgery was evaluated by a prospective study involving 21 institutions from North America, Western Europe, Australia, South Africa and Japan, commissioned by the International Biliary Association (IBA)[57]. Of the 1072 operations included in this audit, 986 (92%) were primary and 86 (8%) were secondary (repeat) procedures with an overall mortality of 1.6% and 2.3% respectively. The details of the surgical procedures in both groups are shown in Figure 5.2 a, b. The mortality after cholecystectomy alone was low (1.1% for the USA cohort, 0.2% for the non-American centres, 0.6% overall), but was substantially higher when common duct exploration was added (5.8% for the USA cohort, 3.5% for the other centres, 4.4% overall). The incidence of retained stones was 4.5% but a negative bile duct exploration rate of 18.5% was observed. In this study there were no instances of iatrogenic bile duct damage but it should be stressed that all the participating centres have a special interest in the biliary tract field. These results, though better than those encountered in the average general hospital, still leave room for improvement and clearly indicate that exploration of the common bile duct should not be undertaken lightly and

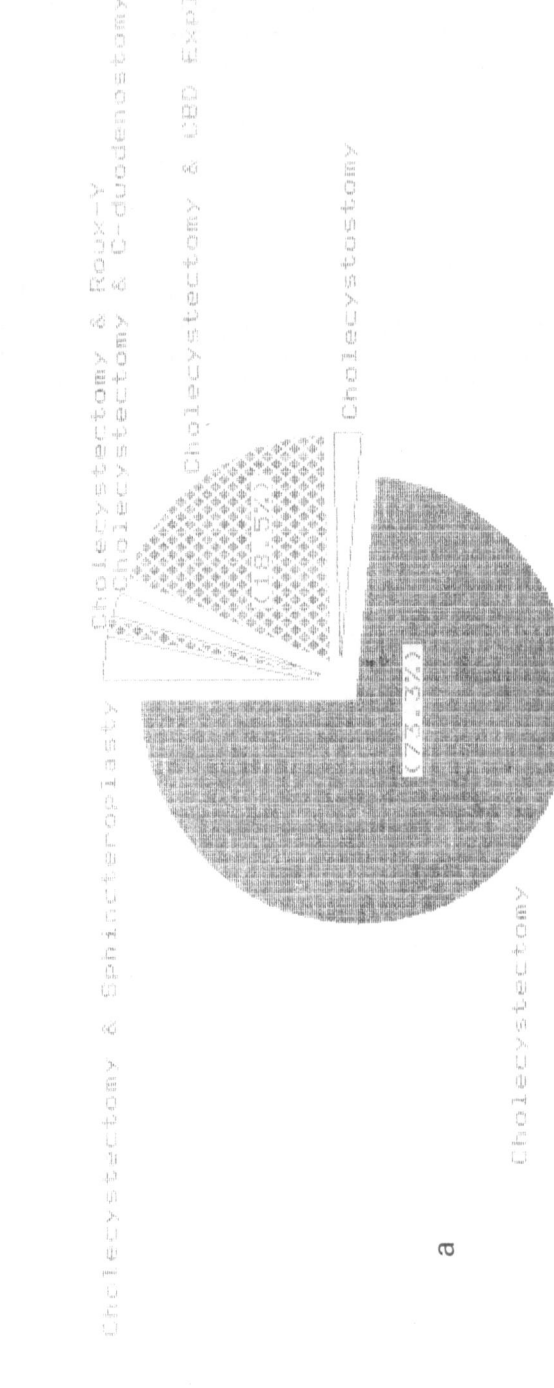

Figure 5.2 Relative incidence of surgical procedures in the prospective study carried out by the International Biliary Association involving 21 different centres: (a) primary operations, (b) secondary procedures

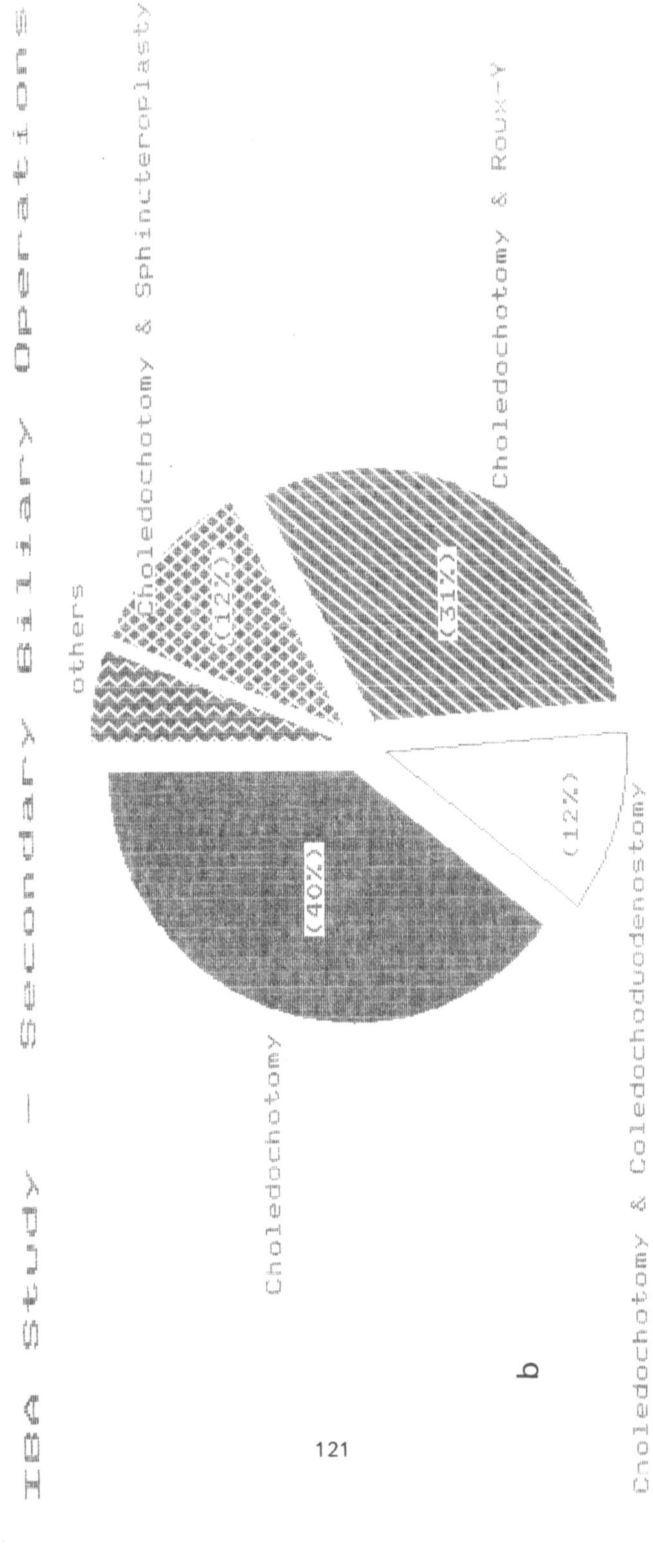

IBA Study — Secondary Biliary Operations

Choledochotomy & Sphincteroplasty

Choledochotomy & Roux-Y

others

(12%)

(31%)

(12%)

(40%)

Choledochotomy

Choledochotomy & Coledochoduodenostomy

b

Figure 5.2

that other options, such as endoscopic papillotomy, should be considered at least in some patients[58,59].

Uncomplicated gallstones

The treatment of symptomatic gallstones is by elective cholecystectomy. The decision to explore the common bile duct in these cases rests on the findings of a properly conducted transcystic operative cholangiogram. One of the strongest arguments for routine operative cholangiography is that this intra-operative investigation reduces the negative exploration rate. There is no indication for cholecystolithotomy which has been reported in some patients with functioning gallbladders. In one follow-up study on 53 patients treated in this way, the vast majority reformed stones[60]. This finding confirms the results of earlier studies which demonstrated an unacceptably high rate of recurrence of both symptoms and stones[61].

Opinion on the need for the insertion of a drainage tube leading to the gallbladder fossa remains divided. It would seem that the argument against drainage has been strengthened by the results of several prospective clinical trials[62–65] since these have either failed to show a difference between the drained and the undrained groups, or indicated that drainage increases the postoperative sepsis and morbidity. However, all of these studies have one severe limitation which precludes safe conclusions. This relates to the small number of patients entered in the trial (highest number being 300). The incidence of unexpected bile leakage after elective cholecystectomy without common bile duct exploration averages 0.5%. It is therefore obvious that with the number involved, it is impossible to detect a significant difference. It seems likely that for the vast majority of patients undergoing elective cholecystectomy, it matters little if drains are inserted or not. However, one in every 200 patients will develop a postoperative bile leak which may not be noticed if the surgeon omitted to insert a subhepatic drain.

Acute cholecystitis

The surgical management depends on whether the inflammatory condition is progressive and life-threatening, or the cholecystitis is mild or resolving.

The indications for emergency surgical intervention are outlined in Table 5.2. The objectives depend on the operative findings removal of the inflamed, perforated or gangrenous gallbladder, closure of any biliary–enteric fistula, peritoneal toilet and lavage with saline–antibiotic solution (tetracycline or cephalosporin). The presence of calculi in the extrahepatic biliary tract is excluded by operative cholangiography. In patients with a tense non-per-forated empyema, preliminary decompression of the gallbladder contents is performed by means of a Mayo–Ochsner suction trocar cannula inserted through a purse string at the fundus. The cholecystectomy is best performed in a retrograde fashion (fundus first) as this permits an easier identification of the cystic duct junction with the common bile duct and thereby reduces the risk of bile duct damage. In poor risk patients with haemodynamic instability or septicaemic shock, excision of the gangrenous patch of gallbladder wall with removal of the gallstones and cholecystostomy with an

Table 5.2 Absolute indications for emergency surgical intervention in patients with acute cholecystitis

Progression of the disease despite adequate conservative treatment. Failure to improve within 24 hours is an indication for surgical treatment, particularly in patients above 60 years of age.

Presence of an inflammatory mass in the right hypochondrium, particularly if enlarging and in the elderly.

Established generalized peritonitis.

Detection of gas in the gallbladder and biliary tract.

Development of intestinal obstruction.

F22–24 tube is performed together with peritoneal toilet and lavage. A cholecystostomy may be a safer option than cholecystectomy if the dissection of the gallbladder is considered too risky due to the presence of severe inflammatory oedema which obscures the normal anatomy, particularly if the surgeon lacks experience with this condition. In either event a chole- cystectomy is advisable at a later stage because of the risk of recurrence of stones and symptoms[66]. Moreover, the incidence of carcinoma of the gallbladder in patients who had previously undergone cholecystostomy was reported to be 6.7% in 105 patients[67]. This is substantially higher than the general incidence of gallbladder cancer. A third option which has been reported recently in the management of patients, in whom formal chole- cystectomy is considered hazardous, is subtotal cholecystectomy[68]. In this procedure, the posterior wall of the gallbladder is left *in situ*, attached to the liver bed, and the cystic duct is secured from within the gallbladder lumen by a purse string suture. However, experience with this operation is limited and the long-term results are not known.

Two options are available in the treatment of mild or resolving acute cholecystitis: interval (delayed) or early cholecystectomy. The interval approach entails conservative management of the acute episode with dis- charge after resolution of the attack, and subsequent readmission some 2–3 months later for elective cholecystectomy. Early cholecystectomy is being increasingly employed in the management of acute cholecystitis, and must be distinguished from emergency cholecystectomy. Following initial con- servative management, the diagnosis is confirmed by the appropriate imaging tests, and the patient is then operated on the next available theatre list (during the same hospital admission). The results of several prospective clinical trials comparing early versus interval cholecystectomy[69–74] have shown clear ben- efit from early cholecystectomy. Patients treated by early cholecystectomy spend, on average, 10 days less in hospital than those managed by the orthodox interval cholecystectomy approach, there being no difference in the overall mortality, morbidity and missed stone rate between the two groups. In addition, interval cholecystectomy incurs a number of disadvantages which include failure of medical treatment in 13%, premature readmission with a further attack whilst waiting for elective cholecystectomy (13%) and patient defaulting after discharge (10%). Despite these results, some surgeons remain sceptical of the safety in terms of bile duct injury when cholecystectomy is performed early during the course of acute cholecystitis. Another argument quoted against early cholecystectomy is the high misdiagnosis rate[75,76]. However, with the use of modern imaging tests, the reported misdiagnosis rate can be reduced to 3%[74]. It has averaged 4.5% in the Ninewells series.

Ductal calculi

The management of patients with ductal calculi remains problematic and controversial. Increasing experience with newer methods of treatment (e.g. interventional endoscopy) has challenged and in some instances replaced surgical intervention because of their proven efficacy, cost-effectiveness and low mortality. Nonetheless, the situation has been compounded by extravagant claims borne of poorly audited series reported without an adequate period of follow-up. It is indeed unfortunate that prospective controlled trials have featured little in this area of management of patients with biliary tract disease. The problem is best addressed by considering the management of patients in light of the clinical problem with which they present:

(1) Patients with symptomatic ductal calculi and a gallbladder.

(2) Patients with ductal calculi discovered during elective cholecystectomy.

(3) Missed ductal calculi discovered soon after cholecystectomy (residual).

(4) Ductal calculi diagnosed beyond 2 years of cholecystectomy (recurrent).

(5) Intrahepatic calculi.

The traditional management of patients with symptomatic ductal calculi (usually jaundice with or without cholangitis) is by surgical intervention under antibiotic cover. A cholecystectomy is performed and the common bile duct explored by the supraduodenal approach and the stones removed by means of biliary balloon catheters, stone-grasping forceps or Dormia basket preferably under visual guidance with the choledochoscope. A completion check by a choledochoscopic inspection and/or T-tube cholangiogram is an essential safeguard against residual stones. A size F16–18 T-tube is inserted in the bile duct and the choledochotomy incision closed. The long limb of the T-tube is exteriorized along a straight path through a separate stab wound in the right flank. In patients with multiple ductal calculi, grossly dilated duct (> 2 cm) and in the presence of papillary stenosis (choledocho duodenal junctional stenosis), a drainage operation is indicated: choledocho-duodenostomy or transduodenal sphincteroplasty. The latter carries a significant risk of pancreatitis and involves a sizeable duodenotomy. A transection choledochoduodenostomy (Figure 5.3) is preferable to the side-to-side anastomosis as it provides dependent drainage and avoids the complication of the inspissated sump syndrome[77].

An alternative approach consists of endoscopic removal of the stones by papillotomy[58,59,78] or balloon dilatation of the papilla[79,80]. Small stones usually pass spontaneously thereafter, but larger calculi require extraction with a Dormia basket or balloon catheters. The endoscopic removal of the ductal calculi is followed by an elective cholecystectomy whenever the condition of the patient permits. To date, this approach has been largely restricted to the elderly and poor risk patients. However, in view of the enhanced risk when

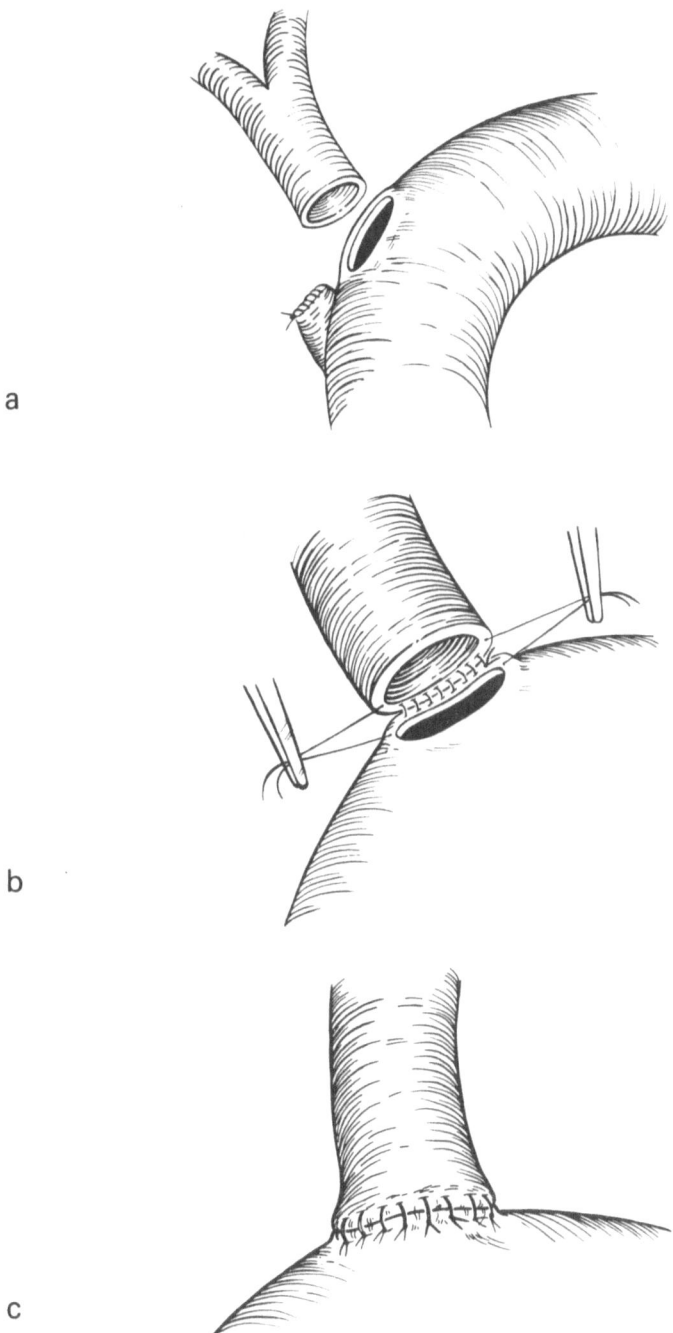

a

b

c

Figure 5.3 Transection choledochoduodenostomy. The bile duct is mobilized and transected as it enters the head of the pancreas (a). It is then re-implanted into the duodenum at the junction of the second with the third part of this organ (b) and (c). This procedure provides better drainage than the conventional side-to-side technique and avoids the complication of the inspissated sump syndrome

common bile duct exploration is added to elective cholecystectomy, pre-operative endoscopic removal of ductal calculi is likely to be employed more frequently and possibly routinely at least in those centres where this expertise is available.

Patients with asymptomatic ductal calculi discovered during elective chole-cystectomy should have the common duct stones removed. These account for 4–10% of cases and are discovered by routine operative cholangiography[81–83]. In 18% of cases, however, the common bile duct exploration proves negative. Most surgeons would still insert a T-tube before closure of the chole-dochotomy; a few do not. This remains a controversial issue. The main argument for the insertion of the T-tube in these cases is that it permits the performance of a postoperative cholangiogram. On the other hand, a small but definable morbidity and an increased hospital stay are attributable to the insertion of a T-tube. The authors' practice in patients with negative common bile duct exploration is to insert a fine catheter through the cystic duct remnant into the bile duct with closure of the latter (Figure 5.4).

Although the incidence of missed stones in the prospective IBA study was 4.5%, a higher incidence approximating to 10% is encountered in routine clinical practice since many centres do not employ operative cholangiography

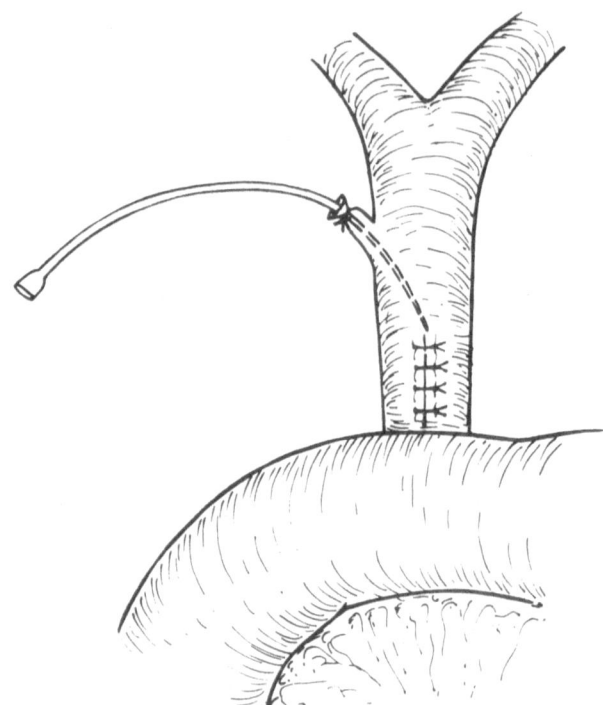

Figure 5.4 Alternative to the use of T-tube in cases with a negative CBD exploration. A fine polyethylene cannula is inserted into the CBD and anchored to the cystic duct by a ligature. The choledochotomy wound is then closed. (Reproduced by kind permission from Cuschieri, A. and Berci, G. (1984). *Common Bile Duct Exploration.* (Boston: Martinus Nijhoff)

routinely and few surgeons are regular users of choledochoscopy. The management of these patients is no longer surgical in the first instance. In the vast majority of cases, the diagnosis of a missed stone is made by the postoperative T-tube cholangiogram. Others become manifest on subsequent investigations some time after discharge because of recurrence of symptoms including the development of jaundice. The management depends on the presence or otherwise of an indwelling T-tube. For those patients in whom the condition is discovered after removal of the T-tube, endoscopic removal is the procedure of choice[84]. Three options are available for patients with an indwelling T-tube: flushing, dissolution and percutaneous stone extraction via the T-tube tract. All these procedures are performed under systemic antibiotic cover. Flushing with heparinized saline or lignocaine saline solution is simple and effective if the stones are small (< 0.7 mm). The flushing is performed by infusing the solution through the T-tube under manometric control such that the pressure in the system does not exceed $25-30 \, cmH_2O$. The efficacy of this simple method of treatment is enhanced when accompanied by pharmacologically induced relaxation of the sphincter of Oddi. In this respect, the results obtained with ceruletide administered as an intravenous infusion during the flushing period have been promising[85]. Cholate infusion dissolved retained cholesterol stones[86] but has been superseded by mono-octanoin which acts more rapidly and is effective in 70% of cases[89]. Percutaneous stone extraction via the T-tube tract was initially performed using a steerable radio-opaque catheter introduced under fluoroscopic control[88]. Once in position, a Dormia basket is advanced through the catheter to snare the ductal stones and withdraw them through the sinus tract. The main disadvantage of this technique is the rather heavy radiation exposure required to direct the manipulations. It has been largely replaced by the flexible choledochoscopic technique which is successful in 90–95% of cases[89–91]. A period of 4–5 weeks from the time of the operation is allowed to elapse to ensure maturation of the T-tube tract. During this time, the patient is allowed home with the tube spigoted but with regular weekly reviews, although some require continuous drainage because of jaundice or episodes of cholangitis. Surgical management of missed stones is reserved for those patients in whom the above methods have failed or complications have developed during or after attempted endoscopic or percutaneous stone extraction.

Recurrent ductal calculi are generally held to be primary stones if they present more than 2 years after cholecystectomy. They are usually associated with gross dilatation of the bile duct in the absence of distal stenosis[92]. However, biliary manometry, contrast selective cholangiography, and choledochoscopic inspection with biopsy of the terminal bile duct, often reveal papillary disease, usually choledochoduodenal junctional stenosis[93]. The preferred treatment is by choledochoduodenostomy, although some favour a sphincteroplasty[94]; or endoscopic papillotomy and stone extraction particularly if the patient is elderly or is considered an operative risk.

Multiple intrahepatic calculi require surgical intervention. Removal may be possible via a standard choledochotomy if the stones are loose and located in the major intrahepatic ducts. Their extraction is best conducted under visual control using the rigid choledochoscope with an attached instrument guide channel through which is inserted either a Dormia basket or a biliary balloon catheter. Thorough irrigation to remove debris is necessary after extraction of the stones. A T-tube is then inserted and a completion cholangiogram performed. An alternative but less favoured technique is the extended choledochotomy. Here the incision in the bile duct is carried up to the region of the bifurcation, and the calculi are cleared with scoops or biliary balloon catheters. Transhepatic lithotomy is necessary when stones are impacted above a strictured intrahepatic duct. The hepatic parenchyma of the affected liver segment is divided down to and including the involved duct. The stones are removed and following irrigation, the stricture is dilated. A silicone T-tube is then inserted into the affected intrahepatic duct and the hepatic parenchyma sutured around it. Hepatic resection is reserved for cases with multiple intrahepatic calculi associated with gross disease of one lobe.

Acute gallstone pancreatitis

The exact timing of biliary surgery for pancreatitis associated with gallstones remain controversial[95]. Currently three different approaches are practised without sufficient evidence for clear superiority of any one regimen. Conventional management entails an interval cholecystectomy during a second admission several weeks after resolution of the pancreatitis. Emergency surgery, defined as intervention within 3 days of the onset of the illness, is advocated to prevent progress of the pancreatic inflammation consequent on ductal obstruction by calculi[48-51]. Others favour an early cholecystectomy approach where the patient is initially treated conservatively during which time the presence of biliary tract disease is established by appropriate tests. The patient is then operated on the next available theatre list during the same admission. The Atlanta trial[49] of emergency versus interval surgical intervention showed no difference in the overall mortality but demonstrated a clear cost benefit in favour of the emergency group. The Dundee trial comparing early with interval cholecystectomy[25] is still in progress. The results to date have shown that approximately 50% of patients randomized to the early group have no evidence of pancreatic inflammation at operation despite an initial hyperamylasaemia exceeding 1200 IU on admission. No significant differences in the postoperative morbidity and mortality have been observed between the two groups. The overall duration of the hospital stay is significantly longer in the interval cholecystectomy group and a number of these patients have developed further attacks whilst waiting for their cholecystectomy. Our experience of the diagnostic accuracy of biliary tract investigations and the surgical pathology found at early elective operation suggests that patients receiving the diagnosis of gallstone pancreatitis on clinical and biochemical grounds comprise two distinct groups. Some have readily identifiable calculous biliary tract disease and a clinical course and operative findings similar to those characterizing biliary stone disease uncomplicated by pancreatitis. Others have gross pathological changes of pancreatitis with a more severe clinical course. This group has been relatively refractory to accurate biliary tract assessment during the acute episode.

Biliary fistulae and gallstone ileus

In the absence of iatrogenic injury to the bile ducts, the vast majority of biliary fistulae arise as a consequence of long-standing calculous disease. A small percentage are the result of intra-abdominal malignancy, usually carcinoma of the hepatic flexure. Most of the naturally occurring fistulae are internal and involve the gallbladder and adjacent hollow organs particularly the duodenum, less commonly the colon and rarely the stomach and small intestine. Isolated instances of external fistulation through the abdominal wall have been reported[96], as have cases involving the portal vein[97] and renal pelvis. The development of a bilioenteric fistula may be followed by serious life-threatening complications including cholangitis with septicaemia and gallstone ileus. The latter results from the impaction of a large stone, usually in the terminal ileum. It accounts for 2% of all cases of intestinal obstruction and is encountered usually in the elderly with females outnumbering males by a ratio of 8:1[98,99]. Plain X-rays of the abdomen may demonstrate gas in the biliary tree and outline the impacted calculus in the right iliac dossa in addition to the usual changes of low small bowel obstruction. The correct management of these patients consists in the surgical relief of the obstruction usually by extraction of the stone through a small enterotomy. Although some advocate fistula repair and cholecystectomy at the same time[99], this is generally considered unwise in these elderly and frail patients. Subsequent surgical treatment for the fistula is only indicated if the patient continues to experience symptoms or develops further complications referable to the biliary tract disease.

In 1948, Mirizzi described a complication of gallstone disease consisting of partial common hepatic duct obstruction from a stone impacted in the cystic duct or neck of the gallbladder with the stone ulcerating directly into the bile duct and the formation of a cholecystocholedochal fistula[100]. Recognition and awareness of this syndrome is important as it renders cholecystectomy extremely difficult and hazardous[101].

INTRA-OPERATIVE DECISION-MAKING IN BILIARY TRACT SURGERY

Although there is no substitute for clinical judgement and experience, reliance on operative findings alone as a basis for operative decisions during biliary tract surgery can result in missed pathology and avoidable mishaps. There are now a number of intra-operative investigative modalities which outline the exact pathological anatomy to the surgeon at the start of the procedure and also provide a means for a completion check as a safeguard against residual disease before closure of the abdomen. The two most important procedures in this respect are operative cholangiography and choledochoscopy (cholangioscopy). Familiarity with these techniques which results from their routine use is necessary for optimal results.

The benefits emanating from routine operative cholangiography during biliary tract surgery have been demonstrated by several reports[102-105], although some surgeons still consider the procedure unnecessary or not cost-effective[106,107]. Other surgeons advocate a selective use for operative cholangiography[108,109]. The initial operative cholangiogram will outline congenital anomalies of the biliary tract and thus reduce the risk of iatrogenic bile duct injury. It demonstrates or confirms the presence of intraductal pathology and therefore the need for exploration of the common bile duct. Although some maintain that established clinical criteria and certain operative findings reliably dictate the need for this procedure, the incidence of negative common bile duct exploration is high (20–40%) when carried out on the basis of these indications alone[110]. One of the main benefits of operative cholangiography is the documented reduction in the number of negative explorations[111]. Furthermore, routine operative cholangiography detects the presence of unsuspected ductal stones in 4–10% of cases[102,103,112].

Following common bile duct exploration, a completion T-tube cholangiogram provides a necessary check against residual ductal calculi and demonstrates free entry of contrast into the duodenum. There are, however, practical difficulties which may militate against a good and reliable completion cholangiogram, and artefacts such as air bubbles and small blood clots may be mistaken for stones. Oedema or spasm at the lower end of the bile duct may prevent the entry of dye into the duodenum. The administration of drugs which relax the sphincter can readily resolve the dilemma. In this respect we have found the intravenous ceruletide (1 μg) to be particularly useful.

The technique of contact selective cholangiography[113] provides great and magnified detail of the lower end of the bile duct and is especially useful for the demonstration of the anatomy of the Vaterian segment of the common bile duct. Used in conjunction with conventional (panoramic) cholangiography during secondary biliary intervention, it results in a diagnostic accuracy rate of 100%. Contact selective cholangiography allows the visualization of distal calculi too small to be identified by conventional cholangiography and is the radiological method of choice for the demonstration of papillary stenosis during surgical intervention[93]. It entails mobilization of the duodenum and head of the pancreas and the insertion of a sterile dental X-ray film.

Although first reported in 1941[114], operative choledochoscopy was not adopted until fairly recently. There are two types of choledochoscopes: the flexible and the rigid. The latter is equipped with the Hopkins rod-lens system and is used in preference to the flexible system because of its superior resolution and depth of field. The key to successful cholangioscopic examination of the biliary tract, particularly the lower end of the bile duct, is mobilization of the duodenum and head of the pancreas. This procedure allows the surgeon to put the second part of the duodenum on the stretch and thereby straightens the lower end of the bile duct[115]. Choledochoscopy should always be used when the common bile duct is explored. The initial inspection is performed when the duct is opened and before any manipulations or instruments are introduced. A careful inspection will then identify stones, tumours, strictures and cholangitis. Extraction of stones can be performed under visual guidance and any suspicious lesion can be biopsied. The rigid choledochoscope is invaluable for the extraction of intraheptic calculi and for the removal of stones impacted in the lower end of the common bile duct. A final inspection by the choledochoscope once the duct exploration is completed, is used instead of or in addition to completion T-tube cholangiography. The value of operative choledochoscopy in the detection of bile duct tumours and in the virtual abolition of missed stones is well documented[116-120].

Biliary manometry is not used by the majority of surgeons during surgery on the gallbladder and bile ducts. It can, however, provide useful information in difficult cases, particularly during secondary biliary intervention. It enhances the diagnostic yield of operative cholangiography[121]. Biliary manometry is extremely useful in the diagnosis of papillary stenosis[122-124] and can differentiate organic obstruction from spasm of the sphincter of Oddi by documenting the pressure response to spasmolytic agents. Estimation of the flow rate through the sphincter at a standard pressure head, usually of 25–30 cmH$_2$O, has been used to diagnose the presence of ductal calculi as an alternative to operative cholangiography[125], but it is less reliable due to a high false negative rate.

References

1. Lieber, M. M. (1952). The incidence of gallstones and their correlation with other diseases. *Ann. Surg.*, **153**, 37–42
2. Cleland, J. B. (1953). Gallstones in seven thousand post-mortem examinations. *Med. J. Aust.*, **2**, 488–90
3. Torvik, A. and Hoivik, B. (1960). Gallstones in an autopsy series. Incidence, complications and correlations with carcinoma of the gallbladder. *Acta Chir. Scand.*, **120**, 168–74
4. Barker, D. J. P., Gardner, M. J., Power, C. and Hutt, M. S. R. (1979). Prevalence of gallstones at necropsy in nine British towns. A collaborative study. *Br. Med. J.*, **2**, 1389–92
5. Opit, L. T. and Grenhill, S. (1974). Prevalence of gallstones in relation to differing treatment rates for biliary disease. *Br. J. Prevent. Soc.*, **28**, 269–72
6. Godfrey, P. J., Bates, T., Harrison, H., King, M. B. and Padley, N. R. (1984). Gallstones and mortality: a study of all gallstone related deaths in a single health district. *Gut*, **25**, 1029–33
7. Bunker, J. P. (1970). Surgical manpower: a comparison of operations and surgeons in the United States and in England and Wales. *N. Engl. J. Med.*, **222**, 135–9
8. Vayda, E. (1970). A comparison of surgical rates in Canada and in England and Wales. *N. Engl. J. Med.*, **289**, 1224–34
9. Bateson, M. C. (1984). Gallbladder disease and cholecystectomy rate are independently variable. *Lancet*, **5**, 621–4
10. Rosenberg, L., Shapiro, S., Sloane, D., Kaufman, D. W., Miethinen, O. S. and Stolley, P. D. (1980). Thiazides and acute cholecystitis. *N. Engl. J. Med.*, **303**, 546–8
11. Van der Linden, W., Ritter, B. and Edlund, G. (1984). Acute cholecystitis and thiazides. *Br. Med. J.*, **2**, 654–5
12. Moynihan, B. G. A. (1908). An address on inaugural symptoms. *Br. Med. J.*, **2**, 1579–1601
13. Mayo, W. J. (1911). Innocent gallstones, a myth. *J. Am. Med. Assoc.*, **56**, 1021–4
14. Gracie, W. A. and Ransohoff, D. F. (1983). The silent gallstone; requiescat in peace. In Delaney, J. P. and Varco, R. L. (eds.) *Controversies in Surgery* II. Vol. 2, pp. 361–71. (Philadelphia: W. B. Saunders)
15. Ransohoff, D. F., Gracie, W. A., Wolfsen, L. B. and Neuhauser, D. (1983). Prophylactic cholecystectomy or expectant management for silent stones. *Ann. Intern. Med.*, **99**, 199–204
16. Diehl, A. K. and Beral, V. (1981). Cholecystectomy and changing mortality from gallbladder cancer. *Lancet*, **2**, 187
17. Schottenfeld, D. and Winawer, S. J. (1983). Cholecystectomy and colorectal cancer (Editorial). *Gastroenterology*, **85**, 966–7
18. Wenkert, A. and Robertson, B. (1966). The natural course of gallstone disease. Eleven-year review of 781 non-operated cases. *Gastroenterology*, **50**, 376–81

19. Bhansali, S. K. (1985). Preoperative complications of gallstones and their relevance to treatment and prognosis: experience with 451 cases. *Am. J. Gastroenterol.*, **80**, 648–54

20. Kune, G. A. and Birks, D. (1970). Acute cholecystitis. An appraisal or current methods of treatment. *Med. J. Aust.*, **2**, 218–21

21. Thornell, E., Jivegard, L., Bukhave, K., Rask-Madsen, J. and Svanvik, J. (1986). Prostaglandin E_2 formation by the gallbladder in experimental cholecystitis. *Gut*, **27**, 370–3

22. Lou, M. A., Mandel, A. K. and Alexander, H. L. (1978). Bacteriology of the human biliary tract and the duodenum. *Arch. Surg.*, **112**, 965–7

23. Pitluk, H. C. and Beal, J. M. (1979). Choledocholithiasis associated with cholecystitis. *Arch. Surg.*, **114**, 887–8

24. Stryker, S. J. and Beal, J. M. (1983). Acute cholecystitis and common duct calculi. *Arch. Surg.*, **118**, 1063–4

25. Mackie, C. R., Wood, R. A. B., Preece, P. W. and Cuschieri, A. (1985). Surgical pathology at early operation for suspected acute gallstone pancreatitis: preliminary results of a prospective clinical trial. *Br. J. Surg.*, **72**, 179–81

26. Ulreich, S., Foster, K. W., Stier, S. A. and Rosenfield, A. T. (1980). Acute cholecystitis: comparison of ultrasound and intravenous cholangiography. *Arch. Surg.*, **115**, 158–60

27. Zeman, R. K., Burrell, M. I., Cahow, C. E. and Caride, V. (1981). Diagnostic utility of cholescintigraphy and ultrasonography in acute cholecystitis. *Am. J. Surg.*, **141**, 446–51

28. Krishnamurthy, G. T. (1982). Acute cholecystitis: the diagnostic role for current imaging tests. *World J. Med.*, **137**, 87–94

29. Hall, A. W., Wisbey, M. L., Hutchinson, F., Wood, R. A. B. and Cuschieri, A. (1981). The place of hepatobiliary isotope scanning in the diagnosis of gallbladder disease. *Br. J. Surg.*, **68**, 85–90

30. Freitas, J. E. and Gulati, R. M. (1980). Rapid evaluation of acute abdominal pain by hepatobiliary scanning. *J. Am. Med. Assoc.*, **224**, 1585–7

31. O'Callaghan, J. D., Verow. P. W., Hopton, D. and Craven, J. L. (1980). The diagnosis of acute gallbladder disease by technetium-99m-labelled HIDA hepatobiliary scanning. *Br. J. Surg.*, **67**, 805–8

32. Ralls, P. W., Coletti, P. M., Halls, J. M. and Siemsen, J. K. (1982). Prospective evaluation of ^{99m}Tc-IDA cholescintigraphy and grey-scale ultrasound in the diagnosis of acute cholecystitis. *Radiology*, **144**, 369–71

33. Glazer, G., Murphy, F., Clayden, G. S. and Lawrence, R. G. (1981). Radionuclide biliary scanning in acute pancreatitis. *Br. J. Surg.*, **68**, 766–70

34. Roslyn, J. J., Pitt, H. A., Mann, L., Fonkalsrud, E. W. and DenBesten, L. (1984). Parenteral nutrition in induced gallbladder disease: a reason for early cholecystectomy, *Am. J. Surg.*, **148**, 58–63

35. Ternberg, J. L. and Kaeting, J. P. (1978). Acute acalculous cholecystitis; complications of other illnesses in childhood. *Arch. Surg.*, **110**, 543–7

36. Long, T. N., Heimbach, D. M. and Carrico, C. J. (1978). Acalculous cholecystitis in critically ill patients. *Am. J. Surg.*, **136**, 30–36

37. Petersen, S. R. and Sheldon, G. F. (1979). Acute acalculous cholecystitis. A complication of hyperalimentation. *Am. J. Surg.*, **138**, 814–17

38. Glenn, F. and Becker, C. G. (1982). Acute acalculous cholecystitis, an increasing entity. *Ann. Surg.*, **195**, 131–6

39. May, R. E. and Strong, R. (1971). Acute emphysematous cholecystitis. *Br. J. Surg.*, **58**, 453

40. Mentzer, R. M. Jr., Golden, G. T. and Chandler, J. G. (1975). A comparative appraisal of emphysematous cholecystitis. *Am. J. Surg.*, **129**, 10–15

41. Thorton, J., Heaton, K. W., Espiner, H. J. and Eltringham, W. K. (1983). Empyema of the gallbladder: reappraisal of a neglected disease. *Gut*, **24**, 1183–5

42. Maki, T., Sato, T. and Saitoh, T. (1962). A study on the activity of beta-glucuronidase in bile in connection with precipitation of calcium bilirubinate. *Tohoku J. Exp. Med.*, **77**, 179–86

43. Nagase, M., Hilasa, Y., Soloway, R. D., Tanimura, H., Setoyama, M. and Kato, H. (1980). Gallstones in Western Japan: factors affecting the prevalence of intrahepatic gallstones. *Gastroenterology*, **78**, 684–90

44. Sato, T., Suzuki, N., Takahashi, W. and Uematsu, I. (1980). Surgical management of intrahepatic gallstones. *Ann. Surg.*, **192**, 28–32
45. Madden, J. L. (1978). Primary common bile duct stones. *World J. Surg.*, **2**, 465–9
46. Maki, T. (1966). Pathogenesis of calcium bilirubinate gallstones. *Ann. Surg.*, **90**, 90–100
47. Rubin, J. R. and Beal, J. M. (1983). Diagnosis of choledocholithiasis. *Surg. Gynecol. Obstet.*, **156**, 16
48. Acosta, J. M. and Ledesma, C. L. (1974). Gallstone migration as a cause of acute pancreatitis. *N. Engl. J. Med.*, **290**, 484–7
49. Stone, H. H., Fabian, T. C. and Dunlop, W. E. (1981). Gallstone pancreatitis. Biliary tract pathology in relation to time of operation. *Ann. Surg.*, **194**, 305–12
50. Kelly, T. R. (1980). Gallstone pancreatitis: the timing of surgery. *Surgery*, **88**, 345–50
51. Acosta, J. M., Rossi, R., Galli, O. M. R., Pellegrini, C. A. and Skinner, D. B. (1978). Early surgery for acute gallstone pancreatitis: evaluation of a systematic approach. *Surgery*, **83**, 367–70
52. Opie, E. L. (1901). The etiology of acute haemorrhagic pancreatitis. *Bull. Johns Hopkins Hosp.*, **12**, 182–8
53. Osborne, D. H., Imrie, C. W. and Carter, D. C. (1981). Biliary surgery in the same admission for gallstone-associated acute pancreatitis. *Br. J. Surg.*, **68**, 758–61
54. Kia, U. and Sheth, M. (1980). Optimal timing of surgical intervention in patients with acute pancreatitis associated with cholecystitis. *Surg. Gynecol. Obstet.*, **150**, 499–501
55. Semel, L., Schrieber, D. and Fromm, D. (1983). Gallstone pancreatitis. Support for a flexible approach. *Arch. Surg.*, **118**, 961
56. Cuschieri, A., Cumming, J. G. R., Wood, R. A. B. and Baker, P. R. (1984). Evidence for sphincter dysfunction in patients with gallstone associated pancreatitis: effect of ceruletide in patients undergoing cholecystectomy for gallbladder disease and gallstone associated pancreatitis. *Br. Surg.*, **71**, 858–88
57. DenBesten, L. and Berci, G. (1986). The current status of biliary tract surgery: an international study of 1072 consecutive patients. *World J. Surg.*, **10**, 116–22
58. Mazzeo, F. J. and Jordan, F. T. (1983). Endoscopic papillotomy for recurrent common duct stones and papillary stenosis. *Arch. Surg.*, **118**, 693
59. Stout, D. J., Sorak, M. V. and Sallivan, B. H. (1980). Endoscopic sphincterotomy and removal of gallstones. *Surg. Gynecol. Obstet.*, **150**, 673–7
60. Norrby, S. and Schonebeck, J. (1970). Long term results with cholecystolithotomy. *Acta Chir. Scand.*, **136**, 711–13
61. Lang, R. C. and Webster, D. R. (1957). Cholecystolithotomy in functioning gallbladders. *Surgery*, **42**, 837–40
62. Gordon, A. B., Bates, T. and Fiddian, V. (1976). A controlled trial of drainage after cholecystectomy. *Br. J. Surg.*, **63**, 278–82
63. Edlund, G., Gedda, S. and Van der Linden, W. (1979). Intraperitoneal drains and nasogastric tubes in elective cholecystectomy. A controlled clinical trial. *Am. J. Surg.*, **137**, 775–9
64. Man, B., Kraus, L. and Motovic, A. (1977). Cholecystectomy without drainage, nasogastric suction and intravenous fluids. *Am. J. Surg.*, **133**, 312–14
65. Budd, D. C., Cochran, R. C. and Fouty, W. (1982). Cholecystectomy with and without drainage. A randomized prospective study in 300 patients. *Am. J. Surg.*, **143**, 307–9
66. Welch, J. P. and Malt, R. A. (1972). Outcome of cholecystostomy. *Surg. Gynecol. Obstet.*, **135**, 717–20
67. Castle, W. N., Wanebo, H. J. and Fechner, R. E. (1982). Carcinoma of the gallbladder and cholecystostomy. *Arch. Surg.*, **117**, 946–8
68. Bornman, P. C. and Terblanche, J. (1985). Subtotal cholecystectomy for the difficult gallbladder in hypertension and cholecystitis. *Surgery*, **98**, 1–6
69. Van der Linden, W. and Sunzel, H. (1970). Early versus delayed operations for acute cholecystitis. *Am. J. Surg.*, **120**, 7–13
70. McArthur, P., Cuschieri, A., Sells, R. A. and Shields, R. (1975). Controlled clinical trial comparing early with interval cholecystectomy for acute cholecystitis. *Br. J. Surg.*, **62**, 850–2
71. Lathinen, J., Alhava, E. M. and Aukes, S. (1978). Acute cholecystitis treated by early and delayed surgery. *Scand. J. Gastroenterol.*, **13**, 673–8

72. Jarviven, J. H. and Hastbacka, J. (1980). Early cholecystectomy for acute cholecystitis. A prospective randomised study. *Ann. Surg.*, **191**, 502–5
73. Van der Linden, W. and Edlund, B. (1981). Early versus delayed cholacystectomy. The effect of a change in management. *Br. J. Surg.*, **68**, 753–7
74. Norrby, S., Herlin, P., Holmin, T., Sjodahl, R. and Tagesson, C. (1983). Early or delayed cholecystectomy for acute cholecystitis? A clinical trial. *Br. J. Surg.*, **70**, 163–5
75. Essenhigh, D. M. (1966). Management of acute cholecystitis. *Br. J. Surg.*, **53**, 1032–8
76. Halaz, S. N. A. (1975). Counterfeit cholecystitis. *Am. J. Surg.*, **130**, 189–92
77. Cuschieri, A., Wood, R. A. B., Metcalf, M. J. and Cumming, J. G. R. (1983). Long term experience with transection choledochoduodenostomy. *World J. Surg.*, **7**, 502–4
78. Cotton, P. B. (1984). Endoscopic management of bile duct stones (apples and oranges). *Gut*, **25**, 587–97
79. Staritz, M., Ewe, K. and Meyer Zum Buschenfelde, K. H. (1982). Endoscopic papillary dilatation, a possible alternative to endoscopic papillotomy. *Lancet*, **1**, 1306–7
80. Stave, R. and Osmes, M. (1985). Endoscopic gallstone extraction following hydrostatic balloon dilatation of stricture in the common bile duct. *Endoscopy*, **17**, 159–60
81. Farha, G. J. and Pearson, R. N. (1975). Transcystic duct operative cholangiography. *Am. J. Surg.*, **131**, 228–31
82. Chatterjee, D. K. and Jones, Wm. (1978). Value of operative cholangiography. *Br. J. Surg.*, **32**, 105–6
83. Berci, G. and Hamlin, J. A. (1982). Unsuspected stones. In Berci, G. and Hamlin, J. A. (eds.) *Operative Biliary Radiology.* pp. 137–79. (Baltimore: William and Wilkins)
84. Safrany, L. (1978). Endoscopic treatment of biliary tract disease. An international study. *Lancet*, **2**, 983–5
85. Cuschieri, A. (1984). Management of retained biliary calculi: relation of sphincter induced by ceruletide. *Br. Med. J.*, **289**, 1582
86. Way, L., Admirand, W. H. and Dunphy, J. E. (1972). Management of choledocholithiasis. *Ann. Surg.*, **176**, 347–59
87. Jarrett, L. N., Balfour, T. W., Bell, G. D., Knapp, D. R. and Rose, D. H. (1981). Intraductal infusion of mono-octanoin. Experience in 24 patients with retained common duct stones. *Lancet*, **1**, 68–70
88. Burhenne, J. J. (1973). Nonoperative retained biliary tract stone extraction. *Am. J. Roentgenol.*, **117**, 388–99
89. Yamakawa, T. (1976). An improved choledocho-fiberscope and non-surgical removal of retained biliary calculi under direct visual control. *Gastrointest. Endosc.*, **22**, 160–5
90. Moss, J. P., Whelan, J. G., Powell, H. W., Dedman, T. and Oliver, W. J. (1976). Post-operative choledochoscopy via the T-tube tract. *J. Am. Med. Assoc.*, **236**, 2781–2
91. Berci, G. and Hamlin, J. A. (1981). A combined fluoroscopic and endoscopic approach for retrieval of retained stones through the T-tube tract. *Surg. Gynecol. Obstet.*, **153**, 237–40
92. Braasch, J. W., Fender, H. R. and Bonneval, M. M. (1983). Refractory primary common bile duct stone disease. *Am J. Surg.*, **139**, 526–30
93. Cuschieri, A., Shaw, J. W. and El-Muhtaseb, H. H. (1985). Evaluation of contact selective cholangiography during secondary biliary intervention. *R. Coll. Surg. Edinburgh*, **30**, 353–7
94. Jones, S. A. (1978). The prevention and treatment of recurrent bile duct stones by trans-duodenal sphincteroplasty. *World J. Surg.*, **2**, 473–85
95. Walt, A. (1983). Editorial comment. *Arch. Surg.*, **118**, 904
96. Knochal, J. P., Cooper, E. B. and Barry, K. G. (1962). External biliart fistula: a study of electrolyte derangements and secondary cardiovascular and renal abnormalities. *Surgery*, **51**, 746–54
97. Stitt, R. B., Heslin, D. J. and Currie, D. J. (1976). Gallstone ileus. *Br. J. Surg.*, **54**, 673–8
98. Svartolm, E., Andren-Sandberg, A., Evander, A., Jarhult, J. and Thulin, A. (1982). Diagnosis and treatment of gallstone ileus. *Acta Chir. Scand.*, **148**, 435–8
99. Day, E. A. and Marks, C. (1975). Gallstone ileus. Review of the literature and presentation of thirty-four new cases. *Am. J. Surg.*, **129**, 552
100. Mirizzi, P. L. (1948). Sindrome del conducto hepatico. *J. Int. Chir.*, **V**, 731–77

101. McSherry, C. K., Ferstenberg, G. and Virshup, M. (1982). The Mirizzi syndrome: suggested classification and surgical therapy. *Surg. Gastroenterol.*, 1, 219

102. Farha, G. J. and Pearson R. N. (1975). Transcystic duct operative cholangiography. *Am. J. Surg.*, 131, 228–31

103. Chatterjee, D. K. and Jones, W. M. (1978). Value of operative cholangiography. *Br. J. Surg.*, 32, 105–6

104. Borge, J. (1977). Operative cholangiography. *Arch. Surg.*, 112, 340–42

105. Chant, A. D. B., Dewbury, K. G., Guyer, P. B. and Goh, H. (1982). Operative cholangiography reassessed. *Clin. Radiol.*, 33, 289–91

106. Skillings, J. C., Williams, J. S. and Hinshaw, J. R. (1979). Cost-effectiveness of operative cholangiography. *Am. J. Surg.*, 137, 26–31

107. Nottle, P. D., Hughes, E. S. R., McDermott, F. T. (1982). Cholecystectomy without routine operative cholangiography. *Aust. N. Zealand J. Surg.*, 52, 484–7

108. Deitch, E. A. and Voci, V. E. (1982). Operative cholangiography: the case for selective instead of routine operative cholangiography. *Am. Surg.*, 48, 297–301

109. Del Santo, P., Kazarian, K. K., Rogers, J. F., Bevins, P. A. and Hall, J. R. (1985). Prediction of operative cholangiography in patients with routine liver function chemistries. *Surgery*, 98, 7–11

110. Bartlett, M. K. and Wadell, W. R. (1958). Indications for common duct exploration. *N. Engl. J. Med.*, 258, 164–8

111. Doyle, P. J., Ward-McQuaid, J. N. and McEwan-Smith, A. (1982). The value of routine peroperative cholangiography – a report of 4000 cholecystectomies. *Br. J. Surg.*, 69, 617–9

112. Hamlin, J. A. and Berci, G. (1982). The fluoro-cholangiogram. In Berci, G. and Hamlin, J. A. (eds.) *Operative Biliary Radiology*. pp. 63–109. (Baltimore: Williams and Wilkins)

113. Slatterly, L. R. and Saypol, G. M. (1952). Intra-abdominal choledochography. Preliminary report of a method of detecting stones in the common bile duct. *Am. J. Surg.*, 94, 229–32

114. McIver, M. A. (1941). An instrument for visualizing the interior of the common duct at operation. *Surgery*, 9, 112–14

115. Cuschieri, A. and Berci, G. (1984). Operative biliary endoscopy. In Cuschieri, A. and Berci, G. (eds.) *Common Bile Duct Exploration*. pp. 55–9. (Boston: Martinus Nijhoff)

116. Tompkins, R. K. and Pitt, H. A. (1982). Surgical management of benign lesions of the bile ducts. *Curr. Problems Surg.*, 19, 321–98

117. Shore, J. M., Morgenstern, L. and Berci, G. (1971). An improved rigid choledochoscope. *Am. J. Surg.*, 122, 567–8

118. Nora, P. F., Berci, G. Rorazio, R. A., Kirhenbaum, G., Shore, J. M., Tompkins, P. K. and Wilson, S. D. (1977). Operative choledochoscopy. *Am. J. Surg.*, 133, 105–10

119. Finnis, D. and Rowntree, T. (1977). Choledochoscopy in exploration of the common bile duct. *Br. J. Surg.*, 64, 661–4

120. Kappas, A., Alexandre-Williams, J., Keighley, M. R. B. and Watts, G. T. (1979). Operative choledochoscopy. *Br, J. Surg.*, 66, 177–9

121. White, T. T. and Bordley, J. N. (1978). One per cent incidence of recurrent gallstones six to eight years after manometric cholangiography. *Ann. Surg.*, 188, 562–9

122. Boeckl, O. (1976). Rationale for primary operations on the papilla of Vater. *Eur. Surg. Res.*, 8, 400–10

123. Mallet-Guy, P. and Rose, D. F. (1956). Peroperative manometry and radiology in biliary tract disorders. *Br. J. Surg.*, 44, 55–8

124. Yvergneaux, J. P., Bauwens, E., Van Outryve, L. and Yvergneaux, E. (1977). Benign stenosis of the papilla of Vater. *Acta Chir. Belgica*, 76, 523–32

125. Besançon, F., Pironneaur, A., Lopez-Macedo, L., Longuet, Y. L. and Debray, C. H. (1965). Technique nouvelle et simple d'exploration opératoire du cholédoque: le débimètre à flotteur perfusé sous pression constante et élevée. *Arch. Mal. App. Dig.*, 54, 59–70

6
Complications of Surgery and Their Treatment

R. S. STUBBS and L. H. BLUMGART

Since the time of the first successful cholecystectomy in 1882 surgery for gallstone disease has become commonplace and today cholecystectomy is probably the most frequently performed elective abdominal operation in most Western countries. The operation, however, is a major one, particularly when it is accompanied by exploration of the common bile duct (CBD), and is attended by not insignificant morbidity and mortality.

The operative mortality and morbidity attendant on any abdominal operation are primarily related to the patient's ability to withstand the trauma and stress of the operation. These will be discussed only briefly in this chapter. It is the complications specifically related to biliary surgery and in particular those related to technical problems which may arise during the operation which will be addressed in some detail.

OPERATIVE MORTALITY

The operative mortality of surgery for gallstone disease is dependent on a number of factors. The most important are the age of the patient, whether the operation is performed electively or as a matter of urgency and whether the common bile duct is explored.

Elective cholecystectomy carries an overall mortality of less than 0.3%[1-3] and even in elderly patients may be achieved with a mortality of the order of 1%[1,4]. Deaths are most commonly associated with pre-existing cardiovascular disease, which may or may not have been apparent on routine preoperative testing. Where surgery is performed as a matter of urgency, usually for acute cholecystitis, the risks are approximately doubled[1] although in elderly patients they may be considerably greater[4]. Here the deaths are usually related to septic complications superimposed on pre-existing cardiovascular disease. Where stones are present in the bile ducts and elective cholecystectomy is accompanied by exploration of the common bile duct (CBD) the mortality is of the order of 2–3%[1-3]. Once again the risks are largely related to age and pre-existing cardiovascular disease. Mortality is, however, also dependent on the mode of exploration of the CBD. Supraduodenal exploration carries a mortality of approximately 2–3%[1-3] whereas transduodenal exploration with sphincterotomy or sphincteroplasty carries a somewhat higher mortality of 6–8% because of the additional risk of duodenal fistula and postoperative pancreatitis[3,5-7]. A combined approach of both supraduodenal and transduodenal exploration may be particularly hazardous, especially in the elderly[3,7]. For this reason it would seem preferable to remove a calculus *impacted* at the lower end of the CBD by initial transduodenal exploration, rather than by resorting to this method only after prolonged attempts at its removal via the supraduodenal route.

MORBIDITY RELATED TO ABDOMINAL SURGERY

Chest infection is perhaps the most frequent single complication occurring after abdominal surgery and is related to pre-existing lung disease, a history of smoking and poor postoperative respiratory excursion. Although common, it is unusual for it to be a severe problem and it can usually be adequately treated with physiotherapy alone although in some instances antibiotics will be required.

Wound infection after biliary surgery is relatively common and relates largely to the presence of bacteria in the bile. Although bile should ordinarily be sterile it contains organisms in up to 30% of patients with gallbladder stones and in as many as 70% of patients with common duct stones[8]. Unless prophylactic antibiotics are administered preoperatively wound infection occurs in some 15–20% of patients after simple cholecystectomy and in as many as 30% of patients following exploration of the common bile duct[9,10]. In both these instances wound infection rates can be reduced to the order of 3–5% by as little as a single dose of an appropriate prophylactic antibiotic[9,10]. Where wound infection does occur it is usually adequately treated by drainage alone. On occasions, however, deep-seated and spreading infections will require the use of antibiotics and even further surgery.

Subphrenic abscess and septicaemia are two other infective complications which may occasionally follow cholecystectomy or exploration of the common bile duct. Their incidence might also be expected to be reduced with the use of prophylactic antibiotics.

Thromboembolic complications with deep venous thrombosis and pulmonary embolus can of course occur after any major surgical procedure. Attempts to reduce the incidence of these serious complications can be made with the use of compression stockings[11,12], intermittent compression devices[13,14] or subcutaneous heparin[15,16]. The cardiovascular complications of myocardial infarction and cerebrovascular accident are also seen occasionally following abdominal surgery, particularly in patients with a previous history of cardiovascular disease.

MORBIDITY RELATED SPECIFICALLY TO BILIARY SURGERY

A number of important complications may occur which relate specifically to cholecystectomy. These include bile duct injury, arterial injury with subsequent haemobilia, acute pancreatitis and a miscellaneous group of complications which lead to what can best be called post cholecystectomy problems. Each of these will now be considered in turn.

Bile duct injuries

The most serious surgical complication to follow cholecystectomy is injury to the biliary tree. Figures available from surveys conducted in Sweden, Finland, Germany and France suggest that the incidence is approximately 1 per 500 cholecystectomies[17-20]. Kune and Sali suggest that the incidence is a little higher at approximately 1 per 300–500 gallstone operations[21]. The seriousness of this complication relates in part to problems of biliary fistula and uncontrolled sepsis, and in part to the technical difficulties of successfully repairing bile duct injuries. Failure to restore unobstructed biliary drainage leads to inevitable sequelae of hepatic fibrosis, cirrhosis, portal hypertension and eventual liver failure. For these reasons it is advisable that early repair be carried out by a surgeon experienced in the management of these injuries.

Causative factors

The precise reason for bile duct injury in any particular instance is not usually identifiable. However, a number of contributing factors may be implicated.

Anatomical variations – Anatomical variations in the extrahepatic biliary tree and the adjacent hepatic arteries are numerous and occur frequently. Indeed, less than 50% of individuals display a commonly described pattern of biliary and vascular anatomy[22]. The common variations in the anatomy of the biliary tree are shown in Figure 6.1. Detailed accounts of these anomalies are well documented elsewhere[22,23]. Knowledge of them is essential for all surgeons performing cholecystectomy if bile duct injuries are to be minimized.

Pathological features – The extensive oedema in the region of the porta hepatis and Calot's triangle which may accompany acute cholecystitis and the considerable fibrosis which sometimes occurs in this area following repeated episodes of cholecystitis can make dissection in Calot's triangle exceedingly difficult and hazardous. In such cases the gallbladder is best dissected in an antegrade or fundus first manner with slow and cautious dissection close to its wall. Excessive traction on the gallbladder should be avoided in order to prevent avulsion from the artery or duct, and to prevent tenting of the common bile duct/common hepatic duct junction which might lead to excision or ligation across a segment of the duct. Using this method of antegrade cholecystectomy most cases can be safely dissected. Should difficulty be encountered as the neck of the gallbladder is approached, attempts at cholecystectomy should probably be abandoned in favour of partial cholecystectomy through Hartmann's pouch.

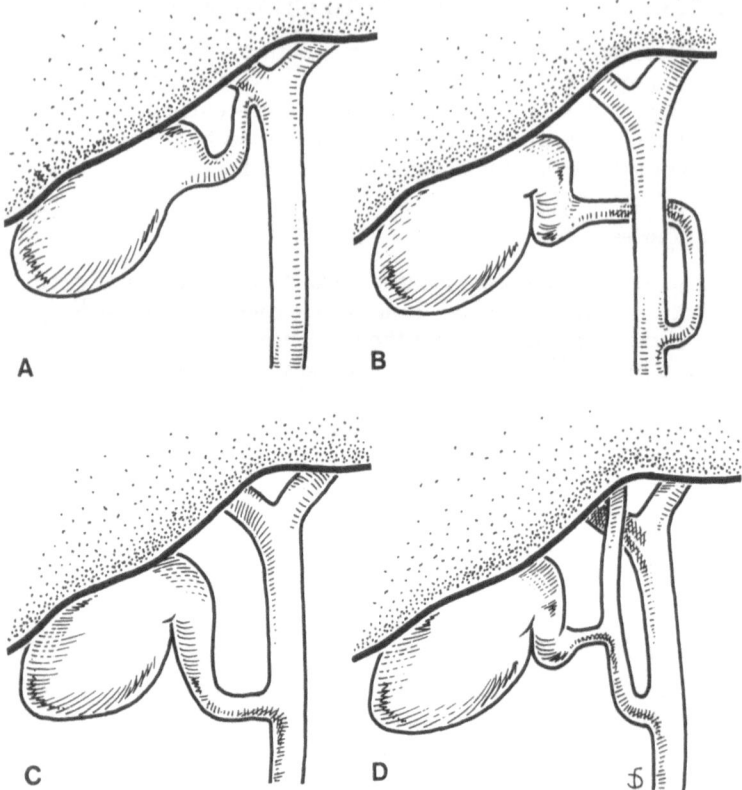

Figure 6.1 The cystic duct joins the common hepatic duct at an angle and on its right side in approximately 65% of cases. In the remainder it can enter the main right hepatic duct (A) or take a variable course around the common hepatic duct before joining it (B,C). The cystic duct may join a right hepatic sectoral duct which may itself join the common bile duct at a variable level and site (D)

Technical factors – While the experience of the surgeon is undoubtedly an important factor in determining the likelihood of injury to the bile duct during cholecystectomy, it is by no means only the inexperienced or inadequately trained surgeon who is likely to inflict such an injury. Indeed Bengmark has reported that surgeons of intermediate experience are most likely to inflict injury on the bile duct[24]. Furthermore, although cholecystectomy varies considerably in the ease with which it is performed, it is certainly not the case that the bile duct is more often injured in the course of a difficult cholecystectomy. Indeed frequently the damage occurs during a so-called straightforward cholecystectomy[25,26].

A number of technical points are noteworthy. Good assistance is important and incisions must be appropriately sited and be of adequate length to permit good visualization. Early demonstration of the cystic artery and cystic duct is desirable and the cystic artery should be ligated close to the gallbladder wall so as to avoid hepatic arterial injury. At greatest risk of damage are the right hepatic artery, and an accessory right hepatic artery which arises from the superior mesenteric artery in some 16% of patients[27]. When present this accessory artery commonly lies on the right in the groove between the portal vein and the common bile duct and is liable to damage during dissection and ligation of the cystic duct. Should bleeding occur during operation its control must be precise rather than by blind application of artery forceps, haemostatic clips or sutures. Haemorrhage should be controlled initially either by direct pressure by means of a pack or by pressure with the finger and thumb on the hepatic artery at the free edge of the lesser omentum. Following this the offending vessel can usually be identified, dissected and precisely controlled.

Some authors argue that the junction of the cystic duct with the common hepatic duct should be clearly demonstrated and ligated even to the extent of separating a cystic duct which is adherent to the common bile duct over some little distance[21]. This is not only unnecessary but potentially dangerous. It is preferable to leave some cystic duct remnant. Such practice is less liable to injure the blood supply to the bile duct which runs in three columns, one posterior and two lateral. The importance of this relates to the suggestion that damage to these vessels may result in ischaemia of the bile duct with consequent necrosis and stricture formation[28]. The likelihood of this event would obviously be increased by undue dissection of the common bile duct during cholecystectomy or prior to choledochotomy.

In view of the frequency of anomalies of the biliary tree peroperative cholangiography would seem a valuable adjunct to cholecystectomy. Based on our own experience that the majority of patients who have suffered bile duct injury did not have peroperative cholangiography performed at the time of cholecystectomy[29] we believe adoption of its routine use might result in a reduction in the numbers of bile duct injuries.

Clinical presentation

While damage to the biliary tree may be recognized at the time of the original operation, it is more usual for it to become evident either early in the postoperative period or some months later when a biliary stricture is established. The clinical presentation may be of excessive biliary drainage from the wound or drain site in the early postoperative period or, alternatively, of a localized or generalized peritonitis resulting from an intra-abdominal collection of bile. In other instances there is a history of postoperative biliary drainage and fever, with or without a subphrenic abscess, following which the patient became free of symptoms for some months before developing recurrent cholangitis. In still other patients steadily progressive obstructive jaundice may be the first sign of bile duct injury. Although this usually develops immediately after cholecystectomy it may come on some weeks or months after the initial operation.

On physical examination jaundice is usually apparent although it may be intermittent or even absent depending on whether the bile duct obstruction is complete or partial and whether or not a biliary fistula is present. Hepa-

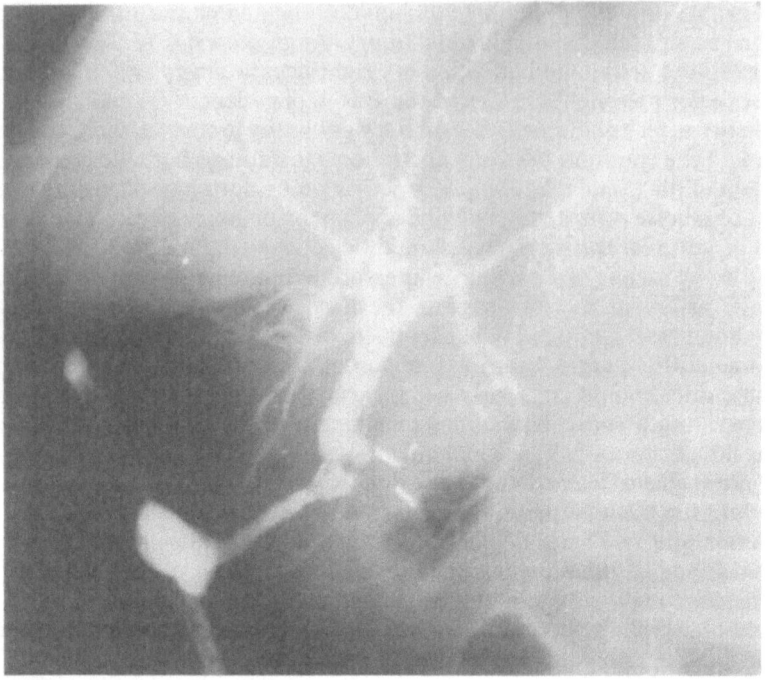

Figure 6.2 Tubogram outlining the proximal biliary tree in a 66-year-old lady demonstrating complete obstruction of the common hepatic duct (type I stricture). Four months previously she had undergone a cholecystectomy which was complicated by a post operative subphrenic abscess and bile collection which was drained percutaneously and resulted in a total external biliary fistula. Subsequent repair of the bile duct injury was achieved by hepaticojejunostomy Roux-en-Y

tomegaly usually indicates long-standing obstruction. Splenomegaly is seen as a late result, particularly after a number of unsuccessful attempts at biliary repair. It follows the development of secondary biliary fibrosis/cirrhosis and portal hypertension, although the possibility of direct damage to or thrombosis of the portal vein should be considered.

Confirmation of damage to the biliary tree is accomplished by radiology. This should provide precise demonstration of the level and extent of the damage, particularly in the proximal portion of the bile duct. Such information is essential before any sensible plan of management can be formulated.

Radiology and other investigations

When there exists an external fistula or a tube is *in situ*, contrast medium can be injected to outline the biliary tree (see Figure 6.2). Ultrasonography, while excellent for demonstrating dilatation of the intrahepatic ducts, is of little value for giving precise information regarding the extent of the stricture and is of no value if the ducts are not dilated. Endoscopic retrograde chol-

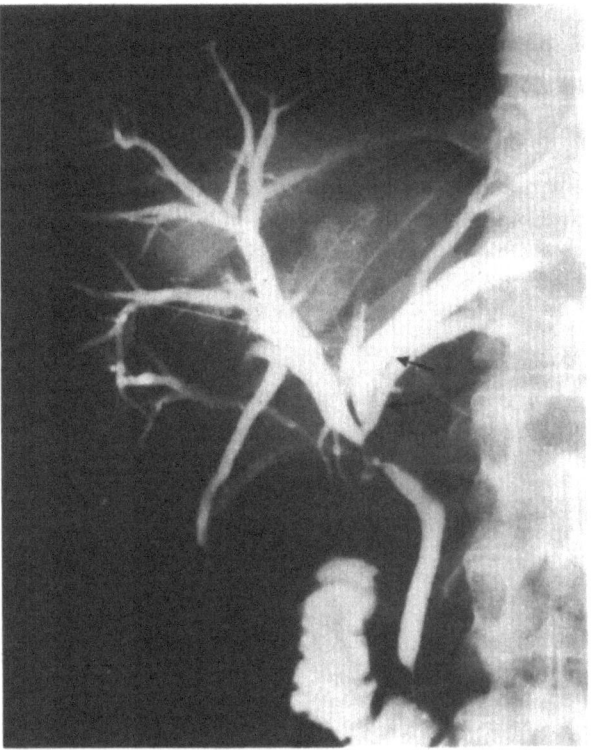

Figure 6.3 Percutaneous transhepatic cholangiogram (PTC) demonstrating a tight stricture at the confluence of the bile ducts with dilatation of intrahepatic ducts (type III stricture). The left hepatic ducts (segment II and III) are anomalous in that they enter separately at the confluence making repair more difficult. The patient, a 26-year-old lady, suffered recurrent cholangitis following a difficult cholecystectomy and exploration CBD. Subsequent, successful reconstruction was achieved by hepaticojejunostomy Roux-en-Y

angiography (ERC) is also of limited value in most instances of bile duct stricture since usually only the lower bile duct will be shown. Percutaneous transhepatic cholangiography (PTC) is the key investigation (see Figure 6.3). Risks of cholangitis and bile leakage have largely been overcome with the introduction of the fine needle[30] provided antibiotic cover is used and the ducts are not overfilled. Care must be taken to outline all branches of the intrahepatic biliary tree, particularly in high bile duct stricture and in cases of recurrent stricture. This may require numerous passes of the needle because of loss of communication between the left and the right ductal systems as a result of high stricture. It is particularly important to display the confluence of the bile ducts (if intact) and the left ductal system since this information is important for deciding operative strategy.

Where there is suspicion of vascular damage either from the history or the presence of a palpable spleen or oesophageal varices then arteriography and portography are important. The latter is usually obtainable by examination of late phase films after splenic arterial injection but on occasions direct percutaneous splenoportography may be required.

It is important to appreciate that unilateral bile duct and/or portal venous obstruction can lead to segmental liver atrophy[31], the radiological signs of which include crowding and irregularity of the smaller biliary radicals and arteries within the affected area. Evidence of atrophy may also be seen on CT scanning and HIDA isotope scanning. A biliary bypass to even widely dilated ducts in an atrophic segment may not on its own result in relief of jaundice but is nevertheless necessary as part of a reconstructive procedure if recurring cholangitis is to be avoided.

HIDA isotope scanning can be of value in the assessment of bile duct

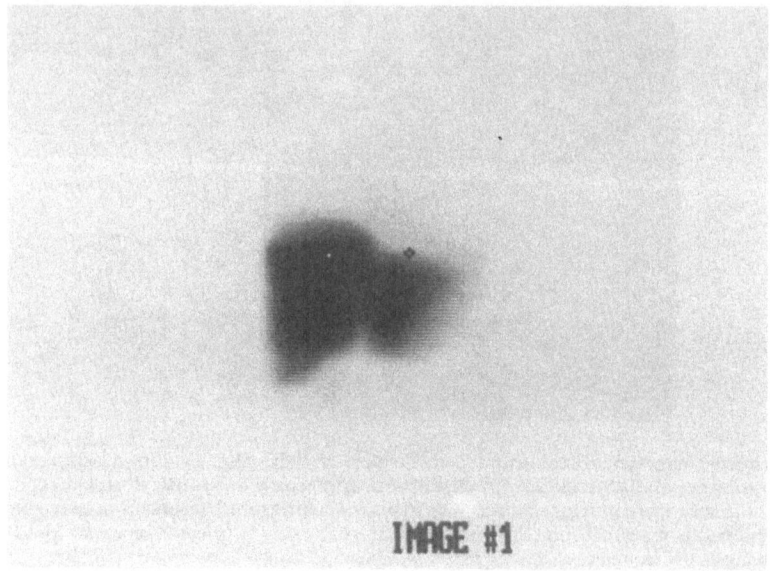

Figure 6.4 HIDA scan of a patient with complete obstruction at the confluence of the bile ducts. No excretion into either common bile duct or duodenum is seen 40 min after i.v. injection of ^{99m}Tc-labelled HIDA. Normally HIDA should appear in the duodenum within 15–20 min

strictures (see Figure 6.4) and in particular of the functional assessment of incomplete strictures and of previous anastomoses and reconstructive attempts[32]. It permits a dynamic and quantitative assessment of liver function and of the clearance of bile across strictures or anastomoses. Its advantages are that unlike PTC it is non-invasive and will yield information even in the absence of a dilated biliary tree. Furthermore, the functional assessment which it gives is of particular value in complex cases.

Classification of strictures

Bismuth has proposed an anatomical classification of bile duct strictures which is of value when methods of repair and results of reconstruction are considered[33] (see Figure 6.5).

144

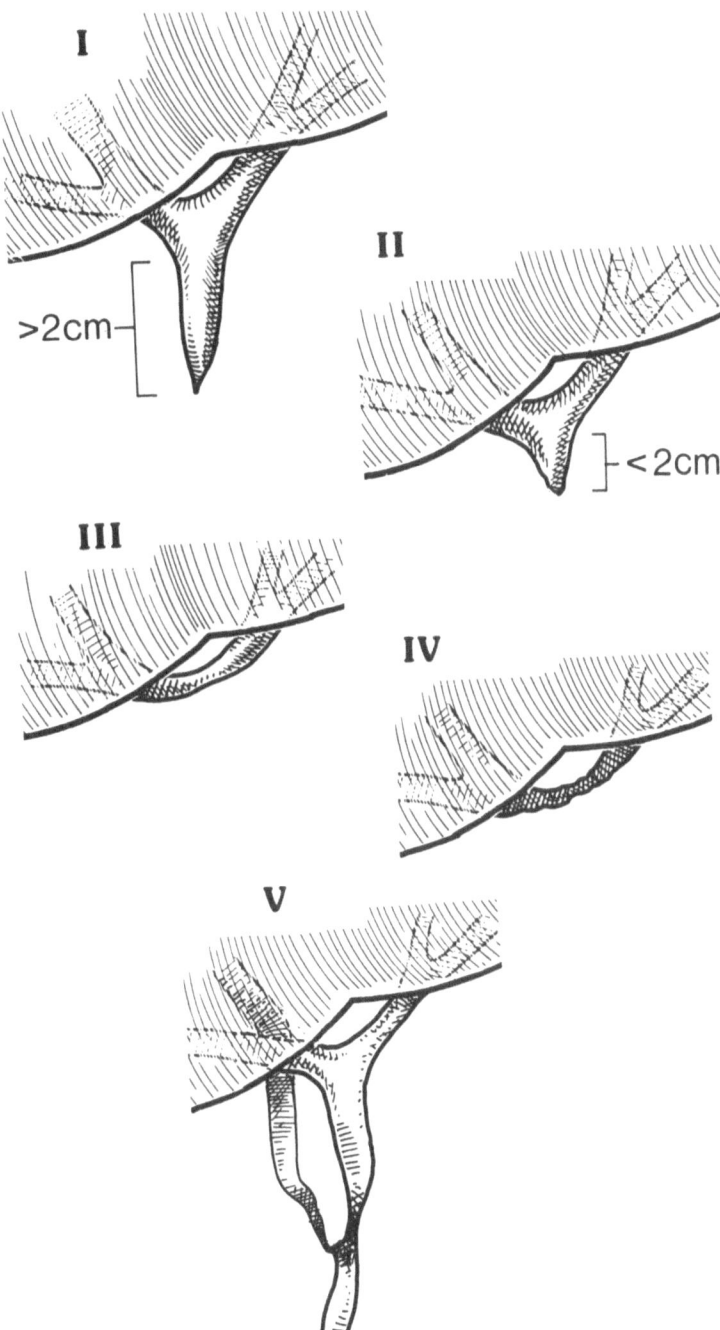

Figure 6.5 Classification of benign bile duct strictures proposed by Bismuth (see text)

Type I   Low common hepatic duct stricture
            Hepatic duct stump > 2 cm

Type II   Mid common hepatic duct stricture
            Hepatic duct stump < 2 cm

Type III   High stricture. No common hepatic duct
            Confluence intact

Type IV   Destruction of hilar confluence
            Right and left ducts separate

Type V   Involvement of right sectoral branch alone or together with the
            common duct

Clinical interpretation

The discovery on cholangiography of an area of stenosis or incomplete stricture is not itself an indication for surgery. An established internal fistula may provide good long-term drainage and even quite severe degrees of stenosis on cholangiography may be accompanied by little in the way of symptoms and near normal liver function tests. The decision when or whether to operate rests largely on the development of the complications of biliary obstruction (cholangitis and impaired liver function) which is left unchecked will result in chronic changes of hepatic fibrosis/cirrhosis and consequent portal hypertension and liver failure.

Preoperative management

Except in the case of injury recognized at the time of cholecystectomy, or in patients in whom emergency operation is dictated by peritonitis, there is no hurry to proceed to surgical reconstruction. Full investigation should be carried out to determine the level and extent of damage and the patient should be allowed time to be brought to optimal condition for surgery. This entails treatment of infection, correction of anaemia and coagulation defects, and assessment of nutritional status. In our experience nutritional support frequently requires the use of intravenous feeding. Where an external biliary fistula is present fluid and electrolyte disturbances will require correction. Prophylactic antibiotics prior to surgery or any invasive investigation of the biliary system are advisable for the prevention of bacteraemia and septicaemia as almost all these patients will have infected bile.

Treatment

The aim of surgery for the treatment of bile duct injuries is to restore biliary–enteric continuity without obstruction. Only if this is achieved will a lasting solution to the problem be obtained. Where complications of bile duct injuries exist, such as biliary peritonitis, subphrenic or subhepatic abscess, haematemesis or liver failure, these will usually require treatment prior to and on a separate occasion from definitive biliary repair. In this regard localized collections and abscesses are probably best managed percutaneously and definitive surgery delayed until all signs of infection have settled.

The precise operative management varies depending upon whether the injury is recognized at the time of the cholecystectomy, presents in the postoperative period or occurs as a late event.

Injuries recognized at the time of operation – Whatever the site or nature of the injury, primary repair should carry two basic and important objectives. The first is maintenance of ductal length below the hilus without sacrifice of tissue and the second, avoidance of uncontrolled postoperative bile leakage. In the event that the surgeon feels unable, for any reason, to achieve these objectives it is probably preferable that he resort to external biliary drainage by means of a tube placed above the injury and refer the patient for specialist treatment than that he complicate the situation by an attempt at repair which may cause further damage to the proximal ducts with consequent loss of tissue and a more difficult ultimate repair.

If repair is to be undertaken the damaged area and bile ducts on either side should be carefully dissected to define the extent of the injury. Operative cholangiography may be helpful at this time. In general, the injury may be high, close to the hilus of the liver, or low, in the supraduodenal area involving the confluence of the common bile duct and cystic duct. The injury may be partial, with maintenance of mucosal continuity along a portion of the bile duct wall or, more usually, complete, with either transection or excision of a portion of common duct. The latter is particularly liable to occur where the bile duct is small and is mistaken by the surgeon for the cystic duct. In this situation primary repair is likely to be difficult and restricturing is liable to occur. However, a subsequent repair, in the presence of dilated ducts, will most likely be successful, provided it is performed by an experienced surgeon.

If the bile duct has been transected and the injury is not too high, providing the ends can be apposed without tension, an end-to-end anastomosis over a T-tube may be performed with fine, interrupted, absorbable sutures. Where this is done the duodenum should be fully mobilized prior to anastomosis so as to minimize tension. The limb of the T-tube should not be brought out through the anastomosis, but rather distal to it. Many such anastomoses will restricture, with a need for subsequent repair (see Figure 6.6). For this reason it is preferable in the case of a high injury to perform initial repair by hepaticojejunostomy Roux-en-Y. This is more likely to give good long-term results[34].

Lateral injuries, though less common, are important to recognize as it may be possible to achieve repair by direct suture of the defect over a T-tube. Where the lateral injury is more extensive and cannot be closed in this manner a Roux-en-Y jejunal loop may be used to provide a serosal patch. A T-tube should be placed across the defect and its long limb led through the Roux loop and developed as a transjejunal tube to the skin. By this means postoperative tubography can be performed to look at the repair and when the T-tube is removed there is the additional advantage of a fistula to the adjacent jejunum. This method may occasionally be very useful, particularly for an inexperienced surgeon in difficulty. An alternative, of which we have no experi-

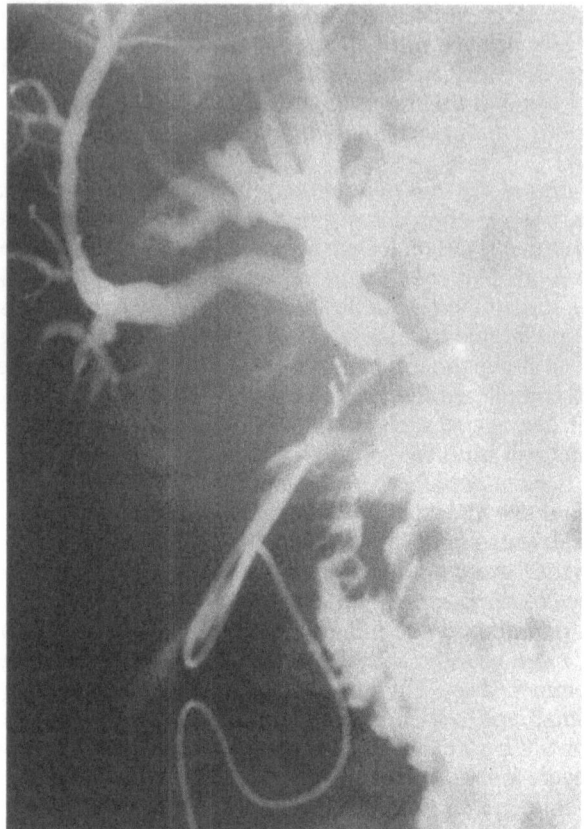

Figure 6.6 Tubogram demonstrating primary repair of a bile duct injury by end-to-end anastomosis over a T-tube. Stricturing is beginning to occur and a hepaticojejunostomy Roux-en-Y was required 3 months later

ence, is the use of a venous patch or even interposition graft as has been suggested by a number of authors[35–37].

The frequency with which immediate repair of the bile duct is effective and long-lasting is difficult to ascertain as many of these injuries may never come to the attention of specialist units or be reported. Although it has been suggested that the restricture rate is as high as 50 or 60%[19,20] the evidence for this is not strong and almost certainly there has been a considerable underestimate of the number of bile duct injuries occurring in non-specialist units and for which successful immediate repair has been achieved.

Injuries recognized in the immediate postoperative period – Injuries not recognized at the time of the original operation present in three possible ways. Firstly, an *external biliary fistula* through either the wound or a drain site may develop. The essential of management is not to re-operate quickly but rather to wait, treat infection, nourish the patient and carry out fistulography. Should this latter reveal continuity between the biliary system and the gastrointestinal tract, a prolonged period of drainage, if well managed, may well result in spontaneous closure of the fistula. Early repair is not required as the patient is not jaundiced and the adverse pathophysiological features associated with cholestasis are not present. Any attempt at repair at this time would be difficult as the bile duct will usually not be dilated and this will hamper efforts to achieve a good and lasting anastomosis. A cautious and expectant approach is preferable since even ultimate closure of the fistula with the development of jaundice is usually associated with proximal ductal dilatation which will afford easier and better subsequent repair. Should fluid loss from the fistula prove unmanageable, the external fistula can after some weeks be converted to an internal fistulojejunostomy[38].

Secondly, presentation in the postoperative period may be with biliary *peritonitis*. This is a serious and usually dangerous condition, especially if the bile is infected and urgent surgery is required to save life. Definitive repair is seldom possible because the bile ducts are collapsed, and the tissues deeply stained with bile and friable. External drainage is the best initial approach and this may be carried out through a Roux-en-Y loop of jejunum, the external drainage tube simply being lead across in a transjejunal fashion to the skin. Such a procedure achieves control of the bile leak, initially as an external fistula and subsequently, potentially at least, internally. The almost certain stenosis at a later date and necessity for a further operation should be accepted. Once again, this will usually be performed in the presence of dilated proximal ducts which will make for an easier and better repair.

Finally, as the third method of presentation, the patient may become progressively *jaundiced* some interval of time following cholecystectomy. In this case the injury should be managed as outlined below.

Injuries presenting at an interval after initial operation – The basic principle guiding the management of late biliary stenosis and stricture is to re-establish mucosal continuity between the biliary tree and digestive mucosa. A mucosa-to-mucosa anastomosis is the surest way to prevent recurrence of the stricture. This requires on the one hand exposure of healthy proximal bile duct and on the other preparation of a suitable segment of digestive mucosa for anastomosis. The latter is relatively easy to achieve either with the use of the distal end of the strictured bile duct or by preparation of a Roux-en-Y loop of jejunum. The use of the distal stump of bile duct to perform an end-to-end anastomosis was used for a long time by some authors[39,40]. However, the difficulty in obtaining good mucosa-to-mucosa anastomosis without undue tension makes the results of this approach less satisfactory than those of a biliary—enteric anastomosis[34,41]. Thus in the vast majority of cases, biliary—enteric anastomosis is the preferable procedure. The precise approach to be advised is dictated principally by the level of the stricture. If this is in the retropancreatic portion or immediate supraduodenal portion of the bile duct then choledochoduodenostomy, either side-to-side or end-to-side, is an ideal procedure and usually provides excellent results providing the common bile duct is dilated. Such strictures, however, are uncommon after cholecystectomy, being more often encountered following partial gastrectomy. Postcholecystectomy strictures almost always involve the common hepatic duct and for this reason are more difficult particularly when close to the hilus of the liver. These must be dealt with by hepticojejunostomy (see Figure 6.7). Should the stricture involve the confluence of the right and left ducts (Bismuth type III or IV) or extend into these ducts, the problem is much more difficult and good results are not easily obtained.

The critical and most difficult step in the operation is the exposure of healthy proximal bile duct mucosa. It is most important that this be found and that the anastomosis is not performed through fibrous tissue. Furthermore, it is important that the proximal bile duct(s) which are exposed and used for anastomosis drain all areas of the liver if a segmental obstruction and recurring cholangitis are not to result.

A variety of approaches to the proximal hepatic duct(s) in order to expose mucosa may be used depending on the site and extent of the stricture. A staged approach may be required because of abscesses, gastrointestinal haemorrhage (due to erosive gastritis or oesophageal varices) or because of poor general condition of the patient. It is certainly unwise to attempt definitive repair in the presence of severe local sepsis or while significant GI bleeding is in progress. In these instances it is better to drain purulent or bile collections, perhaps by percutaneous methods, and establish an external fistula thereby allowing improvement in the general condition of the patient prior to definitive repair of the stricture[42,43]. In patients with portal hypertension with major bleeding an initial portasystemic anastomosis may be required.

Operative approach – Identification and exposure of healthy bile duct proximal to the stricture is the key step in the operative procedure. This is often difficult and a systematic and patient approach is necessary. In all instances a generous incision should be used. The use of a bilateral subcostal incision with a 'gallows' type retractor gives excellent access. Exposure must be full and all adhesions separated. An important feature is the early division of the falciform ligament right back to the diaphragm and the freeing of the liver from any adhesions to the diaphragm. A firm tie is placed on the divided ligamentum teres so that it may be elevated and used as a retractor. A number of different approaches may be used to identify proximal bile duct depending on the circumstances and the nature of the stricture.

For Bismuth type I and II strictures the common hepatic duct can usually be approached directly from the region of the scar of the gallbladder fossa and by proceeding to the left. The duct is generally to be found lateral to the pulsation of the hepatic artery and its identification can be aided by aspiration of bile with a syringe and needle or by following the tract of a previous external biliary fistula. Once identified, the anterior wall of the common hepatic duct stump should be dissected so as to expose the stricture and a length of duct of at least 1 cm. Adhesions posteriorly to the damaged duct are often very dense and it is not always necessary to dissect these completely and indeed to do so may be dangerous. Once exposed, the bile duct should be opened between stays. In some instances it can be completely transected but in others the incision may simply be extended proximally for a centimetre

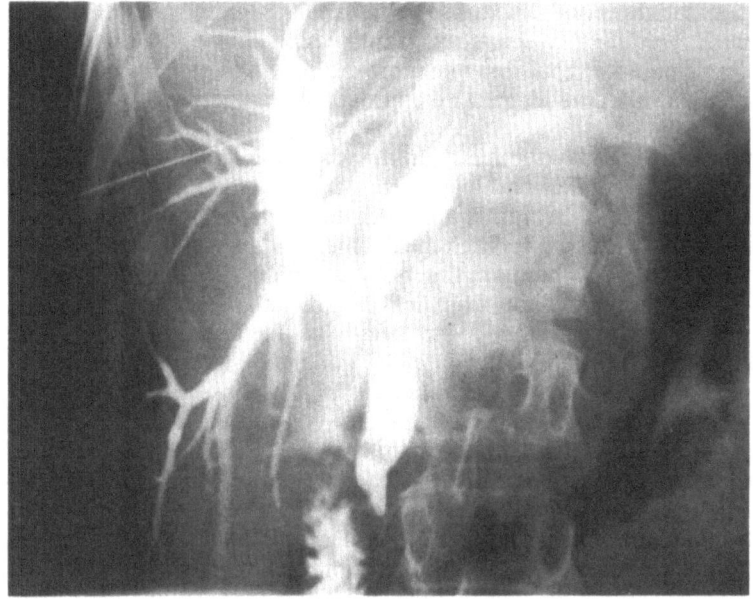

a

b

Figure 6.7 (a) PTC in a 45-year-old lady showing a tight stricture at the confluence of the bile ducts with stones above and below this point. Nine years previously she had undergone cholecystectomy at which time a bile duct injury had occurred necessitating a repair 1 week later by end-to-end anastomosis. (b) Tubogram demonstrating the repair in this patient by hepaticojejunostomy Roux-en-Y. The patient remains well and symptom-free 3 years later

or so in a 'fishmouth' fashion so as to expose healthy mucosa for repair. In Bismuth type III or IV strictures, identification of the strictured area and of a suitable duct for repair may be more difficult than outlined above. In these instances a variety of alternative approaches is available.

Approach to the left hepatic ducts – In the vast majority of high biliary strictures adequate exposure of the bile ducts may be made by dissecting the left main hepatic duct using an approach based on the anatomical studies of Couinaud[44-46]. In this approach the ligamentum teres is elevated as previously described and the base of the quadrate lobe is identified between the gallbladder fossa and the umbilical fissure. The width of the base of the quadrate lobe approximates the length of the left hepatic duct. Even in instances where there is a pyramidal quadrate lobe and the base is short, there is always a length of extrahepatic bile duct on the left side (see Figure 6.8). Splitting of the bridge of tissue between the quadrate lobe and the left lateral segment is often helpful in allowing exposure. Once the inferior border of the quadrate lobe is exposed incision in the connective tissue where Glisson's capsule fuses with the peritoneum of the lesser omentum (the hilar plate) should be made. This incision is deepened and the structures of the left portal triad are lowered from the inferior surface of the quadrate lobe and exposed for dissection[44] (see Figure 6.9). Once this manoeuvre ('lowering of the hilar plate') is performed the dissection can be proceeded with to the right side and usually the confluence is easily exposed. Even in instances where

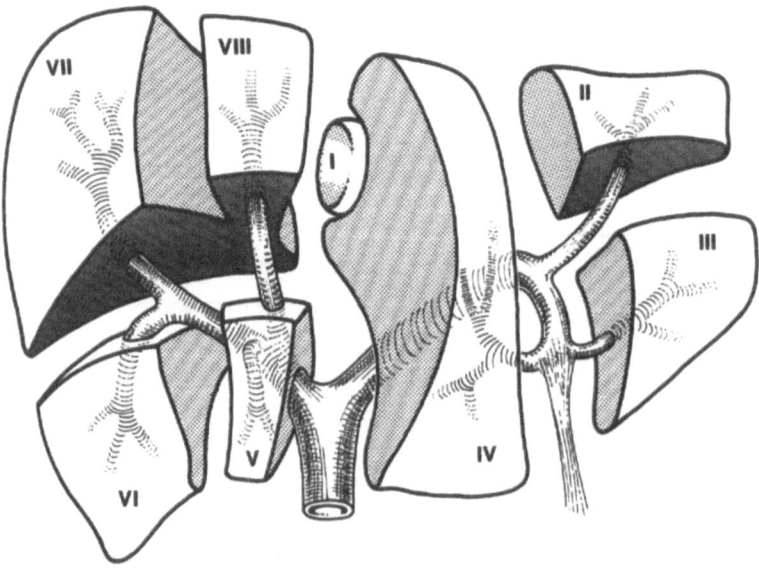

Figure 6.8　Segmental structure of the liver. Note that the left portal triad is always extrahepatic beneath the quadrate lobe (segment IV). From Blumgart, L. H. and Kelley, C. J. (1984). *Br. J. Surg.*, **71**, 257–61, by permission of the publishers, Butterworth and Co.

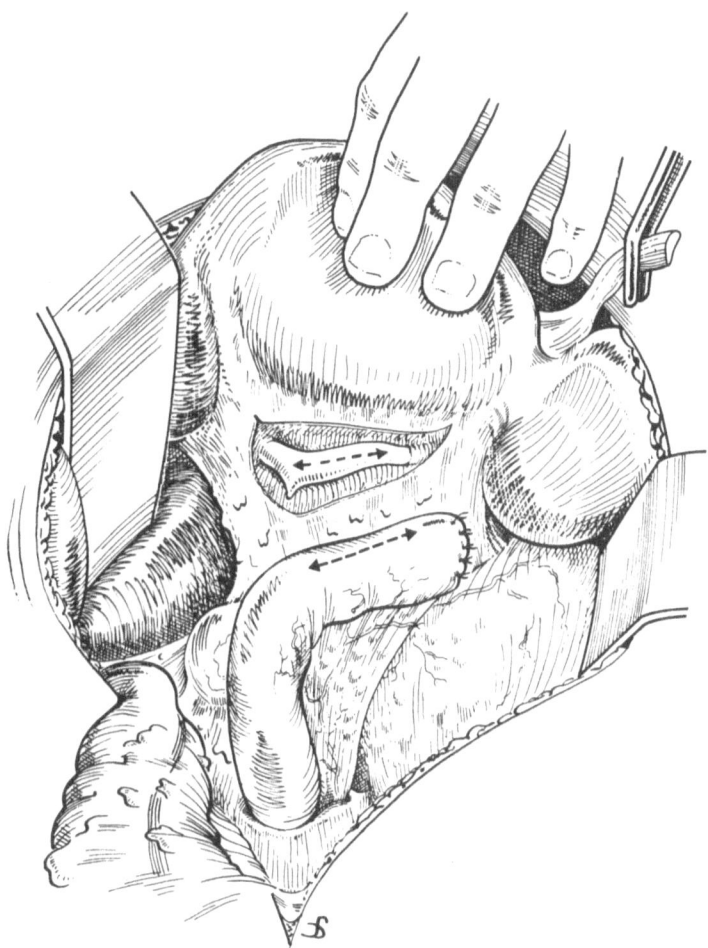

Figure 6.9 Exposure of the left hepatic duct and the confluence by incision of the peritoneal reflection at the base of the quadrate lobe. The duct becomes visible as the hilar plate is lowered (see text). A Roux-en-Y loop has been prepared for the anastomosis and the dotted lines on the duct and jejunum indicate the lines of incision. From Blumgart, L. H. and Kelley, C. J. (1984). *Br. J. Surg.*, **71**, 257–61, by permission of the publishers, Butterworth and Co.

the stricture extends into the confluence, there is usually a bridge of intact mucosa crossing the upper part of the confluence, which permits dissection to the right and exposure of the right hepatic duct. After adequate exposure has been achieved, the left hepatic duct is incised longitudinally to disclose healthy mucosa for repair.

On occasions this approach may be difficult and dangerous either as a result of dense adhesions or because of a hypertrophied quadrate lobe which overhangs the area of the left duct. Alternatively, the extrahepatic length of the left hepatic duct may be too short for adequate exposure. In these instances repair may be effected by dissection of the left hepatic duct in the umbilical fissure (segment III duct) as originally described by Soupault and Couinaud[45]. Although more often required and useful in patients with malignant disease, this approach may be of value in selected cases of benign disease.

Segment III duct approach – The left duct divides deep within the umbilical fissure into major branches, one of which courses forward to the anterior portion of the left lateral segment (segment III) and another backwards into the posterior portion (segment II). Anastomosis to the segment III duct is usually possible after dissection in the umbilical fissure and can be used in difficult cases of benign stricture provided there is communication between the left and the right ductal systems. If this is not present use of the segment III duct would leave an obstructed right lobe to be a potential source of recurring cholangitis. In this approach the ligamentum teres is elevated and the bridge of liver tissue between quadrate lobe and segment III is divided. While the liver is then held up so that its inferior surface may be seen the

a

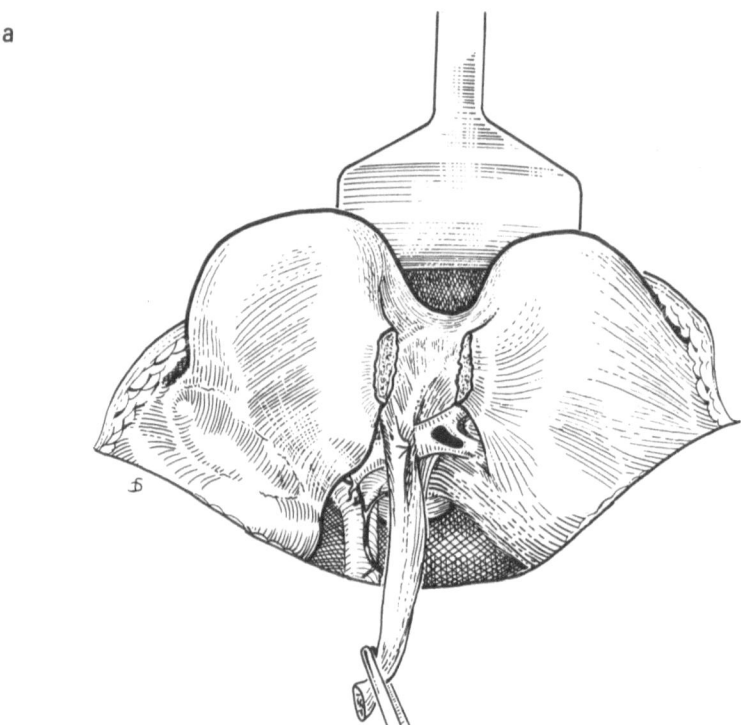

Figure 6.10 Exposure of the segment III duct. (a) The ligamentum teres is elevated and the bridge of tissue between the quadrate lobe and the left lateral segment has been divided to expose the base of the umbilical fissure. (b) The liver is held upwards while the ligamentum teres is pulled downwards. Prolongations at the base of the ligamentum teres are identified and ligated (see text). (c) The segment III duct is exposed and incised ready for anastomosis

b

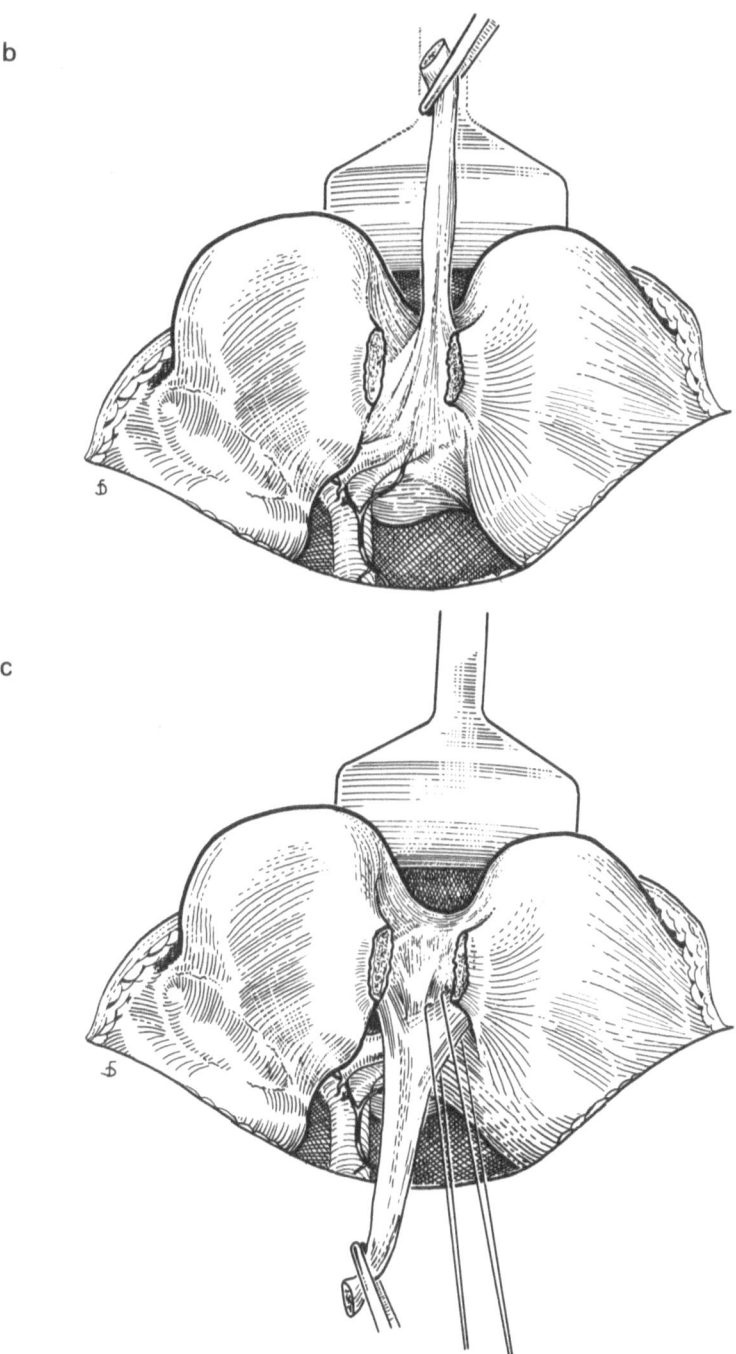

c

Figure 6.10

ligamentum teres is pulled downwards. If the upper surface of the ligament is now dissected, it will be found that a small number of extensions pass into the liver at the base of the ligament (which is itself attached to the left branch of the portal vein). The extensions to the left of the ligament in the umbilical fissure are individually divided between ligatures. If exposure is inadequate a small split of the liver substance can be made just to the left of the falciform ligament with diathermy or finger fracture technique. The segment III duct will be found lying relatively superficially within the liver to the left of the ligamentum teres[45,46] (see Figure 6.10). Needle aspiration may assist in its identification. The duct is then opened longitudinally over 2–3 cm and prepared for anastomosis.

Liver split and liver resection procedures – Additional manoeuvres are sometimes required for adequate exposure of the bile ducts for repair. This is particularly the case in type IV biliary strictures where the confluence is obliterated. In these instances additional exposure may be obtained by splitting liver tissue in the umbilical fissure or in the line of the scar of the gallbladder fossa or both[47]. Liver split in both these sites allows upward mobilization of the entire quadrate lobe with improved access to the left and right hepatic ducts. On rare occasions resection of liver tissue may be necessary for exposure of the bile ducts. This will usually take the form of excision of part of the quadrate lobe or occasionally of a portion of the left lateral segment for intrahepatic hepaticojejunostomy as described by Longmire and Sandford[48]. In general these approaches, and particularly the latter, are dangerous and should seldom be utilized in cases of benign stricture.

Technique of mucosa-to-mucosa suture – Once the bile duct has been prepared for anastomosis, a 70 cm Roux-en-Y jejunal loop is constructed and brought up, preferably in retrocolic fashion, to lie in the subhepatic area. Anastomosis is then performed in a single layer of interrupted 3/0 Vicryl sutures by a technique described by Voyles and Blumgart[49]. The important point in making all high anastomoses is the early placement of the anterior layer of suture in the proximal duct prior to any attempt to place the posterior row. This manoeuvre ensures precise placement of the anterior row of sutures in the duct which is otherwise difficult if the posterior layer has been inserted and tied. Providing the ducts are dilated and a good mucosa-to-mucosa anastomosis is achieved we no longer employ the use of anastomotic stents. If, however, technical difficulty is experienced we prefer to employ a trans-jejunally placed silicone tube across the anastomis so as to provide access for subsequent anastomotic dilatations should these be required.

Mucosal graft operation – In 1969 Smith described his method of jejunal mucosal graft for treating the high stricture in which dissection in the area of the hilus is thought to be impossible or where mucosa-to-mucosa anastomosis cannot be achieved[50,51]. By this technique jejunal mucosa is pulled up through the stenosis by means of a transhepatic tube. The object of the procedure is that apposition of jejunal to biliary mucosa is achieved for subsequent healing without fibrosis. The procedure is claimed to be easier

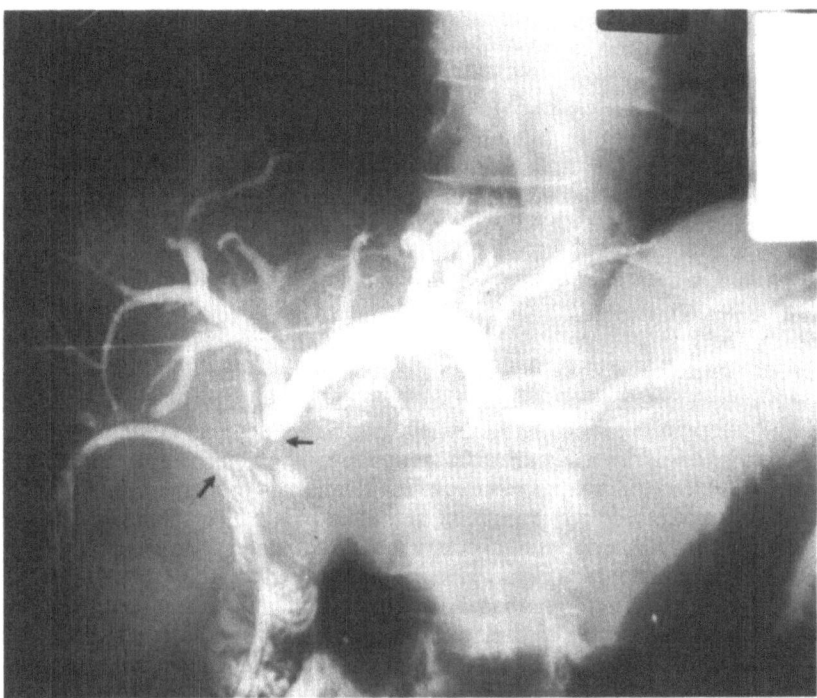

Figure 6.11 Combined PTC and tubogram in a patient who had undergone a 'mucosal graft' hepaticojejunostomy for a recurrent benign bile duct stricture. The mucosal graft has been to a right sectoral duct (left arrow) leaving the remainder of the liver obstructed (right arrow). The patient continued to suffer from recurrent cholangitis and was subsequently treated with a mucosa-to-mucosa anastomosis to the segment III duct. From Blumgart, L. H., Kelley, C. J. and Benjamin, I. S. (1984). *Br. J. Surg.*, 71, 836–43, by permission of the publishers, Butterworth and Co.

than formal anastomosis as no sutures are inserted. It should be emphasized that this procedure has been advocated for cases in which suture anastomosis is thought to be impracticable[21,51,52]. However, the operation is by no means easy in the densely fibrotic liver or where there is secondary biliary cirrhosis since when the ducts are small, passage of a transhepatic tube may not be possible and it is easy to produce false passages. Furthermore, the method is blind and the dome of mucosa pulled up into the hepatic ducts may cause obstruction of important branches of the intrahepatic ductal system resulting in segmental obstruction[53,54] (see Figure 6.11). In addition the mucosa may pull away in the postoperative period and the whole jejunal loop may become detached and lie at a distance from the hilus. Finally doubts must be expressed as to those cases in whom it has been reported that dissection of the bile duct mucosa for anastomosis is impossible. We believe a precise mucosa-to-mucosa anastomosis is possible in almost every case using the techniques described above. In 20 patients referred to the Hepatobiliary Unit, Royal Postgraduate Medical School, London, in whom a previous mucosal graft procedure had been done because an anastomosis had been said to be impossible, subsequent suture anastomosis was possible in all but one and in some patients with ease[54]. Bismuth has reported 180 consecutive cases, many of them of a serious nature, in whom mucosal suture had been possible and mucosal graft procedures never necessary[33]. Unless carried out bilaterally the procedure of mucosal graft is totally unsuitable for type IV strictures where there is separation of the left and right ductal systems. In these instances an approach to the left duct as described above, with or without liver split or resection, is usually necessary.

Portal hypertension and biliary stricture – Patients with biliary stricture may develop portal hypertension as a result either of the development of secondary hepatic fibrosis and cirrhosis or of direct damage to the portal vein or occasionally of coincidental liver disease. The type of patient who develops this complication usually has a high stricture and a history of multiple unsuccessful attempts at repair. Management of such patients is extremely difficult and carries a high mortality[54-58]. In general, attempts at biliary repair should be made. However, in cases where severe haemorrhage is encountered at the time of operation, biliary repair is best deferred until such time as portal hypertension has been brought under control by a portasystemic anastomosis, usually in the form of a distal splenorenal shunt. Variceal bleeding before or after biliary repair is managed on its merits by injection sclerotherapy, oesophageal transection or portasystemic shunting. In this group of patients and particularly those with severely compromised liver function, percutaneous transhepatic biliary drainage or percutaneous balloon dilatation may be advisable prior to or in place of a surgical procedure.

Percutaneous dilatation – Following the development of transluminal balloon angioplasty a similar technique of percutaneous balloon dilatation of biliary strictures has become a possibility[59]. While it should not be used as a substitute for a good biliary–enteric anastomosis, except perhaps in elderly patients, it can be an extremely valuable adjunct to surgery in selected cases. We reserve its use for those few patients with recurrent stricture in whom a satisfactory mucosa-to-mucosa anastomosis cannot be achieved. In such cases we perform a hepaticojejunostomy Roux-en-Y and leave a tube across the anastomosis exiting from the abdominal wall via the blind end of the Roux loop. This tube is placed for the provision of percutaneous access to the anastomosis for subsequent balloon dilatation.

Results of surgery

A large number of factors influence the prognosis and outcome of biliary repair. Of these the most important are undoubtedly the age of the patient, the level or absence of irreversible liver damage, portal hypertension and the number of previous attempts at surgical repair. Ultimately, it is the adequacy of surgical repair which is of over-riding importance in determining long-term prognosis. While untreated cases have progressively deteriorating liver function and an eventually fatal outcome, so too do those in whom surgical treatment achieves only partial relief of obstruction.

Postoperative morbidity and mortality following reconstructive surgery for bile duct stricture is relatively high, particularly in the complex cases where there have been previous attempts at repair[54]. The common complications include subphrenic, subhepatic or pelvic abscess, wound infection, cholangitis, septicaemia, secondary haemorrhage, biliary fistula and pulmonary complications. Mortality is very difficult to assess because, in existing reports, there has been no uniform method employed. For example, some reports do not clearly define operative mortality and whether this includes all hospital mortality. This is important as some patients die *before* operation and others die postoperatively as a result of complications from variceal bleeding. In addition some series do not differentiate high from low strictures, or the mortality of one operative procedure as against another, nor even allow for the effects of multiple operations. Thus, although operative mortality is reported as being between 5 and 8%[58,60,61], this is highly dependent on the proportion of complex and high risk patients in the series. Deaths are usually attributable to uncontrolled haemorrhage, hepatic or renal failure, or a combination of these features. In the Hammersmith series of 78 patients, the overall 30-day hospital mortality was 11.5% which included one death due to bleeding oesophageal varices before operation could be undertaken. The operative mortality for all procedures including surgery for drainage of abscesses, shunt procedures for control of bleeding and biliary repair was 8.3%. There were no deaths in 58 patients treated by hepaticojejunostomy nor in three treated by choledochoduodenostomy. Two patients with complex high strictures treated early in the series by mucosal graft died. Thus in 63 patients treated by stricture repair alone the operative mortality was only 3.2%[54]. In a total of 84 patients treated to date by stricture repair alone the 30-day operative mortality has been 2.4% (two patients) with there having been no deaths in 82 consecutive cases treated by mucosa-to-mucosa suture. Bismuth has reported a similarly low mortality of 0.6% in a consecutive series of 186 patients with benign stricture, treated by hepaticojejunostomy to the left duct system[33].

Late results are difficult to determine because of the considerable variation in the criteria chosen for assessment. The follow-up usually reported is over 2–3 years[51,62], a period which is almost certainly too short. Bismuth has observed failure of the operation more than 3 years after surgery[33] and for this reason suggests that results should be considered after 5 or even 10 years. He has reported 186 patients, operated on by a left duct approach, with at least a 10-year follow-up. One hundred and twenty were available for reassessment and of these 88% had an excellent result defined as the absence of any biliary troubles[33]. This result is essentially similar to our own, although we have a shorter follow-up[54] and to the estimate of Kune and Sali[21] that 85% of patients with a bile duct injury will be restored to normal health if surgical reconstruction is undertaken by a surgeon experienced in the management of these injuries.

It should be emphasized that bile duct injury during cholecystectomy is a most serious problem. Mortality, both initial and late, is related to preoperative procedures, infection and the evolution of hepatic fibrosis and portal hypertension.

Haemobilia

Brisk bleeding into the gastrointestinal tract via the biliary tree is a dangerous condition which requires precise diagnosis and treatment[63]. It may result from traumatic probing of the intrahepatic ducts during exploration of the CBD or, alternatively, it may develop following injury to the right hepatic artery during cholecystectomy. In this latter case it arises following the rupture into the biliary tree of a false aneurysm[64] (see Figure 6.12). The bleeding may be stuttering in nature but will eventually be massive and life-threatening. The diagnosis of haemobilia should be considered whenever bleeding follows cholecystectomy, or indeed other procedures on the biliary tract, particularly those involving invasive percutaneous techniques. There is usually right upper quadrant pain and jaundice. The investigation of such patients is crucial and should entail an upper GI endoscopy. This may fail to show any trace of bleeding, but blood may be seen issuing from the papilla. Selective hepatic arteriography should be performed by an experienced embolization of the feeding artery and aneurysm[65,66]. Embolization or ligation of the *main or even right hepatic artery* may not be successful because of the existence of and rapid development of a collateral circulation[67] which will continue to feed the aneurysm. Selective embolization is unquestionably the

a

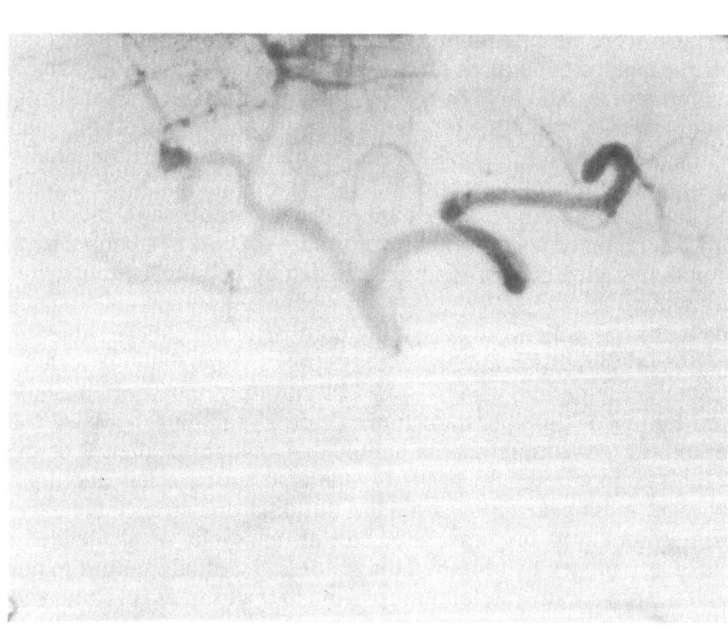

Figure 6.12 Arteriogram in a patient who presented with haemobilia 1 year after cholecystectomy. (a) The coeliac arteriogram shows a false aneurysm related to the right hepatic artery. (b) A selective study demonstrated the aneurysm more clearly and (c) a radiograph taken 10 seconds after the injection of contrast medium showed extravasation of contrast into the common bile duct and duodenum confirming the diagnosis of haemobilia. From Allison, D. J. (1983). Interventional radiology. In Steiner, R. E. (ed.) *Recent Advances in Radiology and Medical Imaging.*Vol. 7, by permission of the publishers, Churchill Livingstone

b

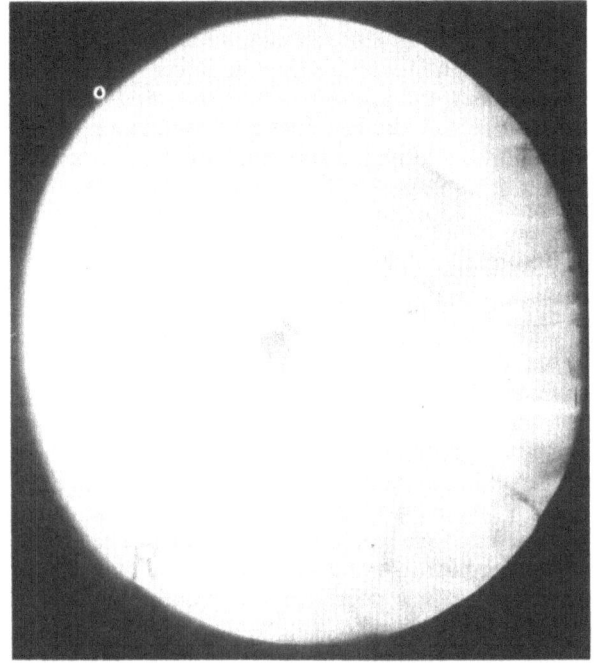

c

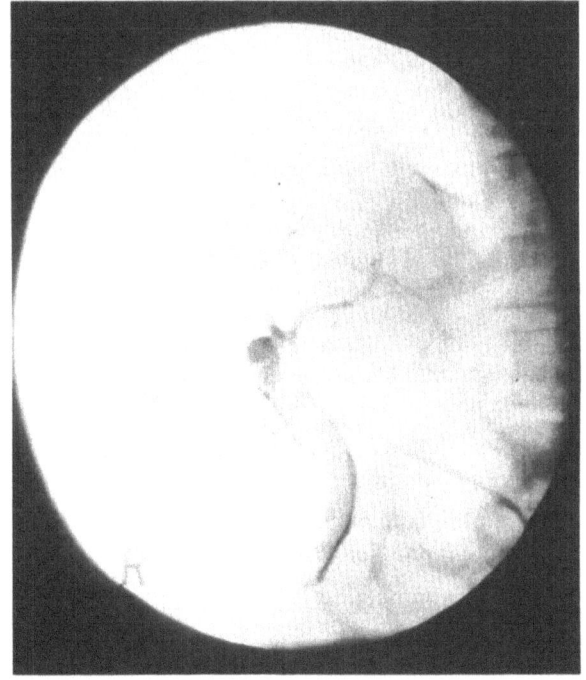

treatment of choice but where this fails emergency surgery will be required. Although in instances where haemobilia follows cholecystectomy, surgical correction may be relatively readily achieved because of the extrahepatic nature of the injury and problem, other structures are placed at risk by this procedure, particularly the bile duct and portal vein. Where haemobilia has an intrahepatic source and embolization is not possible the difficulties are much greater and major hepatic resection may be required.

Acute pancreatitis

Postoperative pancreatitis is an important and serious complication of biliary tract operations with a reported mortality between 30 and 50%[68-71]. A precise incidence is difficult to determine although approximately 5–10% of all cases of acute pancreatitis arise as a postoperative complication, most commonly after biliary tract surgery[69-71]. Acute pancreatitis after simple cholecystectomy is unusual, it being more often seen after exploration of the CBD and especially after sphincterotomy or sphincteroplasty[70,72]. Although various factors have been implicated in its aetiology including trauma, bile reflux, pancreatic ductal obstruction from oedema or long-arm T-tubes, it is probable that reflux of duodenal contents into the pancreatic duct through a damaged or incompetent sphincter is important[72,73]. Deaths are usually associated with late diagnosis[70] and for this reason it is important to consider the diagnosis early if problems develop after biliary tract surgery. The diagnosis is made by the finding of an elevated serum amylase in the appropriate clinical setting. In the absence of specific treatment, management should be supportive and be aimed at the prevention and early treatment of renal and respiratory complications.

Postcholecystectomy problems

While the majority of patients with gallstones are cured following chole-cystectomy, as many as 25%[74], and in one recent report 43%[75], continue to report the occurrence of some symptoms after operation. However, probably only of the order of 5% continue to have significant persistent or recurrent symptoms which require careful further assessment[74]. While the surgical management of such patients may be straightforward, it is frequently difficult and time-consuming. Accurate diagnosis is of course essential for successful management and further laparotomy without a diagnosis is destined to give disappointing results.

Assessment and investigation

Patients with continuing problems following cholecystectomy present with a wide spectrum of symptoms and symptom severity, the precise nature of which influences the extent of investigation considered necessary. In addition abnormalities of liver function tests or of preliminary non-invasive invest-igations (e.g. ultrasound scanning, plain abdominal X-rays) may dictate further assessment of patients with relatively minor symptoms. The commonest presentation is of a patient with persistence of the same symptoms as were experienced prior to cholecystectomy[76]. Although this may suggest unrecognized biliary tract disease (e.g. common bile duct stones or tumour) it is more likely that the cause of symptoms was and remains non-biliary in nature. In general, the more typical are the symptoms prior to chole-cystectomy the more likely they are due to gallstones and that a complete cure will be effected by this operation. Patients with rather ill-defined symptoms, such as those with flatulent dyspepsia, are at greater risk of continuing trouble after surgery. New symptoms which develop immediately following cholecystectomy or after an interval point to an iatrogenic cause.

A full and detailed history of the symptoms may suggest causes other than biliary tract disease but the presence of jaundice, pruritis or rigors is a strong pointer to the presence of biliary problems[77]. While a full physical examination is of course important, it is frequently unhelpful, although careful inspection of the scar may reveal evidence of incisional hernia or a localized area of tenderness suggestive of a neuroma. The lumbar spine should be examined carefully for evidence of spinal disease.

Close scrutiny of previous records, operation notes and X-rays including operative and T-tube cholangiograms may suggest a cause. For example, a finding of multiple small gallstones at cholecystectomy or a history of common duct exploration should raise the possibility of retained stones in the biliary tree, particularly if good postexploratory cholangiography or chole-dochoscopy was not performed. The use of a non-absorbable ligature for the cystic duct may have provided a nidus for subsequent stone formation. A history of difficult duct exploration or the passage of rigid instruments (e.g. Bakes' dilators) through the papilla or a history of transduodenal duct explo-ration should raise suspicion of damage to the papilla or lower common duct.

Initial investigations should include liver function tests, amylase, plain abdominal X-rays and an ultrasound scan of the liver, bile ducts and pancreas. In patients with abnormalities on these or symptoms suggestive of biliary pathology, endoscopic retrograde cholangiopancreatography (ERCP) is the most valuable definitive investigation[77]. In patients with troublesome symptoms, in whom ERCP has been unsuccessful, PTC may be required. Even in patients with a confident ultrasound or cholangiographic diagnosis of residual common duct stones, preoperative duodenoscopy is advisable to carefully inspect the papilla for the possibility of an underlying periampullary tumour.

Endoscopic assessment in this way should also exclude peptic ulceration or other disease, the presence of which does not of course rule out the possibility of concurrent disease in the bile duct or pancreatic duct. Endoscopy may identify the presence of a choledochoduodenal fistula or stenosis of the papilla which may have followed lower common duct instrumentation[78]. Similarly, stenosis at the site of a previous sphincterotomy, spincteroplasty or choledochoduodenostomy, which may be the cause of recurrent cholan-gitis, will be apparent at endoscopy.

The diagnostic yield from endoscopy and ERCP is high when there is a history of jaundice, cholangitis or pancreatitis but in other patients, par-ticularly those in whom symptoms are unchanged by cholecystectomy, it is lower[77]. In our own series, of over 200 cases, abnormalities were most frequently found within the biliary or pancreatic ductal apparatus. The principal causes identified were residual bile duct calculi, unrecognized pancreatic disease and bile duct strictures. Papillary or bile duct tumours and choledochoduodenal fistulas accounted for most of the remaining abnormalities.

Treatment of postcholecystectomy symptoms

Bile duct calculi – In spite of evidence that ductal stones can pass spontaneously[79,80] their removal would be advisable, even in the absence of symptoms, because of the risk of serious complications. A number of options may exist for the removal of such stones (see Figure 6.13). Where a T-tube is present in the bile duct an initial trial of flushing or dissolution with saline or mono-octanoin is worthwhile[81,82]. However, where this is not successful within a week or two it should not be continued. Maturation of the T-tube tract over a period of 6 weeks will permit the employment of percutaneous stone extraction[83] which, in competent hands, is successful in at least 90% of cases and carries minimal morbidity and negligible mortality[84]. Where a T-tube does not exist the options lie essentially between endoscopic sphincterotomy with stone extraction and surgical re-exploration of the bile duct. In expert hands, endoscopic sphincterotomy with complete clearance of ductal stones is achieved in about 85–90% of cases but is less successful with large stones[85,86]. The procedure is, however, attended by a mortality of approximately 1% and a morbidity of 8–10%, principally accounted for by acute pancreatitis and haemorrhage. While this latter complication normally dictates a need for surgery and carries a high mortality, embolization of the bleeding vessel via the gastroduodenal artery is a therapeutic option where the local expertise exists (Professor D. J. Allison, personal communication 1986). The incidence of recurrent stones and papillary stenosis after endoscopic sphincterotomy remains unknown because of limited follow-up data although existing reports give an incidence of between 5 and 10%[87,88]. The overall results of surgical re-exploration for stone are comparable with endoscopy[1,89]. However, whereas the risks of surgery are largely related to age and coincidental disease, this is not the case for endoscopic sphincterotomy. For this reason it is probably preferable to resort to surgery in the younger, fit patients where surgical risks may be expected to be negligible and employ endoscopic sphincterotomy for the elderly and for patients who are regarded as a surgical risk.

Surgical re-exploration is best carried out through a supraduodenal choledochotomy with avoidance of unnecessary instrumentation of the papilla. Both pre-exploratory (either peroperative or preoperative) and post-exploratory cholonagiography or choledochoscopy are essential. For post-exploratory cholangiography, we advocate a technique reported by Gunn *et al.* which utilizes a paediatric urinary catheter positioned initially distally and subsequently proximally at the choledochotomy[90]. With careful technique this usually provides a good cholangiogram and overcomes the problem of air bubbles so frequently encountered when an on-table T-tube cholangiogram is employed. We would also usually combine this with choledochoscopy. It has

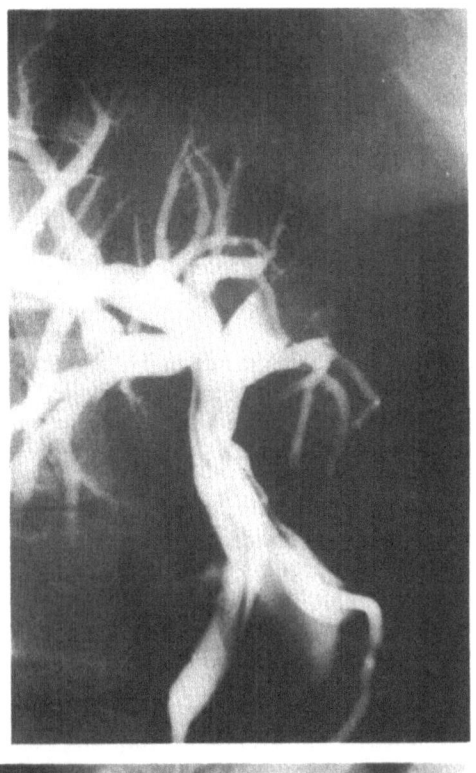

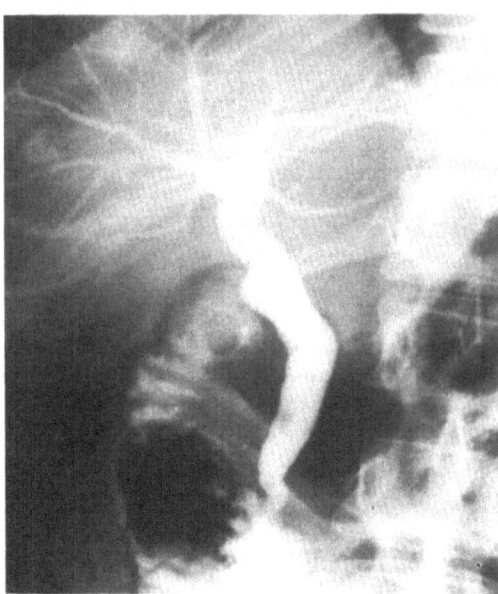

Figure 6.13 (a) Postoperative T-tubogram showing a large retained stone in the left hepatic duct. Its presence had been shown preoperatively by ERCP but attempts to remove it at the time of operation were unsuccessful. A 16F T-tube was placed in the duct and the stone was successfully removed percutaneously 8 weeks later. (b) This patient began to re-experience right upper quadrant pain 8 years after cholecystectomy. Five years later she was investigated and found on ERCP to have several small retained stones in the CBD which were removed by endoscopic sphincterotomy

been our experience, and that of others, that one or both of these techniques reveals further stones in 6–25% of cases after what has been thought to have been a satisfactory duct clearance[91–93]. By this means it should be possible to obtain complete clearance of stones in virtually all cases. In patients with a dilated duct (>15 mm) in whom multiple stones are found, chole-dochoduodenostomy should be considered in order to reduce the likelihood of subsequent stone formation. Where this is done, an anastomosis of at least 2.5 cm should be created if recurrent cholangitis and the so-called 'sump' syndrome are not to be a problem[94,95]. In the event transduodenal exploration is essential for an impacted distal stone a formal sphincteroplasty with mucosa-to-mucosa suture of bile duct to duodenum is preferable to the less precise technique of sphincterotomy. The former is likely to result in a more complete division of the sphincter with less risk of haemorrhage and late stenosis[96].

Tumours – Periampullary or bile duct tumours occasionally present with symptoms persisting after cholecystectomy although such an occurrence should be prevented by full preoperative assessment of all jaundiced patients. However, where they do occur, tumours should be staged as fully as possible with complete cholangiography and assessment of vascular involvement, and restriction or bypass surgery may then be used as indicated. In the older age groups and in high risk patients endoscopic sphincterotomy should be considered for periampullary and low bile duct lesions and endoprosthetic stents should be considered for pancreatic tumours. These may be placed either endoscopically[97] or percutaneously[98] depending on local expertise.

Other biliary disease – Occasionally stones within a cystic duct remnant may cause symptoms and necessitate surgical re-exploration. Sphincter of Oddi incompetence following either surgical or endoscopic sphincterotomy usually leads to duodenobiliary reflux with bile infection and although most patients remain asymptomatic, debris may accumulate and cause recurrent pan-creatitis or cholangitis. This is particularly liable to occur where a degree of stenosis begins to develop at the sphincterotomy site or at the site of an inadequate choledochoduodenostomy. In such patients chole-dochojejunostomy with a long (70 cm) Roux loop should overcome the problem of ascending infection and reflux. Iatrogenic choledochoduodenal fistula may follow rigid instrumentation of the lower duct (e.g. with Bakes' dilators) and be a source of symptoms following cholecystectomy[77]. Although these will usually settle without surgical intervention, in some instances a biliary–enteric bypass may become necessary.

Treatment of non-biliary disease – Wound problems are frequently responsible for postcholecystectomy symptoms. Where an incisional hernia is present this will usually require surgical repair. An area of localized tenderness perhaps relating to neuroma formation is sometimes found and may respond to intercostal nerve block or section. While intra-abdominal adhesions are common after cholecystectomy they very infrequently cause postoperative symptoms. Duodenogastric reflux may occur and be responsible for post-cholecystectomy flatulent dyspepsia. This condition is found in some patients in association with gallstones[99,100] and has recently been reported to be more frequent following cholecystectomy[101,102]. In such cases medical treatment with a coating agent such as sucralfate or aluminium hydroxide together with metoclopramide to enhance gastric emptying may be useful. Recurrent symptoms after cholecystectomy may be the result of acute or chronic pancreatitis. Such an occurrence should prompt a careful search for residual biliary calculi, or injury to the papillary region, particularly when there is no history of excessive alcohol intake or other causal factors.

Patients with no identified cause of pain – Even a thorough assessment of patients with postcholecystectomy symptoms will reveal a significant proportion in whom no organic cause can be found. It has been proposed that many of these patients have a psychosomatic origin for their symptoms and indeed psychological stress acting through the autonomic nervous system may be a factor in some cases[99,103]. A variety of pharmacological provocation tests have been used by some to justify endoscopic or even surgical procedures on the sphincter of Oddi. Encouraging results have been reported with the use of endoscopic manometric pressure studies of the sphincter of Oddi[104] as an indicator of the symptomatic response to endoscopic sphincterotomy or surgical spincteroplasty. These methods, however, require further validation before being widely applied. We have no personal experience of them and at present avoid intervention preferring simple symptomatic and supportive therapy whenever possible.

References

1. McSherry, C. K. and Glenn, F. (1980). The incidence and causes of death following surgery for non-malignant biliary tract disease. *Ann. Surg.*, 191, 271–5
2. Cranley, B. and Logan, H. (1980). Exploration of the common bile duct – the relevance of the clinical picture and the importance of per-operative cholangiography. *Br. J. Surg.*, 67, 869–72
3. Vellacott, K. D. and Powell, P. H. (1979). Exploration of the common bile duct, a comparative study. *Br. J. Surg.*, 66, 389–91
4. Houghton, P. W. J., Jenkinson, L. R. and Donaldson, L. A. (1985). Cholecystectomy in the elderly: a prospective study. *Br. J. Surg.*, 72, 220–2
5. Carter, A. E. (1973). Kocher's periampullary approach for common bile duct calculi. *Br. J. Surg.*, 60, 484–7
6. Braasch, J. W. and McCann, J. C. Jr. (1967). Observation on single section of the sphincter of Oddi. *Surg. Gynecol. Obstet.*, 125, 355–8
7. Peel, A. L. G. (1975). M. Chir. Thesis, University of Cambridge
8. Keighley, M. R. B., Flinn, R. and Alexander-Williams, J. (1976). Multivariate analysis of clinical and operative findings associated with biliary sepsis. *Br. J. Surg.*, 63, 528–31
9. Strachan, C. J. L., Black, J., Powis, S. J. A., Waterworth, T. A., Wise, R., Wilkinson, A. R. *et al.* (1977). Prophylactic use of cephazolin against wound sepsis after cholecystectomy. *Br. Med. J.*, 1, 1254–6
10. Stubbs, R. S. (1983). Wound infection after cholecystectomy: a case for routine prophylaxis. *Ann. R. Coll. Surg. Engl.*, 65, 30–1
11. Allan, A., Williams, J. T., Bolton, J. P. and LeQuesne, L. P. (1983). The use of graduated compression stockings in the prevention of post-operative deep venous thrombosis. *Br. J. Surg.*, 70, 172–4
12. Holford, C. P. (1976) Graded compression for preventing deep venous thrombosis. *Br. Med. J.*, 2, 969–70
13. Hills, N. H., Pflug, J. J., Jeyasingh, K., Boardman, L. and Calnan, J. S. (1972). Prevention

of deep venous thrombosis by intermittent pneumatic compression of calf. *Br. Med. J.*, **1**, 131–5

14. Roberts, V. C. and Colton, L. T. (1974). Prevention of post-operative deep venous thrombosis in patients with malignant disease. *Br. Med. J.*, **1**, 358–60

15. International Multicentre Trial (1975). Prevention of fatal post-operative pulmonary embolism by low dose heparin. *Lancet*, **2**, 45–51

16. Kakkar, V. V. (1978). The current status of low dose heparin in prophylaxis of thrombophlebitis and pulmonary embolism. *World J. Surg.*, **2**, 3–18

17. Viikari, S. J. (1960). Operative injuries to the bile ducts. *Acta Chir. Scand.*, **119**, 83–92

18. Gutgemann, A., Schriefers, K. H., Phillips, R. and Wulfing, D. (1965). Zur rekonstructiven chirurgie des verletzten und strikturierten grossen Gallenganges. *Beitrage Klinisch. Chir.*, **210**, 129–50

19. Bismuth, H. and Lazorthes, F. (1981). *Les Traumatismes Opertoires de la Voie Biliaire Principale.* Vol. 1. (Paris: Masson Ed)

20. Rosenquist, H. and Myrin, S. O. (1960). Operative injury to the bile ducts. *Acta Chir. Scand.* **119**, 92–107

21. Kune, G. A. and Sali, A. (1981). Benign biliary strictures. In *The Practice of Biliary Surgery.* 2nd Edn. (Oxford, London, Edinburgh, Boston, Melbourne: Blackwell Scientific)

22. Northover, J. M. A. and Terblanche, J. (1982). Applied surgical anatomy of the biliary tree. In Blumgart, L. H. (ed.) *The Biliary Tract. Clinical Surgery International.* Vol. 5, Ch. 1. (Edinburgh, London: Churchill Livingstone)

23. Benson, E. A. and Page, R. E. (1976). A practical re-appraisal of the extra-hepatic bile ducts. *Br. J. Surg.*, **63**, 853–60

24. Andren-Sandberg, A., Alinder, G. and Bengmark, S. (1985). Accidental lesions of the common bile duct at cholecystectomy. Pre- and per-operative factors of importance. *Ann. Surg.*, **201**, 328–32

25. Warren, K. W. and McDonald, W. M. (1964). Facts and fiction regarding strictures of the extrahepatic ducts. *Ann. Surg.*, **159**, 996–1010

26. Smith, R. (1979). Obstructions of the bile duct. *Br. J. Surg.*, **66**, 69–79

27. Simon, G. and Hamilton, W. J. (1978). The abdomen. In Simon, G. and Hamilton, W. J. (eds.) *X-ray Anatomy.* pp. 216–55. (London: Butterworths)

28. Northover, J. M. A. and Terblanche, J. (1979). A new look at the arterial blood supply of the bile duct in man and its surgical implications. *Br. J. Surg.*, **66**, 379–84

29. Kelley, C. J. and Blumgart, L. H. (1985). Per-operative cholangiography and post-cholecystectomy biliary strictures. *Ann. R. Coll. Surg. Engl.*, **67**, 93–5

30. Okuda, K., Tanikawa, K., Emura, T., Kuratomi, S., Jinnouchi, S., Urabe, K. *et al.* (1974). Non-surgical percutaneous transhepatic cholangiography – diagnostic significance in the medical problems of the liver. *Am. J. Dig. Dis.*, **19**, 21–36

31. Ham, J. (1979). Partial and complete atrophy affecting hepatic segments and lobes. *Br. J. Surg.*, **66**, 333–7

32. McPherson, G. A. D., Fitzpatrick, M., Benjamin, I. S., Tsikos, D., Lavender, P. and Blumgart, L. H. (1983). Can HIDA scanning provide a functional assessment of biliary–enteric anastomosis? *Br. J. Surg.*, **70**, 306–8

33. Bismuth, H. (1982). Post-operative strictures of the bile duct. In Blumgart, L. H. (ed.) *The Biliary Tract. Clinical Surgery International.* Vol. 5, p. 209. (Edinburgh, London: Churchill Livingstone)

34. Bismuth, H., Franco, D. and Corlette, M. B. (1978). Long term results of Roux-en-Y hepaticojejunostomy. *Surg. Gynecol. Obstet.*, **146**, 161–7

35. Belzer, F. O., Watts, J. McK., Ross, H. B. and Dunphy, J. E. (1965). Autoreconstruction of the common bile duct after venous patch graft. *Ann. Surg.*, **162**, 346–55

36. Ellis, H. and Hoile, R. W. (1980). Vein patch repair of the common bile duct. *J. R. Soc. Med.*, **73**, 635–7

37. Michie, W. and Gunn, A. A. (1964). Bile duct injuries. A new suggestion for their repair. *Br. J. Surg.*, **51**, 96–100

38. Smith, E. E. J., Bowley, N., Allison, D. J. and Blumgart, L. H. (1982). The management of post-traumatic intrahepatic cutaneous biliary fistulas. *Br. J. Surg.*, **69**, 317–8

39. Cattell, R. B. and Braasch, J. W. (1959). Primary repair of benign strictures of the bile duct. *Surg. Gynecol. Obstet.*, **109**, 531–8

40. Lahey, F. H. and Pyrtek, L. J. (1950). Experience with operative management of 280 strictures of the bile ducts. *Surg. Gynecol. Obstet.*, **91**, 25–6
41. Warren, K. W., Mountain, J. C. and Middel, A. I. (1971). Management of strictures of the biliary tract. *Surg. Clin. N. Am.*, **51**, 711–31
42. Cattell, R. B. and Braasch, J. W. (1959). Two-stage repairs of benign strictures of the bile duct. *Surg. Gynecol. Obstet.*, **109**, 691–6
43. Warren, K. W., McDonald, W. M. and Kune, G. A. (1966). Bile duct strictures. New concepts in the management of an old problem. In Irvine, W. T. (ed.) *Modern Trends in Surgery*. 2nd Edn. (London: Butterworth)
44. Hepp, J. and Couinaud, C. (1956). L'abord et l'utilisation du canal hepatique gauche dans les reparations de la voie biliaire principale. *La Presse Medicale*, **64**, 947–8
45. Soupault, R. and Couinaud, C. L. (1957). Sur un procede nouveau de derivation biliaire intra-hepatique. Les cholangio-jejunostomies gauches sans sacrifice hepatique. *La Presse Medicale*, **65**, 1157–9
46. Blumgart, L. H. and Kelley, C. J. (1984). Hepatico-jejunostomy in benign high bile duct stricture: approaches to the left hepatic ducts. *Br. J. Surg.*, **71**, 257–61
47. Blumgart, L. H. (1980). Hepatic resection. In Taylor, S. (ed.) *Recent Advances in Surgery*. Vol. 10, p. 1. (Edinburgh, London: Churchill Livingstone)
48. Longmire, W. P. Jr. and Sandford, M. C. (1949). Intrahepatic cholangiojejunostomy for biliary obstruction – further studies: report of 4 cases. *Ann. Surg.*, **130**, 455–60
49. Voyles, C. R. and Blumgart, L. H. (1982). A technique for the construction of high biliary-enteric anastomoses. *Surg. Gynecol. Obstet.*, **154**, 885–7
50. Smith, R. (1969). Strictures of the bile ducts. *Proc. R. Soc. Med.*, **62**, 131–7
51. Smith, R. (1979). Obstructions of the bile duct. *Br. J. Surg.*, **66**, 69–79
52. Smith, R. (1981). Injuries of the bile ducts. In Smith, R. and Sherlock (eds.) *Surgery of the Gallbladder and Bile Ducts*. 2nd Edn., p. 361. (London, Boston, Sydney, Toronto: Butterworth)
53. Blumgart, L. H. (1978). Biliary tract obstruction – new approaches to old problems. *Am. J. Surg.*, **135**, 19–31
54. Blumgart, L. H., Kelley, C. J. and Benjamin, I. S. (1984). Benign bile duct stricture following cholecystectomy: critical factors in management. *Br. J. Surg.*, **71**, 836–43
55. Adson, M. A. and Wychulis, A. R. (1968). Portal hypertension in secondary biliary cirrhosis. *Arch. Surg.*, **96**, 604–12
56. Ekman, C. A. and Sandblom, P. (1962). Bilio-intestinal anastomosis as a cause of liver cirrhosis with portal hypertension. *Acta Chir. Scand.*, **123**, 383–8
57. Sedgwick, C. E., Poulantzas, J. K. and Kune, G. A. (1966). Management of portal hypertension secondary to bile duct stenosis: review of 18 cases with splenorenal shunt. *Ann. Surg.*, **163**, 949–53
58. Way, L. W. and Dunphy, J. E. (1972). Biliary stricture. *Am. J. Surg.*, **124**, 287–95
59. Toufanian, A., Carey, L. C. and Martin, E. T. Jr. (1978). Transhepatic biliary dilatation: an alternative to surgical reconstruction. *Curr. Surg.*, **35**, 70–3
60. Cattell, R. B. and Braasch, J. W. (1959). General considerations in the management of benign stricture of the bile duct. *N. Engl. J. Med.*, **261**, 929–33
61. Kune, G. A. (1979). Bile duct injury during cholecystectomy. Causes, prevention and surgical repair in 1979. *Aust. N.Z. J. Surg.*, **49**, 35–40
62. Braasch, J. W., Bolter, J. S. and Rossi, R. L. (1981). A technique of biliary tract reconstruction with complete follow-up in 44 consecutive cases. *Ann. Surg.*, **194**, 635–8
63. Sandblom, P., Snegesser, F. and Mirkovitch, V. (1984). Hepatic haemobilia: haemorrhage from the intrahepatic biliary tract, a review. *World J. Surg.*, **8**, 41–50
64. Harlafus, N. N. and Akin, J. T. (1977). Haemobilia from ruptured hepatic artery aneurysm. *Am. J. Surg.*, **33**, 229–32
65. Fagan, E. A., Allison, D. J., Chadwick, V. S. and Hodgson, H. J. F. (1980). Treatment of haemobilia by selective arterial embolisation. *Gut*, **21**, 541–4
66. Kelley, C. J., Hemingway, A. P., McPherson, G. A. D., Allison, D. J. and Blumgart, L. H. (1983). Non-surgical management of post-cholecystectomy haemobilia. *Br. J. Surg.*, **70**, 502–4
67. Bengmark, S. and Rosengren, K. (1970). Angiographic studies of the collateral circulation of the liver after ligation of the hepatic artery in man. *Am. J. Surg.*, **119**, 620–4

68. Peterson, L. M., Collins, J. J. and Wilson, R. E. (1968). Acute pancreatitis occurring after operation. *Surg. Gynecol. Obstet.*, **127**, 23–8
69. White, T. T., Morgan, A. and Hopton, D. (1970). Postoperative pancreatitis. A study of seventy cases. *Am. J. Surg.*, **120**, 132–5
70. Imrie, C. W., McKay, A. J., Benjamin, I. S. and Blumgart, L. H. (1978). Secondary acute pancreatitis: aetiology, prevention, diagnosis and management. *Br. J. Surg.*, **65**, 399–402
71. Ranson, J. H. C., Rifkind, K. M. and Turner, J. W. (1976). Prognostic signs and nonoperative peritoneal lavage in acute pancreatitis. *Surg. Gynecol. Obstet.*, **143**, 209–19
72. Keighley, M. R. B. and Graham, N. G. (1973). The aetiology and prevention of pancreatitis following biliary-tract operations. *Br. J. Surg.*, **60**, 149–52
73. McCutcheon, A. D. (1968). A fresh approach to the pathogenesis of pancreatitis. *Gut*, **9**, 296–310
74. Bodvall, B. (1973). The post-cholecystectomy syndrome. *Clin. Gastroenterol.*, **2**, 103–26
75. Bates, T., Mercer, J. C. and Harrison, M. (1984). Symptomatic gallstone disease: before and after cholecystectomy. *Gut*, **25**, A579, F105
76. Blumgart, L. H. and Lygidakis, N. J. (1982). The postcholecystectomy patient. In Blumgart, L. H. (ed.) *The Biliary Tract. Clinical Surgery International.* Vol. 5, Ch. 9. (Edinburgh, London: Churchill Livingstone)
77. Blumgart, L. H., Carachi, R., Imrie, C. W., Benjamin, I. S. and Duncan, J. G. (1977). Diagnosis and management of post-cholecystectomy symptoms: the place of endoscopy and retrograde choledochopancreatography. *Br. J. Surg.*, **64**, 809–16
78. Hunt, D. R. and Blumgart, L. H. (1980). Iatrogenic choledochoduodenal fistula: an unsuspected cause of post-cholecystectomy symptoms. *Br. J. Surg.*, **67**, 10–13
79. Acosta, J. M. and Ledesma, C. L. (1974). Gallstone migration as a cause of acute pancreatitis. *N. Engl. J. Med.*, **290**, 484–7
80. Kelly, T. R. (1976). Gallstone pancreatitis. Pathophysiology. *Surgery*, **80**, 488–92
81. Wheeler, M. H. (1977). Dissolution of retained choledochal calculi. *Ann. R. Coll. Surg. Engl.*, **59**, 153–7
82. Thistle, J. L., Carlson, G. L., Hoffman, A. F., LaRusso, N. F., MacCarty, R. L., Flynn, G. L., Higuchi, W. I. and Babayou, V. K. (1980). Mono-octanoin, a dissolution agent for retained cholesterol bile duct stones: physical properties and clinical applications. *Gastroenterology*, **78**, 1016–22
83. Burhenne, H. L. (1973). Non-operative retained biliary tract stone extraction: a new roentgenologic technique. *Am. J. Roentgenol.*, **117**, 388–99
84. Burhenne, H. L. (1976). Complications of non-operative extraction of retained common bile duct stones. *Am. J. Surg.*, **131**, 260–2
85. Safrany, L. (1978). Endoscopic treatment of biliary tract diseases. *Lancet*, **2**, 983–5
86. Cotton, P. B. (1980). Non-operative removal of bile duct stones by duodenoscopic sphincterotomy. *Br. J. Surg.*, **67**, 1–5
87. Cotton, P. B. (1984). Endoscopic management of bile duct stones (apples and oranges). *Gut*, **25**, 587–97
88. Rosch, W., Riemann, J. F., Lux, G. and Lindner, H. G. (1981). Long-term follow-up after endoscopic sphincterotomy. *Endoscopy*, **13**, 152–3
89. Girard, R. M. and Legros, G. (1981). Retained and recurrent bile duct stones. Surgical or non-surgical removal? *Ann. Surg.*, **193**, 150–4
90. Myat Thu Ya, Robinson, D. and Gunn, A. A. (1973). Per-operative cholangiography. *Br. J. Surg.*, **60**, 711–2
91. Stubbs, R. S. and Blumgart, L. H. (1984). Exploration of the common bile duct: effect of a change of policy in one surgical unit. *J. R. Coll. Surg. Edin.*, **29**, 76–80
92. LeQuesne, L. P. and Bolton, J. P. (1980). Choledocholithiasis. Incidence, diagnosis and operative procedures. In Maingot, R. (ed.) *Maingot's Abdominal Operations.* 7th Edn., Ch. 66. (Norwalk, Connecticut: Appleton-Century-Crofts)
93. Nora, P. F., Berci, G., Dorazio, R. A., Kirschenbaum, G., Shore, J. M., Tomkins, R. K. and Wilson, S. D. (1977). Operative choledochoscopy. Results of prospective study in several institutions. *Am. J. Surg.*, **133**, 105–9
94. Schein, C. J. and Gliedman, M. L. (1981). Choledocho-duodenostomy as an adjunct to choledocholithotomy. *Surg. Gynecol. Obstet.*, **152**, 797–804

95. Madden, J. L. (1973). Common duct stones: their origin and surgical management. *Surg. Clin. N. Am.*, **53**, 1095–113

96. Jones, S. A. (1973). Sphincteroplasty (not sphincterotomy) in the treatment of biliary tract disease. *Surg. Clin. N. Am.*, **53**, 1123–37

97. Stanley, J., Gobien, R. P., Cunningham, J. and Andriole, J. (1986). Biliary decompression: an institutional comparison of percutaneous and endoscopic methods. *Radiology*, **158**, 195–7

98. Coons, H. G. and Carey, P. H. (1983). Large-bore, long biliary endoprostheses (biliary stents) for improved drainage. *Radiology*, **148**, 89–94

99. Johnson, A. G. (1975). Cholecystectomy and gallstone dyspepsia. *Ann. R. Coll. Surg. Engl.*, **56**, 69–80

100. Johnson, A. G. (1972). Pyloric function and gallstone dyspepsia. *Br. J. Surg.*, **59**, 449–54

101. Cheadle, W. G., Pathi, V., Mackie, C. R. and Cuschieri, A. (1984). Effect of gallbladder function on duodenogastric reflux. *Gut*, **25**, A1138, T20

102. Brough, W. A., Taylor, T. V. and Torrance, H. B. (1984). Role of the pylorus and gallbladder in reflux associated gastritis. *Gut*, **25**, A578, F101

103. Valberg, L. S., Jabbari, M., Kerr, J. W., Curtis, A. C., Ramchand, S. and Prentice, R. S. A. (1971). Biliary pain in young women in the absence of gallstones. *Gastroenterology*, **60**, 1020–26

104. Geenen, J., Hogan, W. J., Toouli, J., Dodds, W. J. and Venu, R. (1984). A prospective randomised study of the efficacy of endoscopic sphincterotomy for patients with presumptive sphincter of Oddi dysfunction. *Gastroenterology*, **86**, 1086

7
Endoscopic Management

D. L. CARR-LOCKE

INTRODUCTION

Endoscopic retrograde cholangiopancreatography (ERCP) has had a dramatic impact on the diagnostic approach to biliary disease and its therapeutic development, endoscopic sphincterotomy (ES), has, in the 10 years since its introduction[1,2], had a similar effect on the management of biliary disease in general and bile duct stones in particular. Where this technique has become readily available it has undoubtedly influenced the surgical approach to bile duct stones as endoscopic treatment has now become a well-accepted mode of therapy for certain categories of patients. There is still a great need, however, to define accurately the place of endoscopic treatment and its associated techniques in the management of bile duct stones in comparison with long-established principles of surgical treatment. The precise documentation of risk factors and how they determine outcome from different modes of therapy is essential to enable clinicians to make rational and logical decisions for their patients with gallstone disease. Many current evaluations comparing endoscopic and surgical therapy are necessarily based on retrospective analyses since results of randomized clinical trials are not yet available. This is bedevilled, however, with the problems of comparing dissimilar groups of patients already selected to undergo widely different forms of treatment. It is essential, therefore, that care is taken to use the most appropriate alternative for comparative assessment. For example, there is little point in quoting surgical morbidity and mortality figures for cholecystectomy when considering similar results for endoscopic sphincterotomy for stones in the bile duct. Preliminary results from the author's own unit will be cited where relevant.

General clinical interest and surgical enthusiasm for ERCP and ES has grown enormously in the UK and in the author's own practice over the last 10 years referrals have grown to over 600 ERCP requests per annum of which more than a quarter are for therapeutic considerations. This has allowed a personal experience of over 700 sphincterotomies up to the end of 1985 and the views expressed in this chapter are based principally on this work with comments derived from collected reports of recognized centres. Endoscopic management encompasses a number of techniques but only *per oral* methods relating to endoscopic sphincterotomy for managing bile duct stones and associated problems will be discussed.

ENDOSCOPIC SPHINCTEROTOMY AND RELATED TECHNIQUES

General considerations

Any centre now offering an ES service for the treatment of bile duct stones must be fully equipped with a suitable array of endoscopic hardware and have access to a radiology suite providing high quality image-intensification and permanent radiographs. The team must be fully cognisant of all the basic procedures and lesser-used techniques as well as potential complications and their management and must include medical, nursing and technical endoscopy staff together with radiography and portering personnel who together allow for smooth running of an ERCP/ES session and facilitate any decisions which need to be made during an examination.

Details of patient preparation, sedation, use of drugs during endoscopy and basic endoscopic technique for ERCP are described in Chapter 4 and provide the basis for proceeding to ES with certain additional considerations. Instrument manufacturers have developed a wide variety of side-viewing duodenoscopes all of which are now fully insulated for electrosurgical use. The newer large channels of 3.7 or 4.2 mm diameter provide a useful extra ability to aspirate duodenal contents easily during procedures as well as allowing placement of larger diameter tubes for nasobiliary and internal drainage. It is essential for the endoscopy staff to explain the nature of the procedure to the patient well beforehand, outlining the purpose, advantages and possible hazards of the examination and therapy. It will happen occasionally that a severe complication, such as haemorrhage, will supervene after ES too rapidly for prolonged explanations to take place with the patient at this stage and forewarning, however small the risk, should be mandatory (as should also be the case for surgical procedures). The patient's coagulation status is always checked and corrected when necessary. Resuscitation facilities should be available and ES should never be undertaken in an institution where a blood transfusion service or surgical staff are not readily to hand to manage complications that may occur. Antibiotics are given in selected patients.

Standard technique

Techniques of performing endoscopic sphincterotomy (ES), or endoscopic papillotomy as it is still termed in some parts of Europe, have remained little changed since their introduction in Germany[2] and Japan[1]. The majority of patients undergoing ES, immediately following diagnostic ERCP which delineates the problem to be treated and allows accurate placement of the instruments within the common bile duct (CBD), will have a vertical or near-vertical incision made from the papillary orifice of the CBD in a cephalad direction along the duodenal wall following the intramural course of the CBD

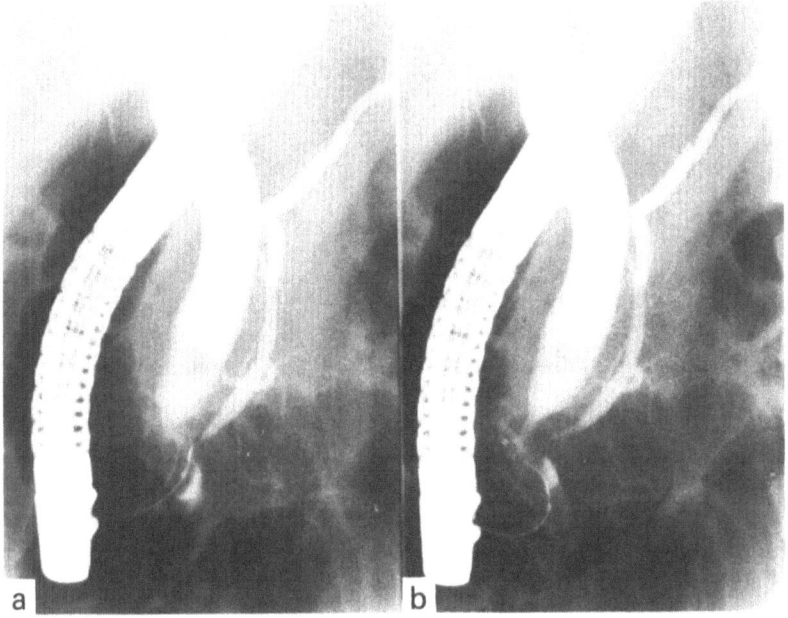

Figure 7.1 Radiograph showing standard sphincterotome in closed (a) and open (b) positions prior to spincterotomy

for a variable length (on average 10–15 mm) depending on local anatomy, degree of bile duct dilatation and size of stone(s) to be removed (Figure 7.1). This effectively ablates the sphincter of Oddi, or choledochal sphincter, and is usually substantially larger than a surgical sphincterotomy being more akin to a surgical sphincteroplasty. The incision is produced by the controlled application of a blended cutting and coagulating diathermy current from a sphincterotome, delivered by a power source specifically designated for endoscopic use which will not exceed 100 watts.

The Demling–Classen-type sphincterotome consists of a catheter of external diameter 1.7 mm within which a wire passes from a control handle, held by the endoscopist or assistant, to the catheter tip where it becomes exteriorized for a variable length (1–3 cm) depending on the exact design. The control handle allows connection to the diathermy source and tension to be transmitted to the distal wire which assumes a 'bow-string' appearance. A wide variety of sphincterotomes have become available in recent years (Figure 7.2), some with well-defined advantages, e.g. more distal placement of the external wire to aid contact when deep cannulation is difficult or impossible; a shortened external wire length to aid contact when access is limited; the addition of a rotating capability and designs specifically made to facilitate practices and whims of the clinician-designer[6]. It is fundamental to good ES technique that complete control of wire tension and diathermy current are maintained at all times by the endoscopist, whether or not the ES incision is

175

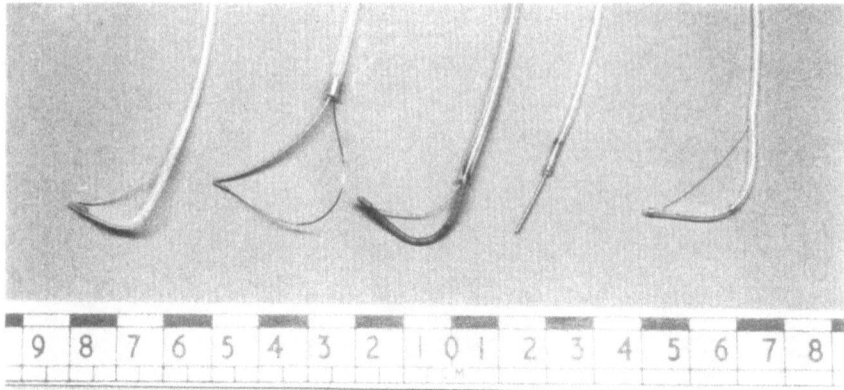

Figure 7.2. Range of sphincterotomes, right to left: standard, needle-knife, rotating, reverse and precut

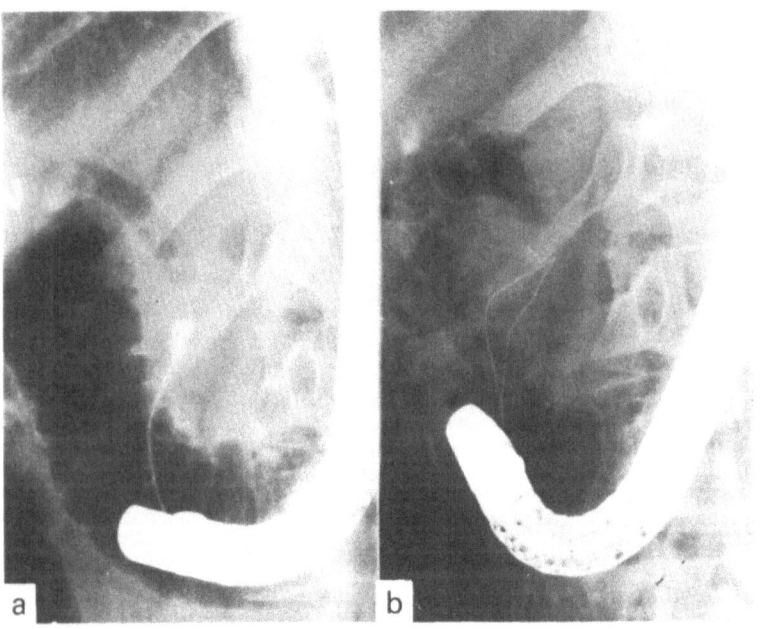

Figure 7.3 Radiograph showing reverse sphincterotome in closed (a) and open (b) positions in patient with Billroth 2 partial gastrectomy

made as a single continuous movement or in incremental steps. More recently developed power units incorporate a timed/pulsed generator which may be safer. Radiographic confirmation of correct sphincterotome placement is mandatory to avoid pancreatic trauma.

Other sphincterotomy methods

Occasionally an experienced operator will find it impossible to insert the standard sphincterotome deeply into the bile duct to initiate an ES and in this situation a preliminary precut or deroofing of the papilla may be made with a suitable 'precut' sphincterotome[7] or straight wire 'needle-knife'[8]. An incision is made in the expected direction of the CBD but it is necessarily a blind procedure and thus carries an increased risk of complications. It will be needed in less than 5% of cases. The needle-knife may also be used to gain entry into the CBD above the papilla to relieve obstruction from an impacted stone by cutting directly through the duodenal wall when the distended intramural duct is clearly identifiable. The choledochoduodenal fistula so created may be left as the definitive 'sphincteromy' or be extended down towards the papillary orifice to produce a more orthodox result.

In patients with a Billroth 2 partial gastrectomy ES is more difficult since the papilla must be approached via the afferent jejunal loop. Increasing experience with ERCP in such patients and success of cannulation with side- or forward-viewing endoscopes has also improved rates of successful ES[9,10]. This has been facilitated by the development of special sphincterotomes and the reverse-type of Sohma sphincterotome would now seem to be the instrument of choice (Figure 7.3).

Stone extraction

It is our and most other centres' practice to attempt stone extraction from the bile duct immediately after ES as this decreases the chances of subsequent complications due to retained stones and removes the necessity of a check ERCP at a later date to confirm spontaneous stone passage. Many stones (especially those less than 10 mm diameter) will pass spontaneously after standard ES but most experts prefer to attempt their immediate extraction using a number of accessory instruments. Although an active extraction policy will be successful in over 90% of attempts, these techniques are not without difficulty and hazard in some patients. The endoscopist must be experienced and confident that the incision is large enough, otherwise bile duct trauma or stone impaction may result. A Dormia-type basket is the most popular device for entrapping stones and removing them either completely, through the patient's mouth on withdrawal of the duodenoscope, if the stone is single (Figure 7.4), or merely into the duodenum, if multiple (Figure 7.5), with repeated passes of the basket. Care must be taken not to exert undue force in this process, to protect patient and endoscope, and to avoid impaction of the basket wires into the stone should release of the stone become necessary. Stone extraction with a Fogarty-type balloon catheter (Figure 7.6) is less traumatic and avoids the possibility of impaction but balloons are currently expensive and insufficiently robust to allow multiple usage. Most units reserve them for special circumstances, e.g. small diameter bile ducts, stone(s) tightly fitting the bile duct and attempts to remove multiple stones simultaneously.

It may be possible to remove small stones without ES, either by relaxing the sphincter of Oddi pharmacologically with lingual application of glyceryl

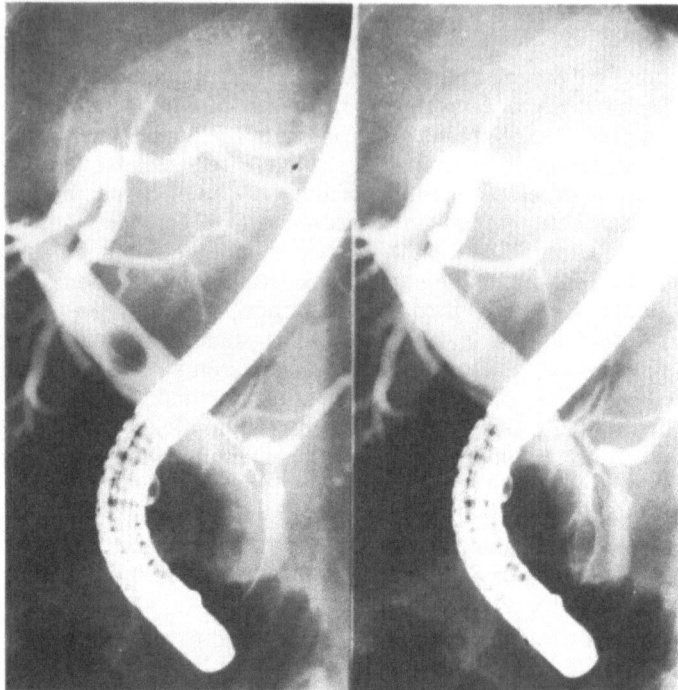

Figure 7.4 Radiograph showing gallstone extraction by Dormia basket

trinitrate[11] (Figure 7.7) or by balloon dilatation of the sphincter[12] but medium-
and long-term results of these procedures are not yet known.

Large and difficult stones (nasobiliary intubation/infusion and lithotripsy)

Some stones may be too large to extract through a standard ES (Figure 7.8),
or there may be a disproportionately narrow lower CBD segment (Figure 7.9)
or unfavourable duodenal or papillary anatomy owing to a large duodenal
diverticulum, previous surgical duodenotomy or sphincter operation. In some
patients surgery will be the most appropriate course of action, but in those
with continuing high risks for surgical bile duct exploration alternative
methods are required. Most endoscopists would now insert a nasobiliary
catheter[13] immediately following failure to clear the bile duct of stones and
where stone impaction seems likely to occur, in order to establish external
bile drainage and so diminish the risk of pain, exacerbation of jaundice and,
most importantly, cholangitis (Figure 7.10). The catheter is a Teflon or
polyethylene tube 3 metres long and usually of seven French gauge external
diameter with a preformed pigtail at its tip and multiple side holes. The pigtail
straightens out over a guide wire for insertion via the duodenoscope across
the papilla (after ES) into the CBD and above the remaining stone(s). The
guide wire is then removed to allow the tip to reshape itself and the endoscope

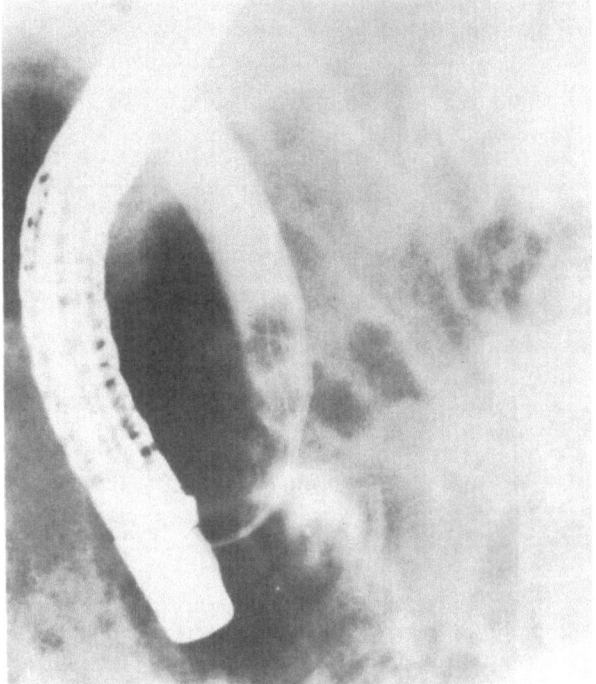

Figure 7.5   Radiograph showing multiple small stone extraction by Dormia basket

is then withdrawn over the catheter leaving a generous loop in the stomach. The tube is re-routed from mouth to nose with a temporary naso-oral overtube and it is connected to a drainage bag. Antibiotics are administered for the duration of tube drainage and cholangiography can be repeated after an arbitrary interval of 24–72 hours to check on spontaneous stone passage as a guide to further therapy. Nasobiliary catheters are tolerated remarkably well for many days and occasionally longer. Loss of bile for prolonged periods can be minimized by connecting the nasobiliary catheter to a separate naso-gastric tube inserted via the other nostril. The technique of nasobiliary drainage is undoubtedly an invaluable adjunct to ES and even when stones are still retained a patient's general condition may be sufficiently improved to allow surgery to be contemplated.

Two additional approaches are currently used for those patients unfit for surgical intervention: nasobiliary infusion and stone fragmentation.

Irrigation with saline[14] or heparinized saline[15] via a nasobiliary tube to displace retained stones is rarely successful for anything but very small stones as has been the experience with T-tubes. Attempts to dissolve or fragment bile duct stones chemically began with ether[16] but side-effects limited its use. The technique was re-introduced when bile salt solutions such as sodium cholate[17] became available but these proved inefficient and potentially hazardous. A semisynthetic vegetable oil, mono-octanoin, was shown to be a

179

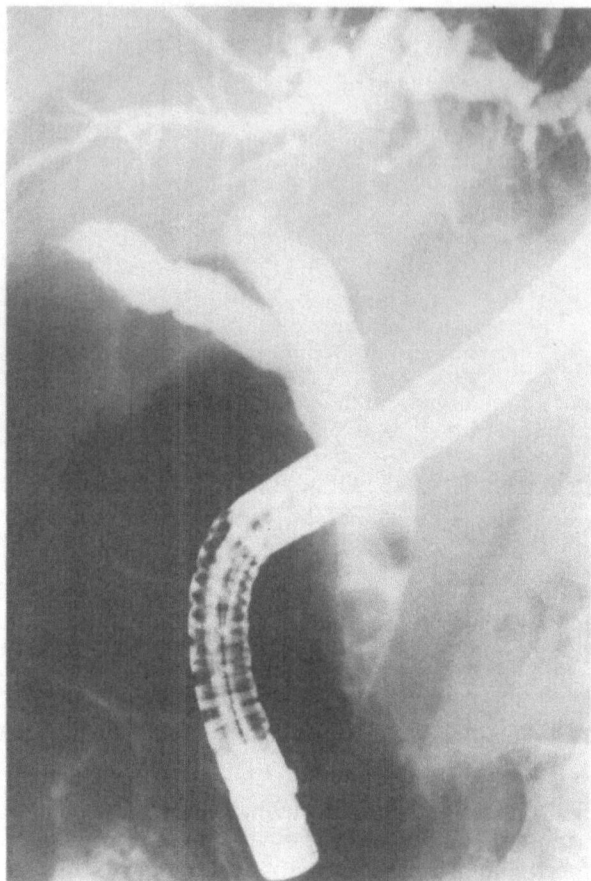

Figure 7.6 Radiograph showing gallstone extraction by balloon catheter (note shrunken empty gallbladder)

more efficient cholesterol solvent than cholate[18]. Mono-octanoin has been used experimentally for the dissolution of bile duct stones since 1977 in the form of the proprietary preparation, Capmul 8210 (renamed Moctanin), which is composed of 70% glyceryl-1-mono-octanoate and 30% glyceryl-1,2-di-octanoate.

Some practical considerations are important when handling this agent. At room temperature Moctanin is a solid anhydrous oil and requires heating to body temperature to become liquid such that sterile filtration can be applied although it has been used in its native form as it possesses bacteriostatic properties. Addition of 10% water reduces viscosity without affecting cholesterol solubilization capacity and may actually improve it[19]. Adequate bile duct drainage during infusion is essential but most patients in this group will have had a sphincterotomy initially, unlike those receiving Moctanin postoperatively via a T-tube. The addition of an overflow manometer allowing

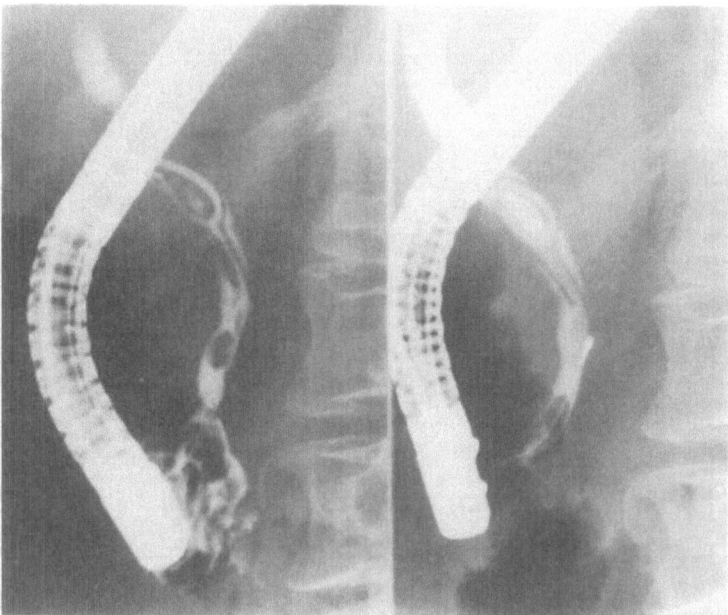

Figure 7.7 Radiograph showing gallstone extraction by basket after lingual GTN without prior sphincterotomy (T-tube *in situ*)

12 cm pressure in the infusion line is a further safeguard against perfusion of an obstructed bile duct. The agent must be kept warm at all times during infusion and we have used the simple arrangement of a standard illuminated light bulb closely positioned near the infusion pump which provides an advantage of close visual supervision of the infusion in progress (Figure 7.11). The warmed oil has a propensity to leak from the smallest break in the infusion tubing, especially at joints, and care must be taken to ensure that the delivery system is kept as closed as possible, also avoiding introduction of infection. Infusion rates of 1–5 ml/h are commonly used and immediately discontinued if pain is experienced by the patient or if sepsis supervenes. Many workers routinely suspend infusion during the patient's meal times.

International results of Moctanin infusion via nasobiliary catheter, T-tube, percutaneous transhepatic catheter and cholecystostomy tube have been collected from 222 clinicians treating 343 patients between 1977 and 1983[20]. Mean age was 66 years (range 17–99), 97% had previously undergone biliary tract surgery and one third had an ES with unsuccessful bile duct clearance. Moctanin therapy was judged to be completely successful without need for further intervention in 25.6%, helpful in facilitating other extraction methods in 8.5% and partially successful in 20.4% when stones were rendered smaller but remained in the biliary tract. Thus the technique was useful in only 54.5%, with complete failure to influence stone size in 36.2% and aborted treatments in 9.3% owing to side-effects. These were present overall in 67%

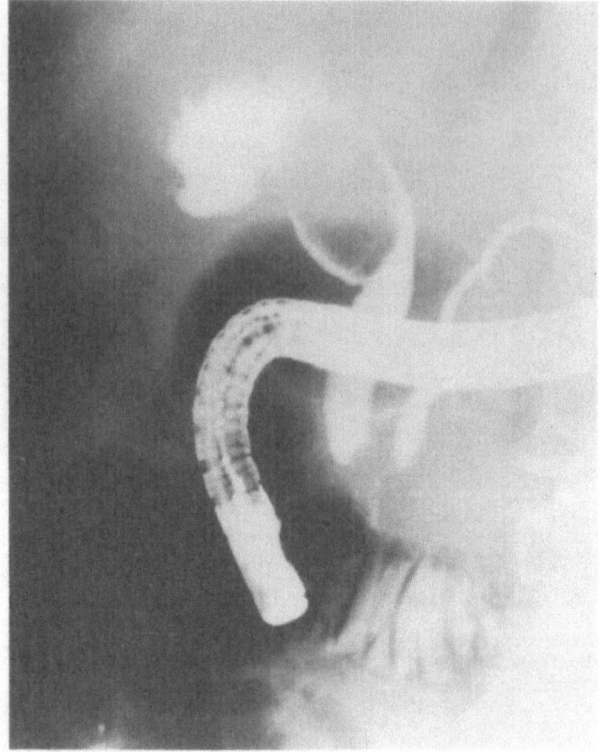

Figure 7.8 Radiograph showing large bile duct stone not amenable to endoscopic therapy

of patients but did not necessitate cessation of therapy in the majority. Abdominal pain was most common, with one form (not dose-related nor due to high infusion pressures) being described as burning and presumably a direct effect of the Moctanin. Nausea, vomiting and diarrhoea were reduced by lowering infusion rates. A variety of serious adverse effects occurred in 5% with haemorrhage from duodenal ulceration, acute pancreatitis, jaundice, pulmonary oedema, acidosis with hepatic encephalopathy, anaphylaxis, septicaemia and leukopenia but, despite advanced age and poor general condition in many of these patients, there were no deaths.

Further improvement in successful dissolution and bile duct clearance has been claimed by the addition of a bile salt/EDTA solution[21,22] but there are no controlled comparative studies. A new generation of solvents based on methyl-tert-butyl-ether (MTBE) is on the horizon for use in man[23] with the potential for dissolving cholesterol stones within a few hours but there are problems with using such compounds and clinical trials must be awaited to decide which of these will be safe and most effective.

Mechanical biliary lithotripsy for stone fragmentation within the bile duct has recently become available with the development of suitably modified Dormia baskets[24-26]. The plastic catheter of the basket is replaced by a metal

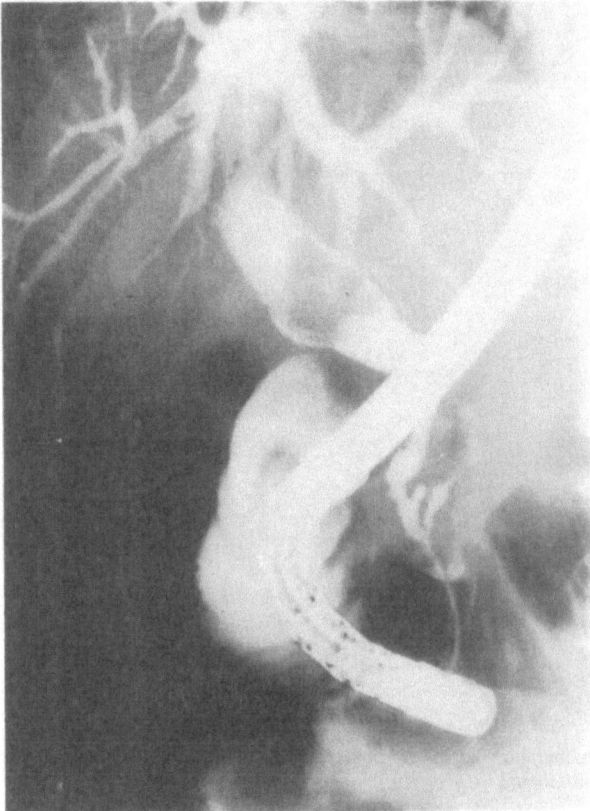

Figure 7.9 Radiograph showing a stone above a narrow bile duct segment not suitable for ES alone

sheath and the standard handle by a strong ratchet device through which a continuously increasing pressure may be applied to the entrapped stone (Figure 7.12) until fracture or shearing occur. Initial reports were enthusiastic with a high success rate for stone fragmentation[24] but subsequent experience in the UK and Europe seems less encouraging. Further prototypes permitting conversion of a standard basket to a crushing type[25] are welcome and may improve success in these difficult cases.

In exceptional circumstances when all endoscopic manoeuvres have failed and surgical intervention is contraindicated the insertion of an endoprosthesis (Figure 7.13) may seem justified to maintain bile flow although no long-term results are available.

More novel techniques have been attempted in the laboratory and to a limited extent in man including electrohydraulic shock waves[27], laser sphincterotomy[28], and ultrasound fragmentation[29,30] but none has yet achieved standards of clinical acceptability, safety or success.

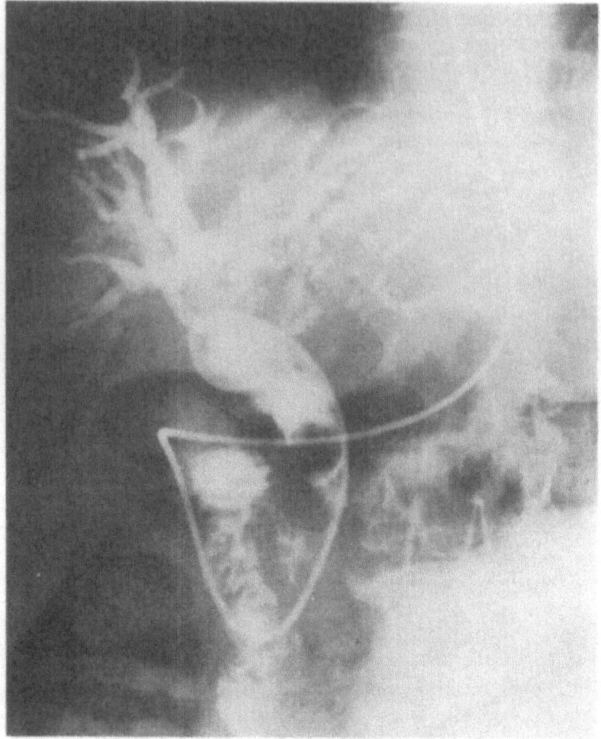

Figure 7.10 Radiograph showing nasobiliary catheter *in situ* with bile duct stone after failed post-ES extraction attempt

INDICATIONS FOR ENDOSCOPIC THERAPY

Patients with bile duct stones present with a variety of clinical problems either alone or in combination, e.g. cholestasis, pain, cholangitis, pancreatitis, or postoperatively on T-tube cholangiography. The popularity of ES in treating patients in all of these categories has become increasingly acceptable to clinicians and has been reflected in the growing numbers of patients referred to our unit, especially by surgeons.

Endoscopic sphincterotomy was initially considered justifiable only in elderly postcholecystectomy patients with recurrent or retained CBD stones, who were at high risk of serious complications from orthodox surgical CBD exploration or re-exploration at a time when few endoscopy centres could offer the technique and criticisms by surgical experts were common[31]. The impressive successes of ES in this group, however, and an expansion of units practising ES together with a low level of complications and a strong patient preference led many centres to widen their indications for the procedure to include younger and fitter postcholecystectomy patients. More recently a range of patients in whom the gallbladder is still *in situ* but in whom CBD stones give rise to the principal clinical problem have also been considered

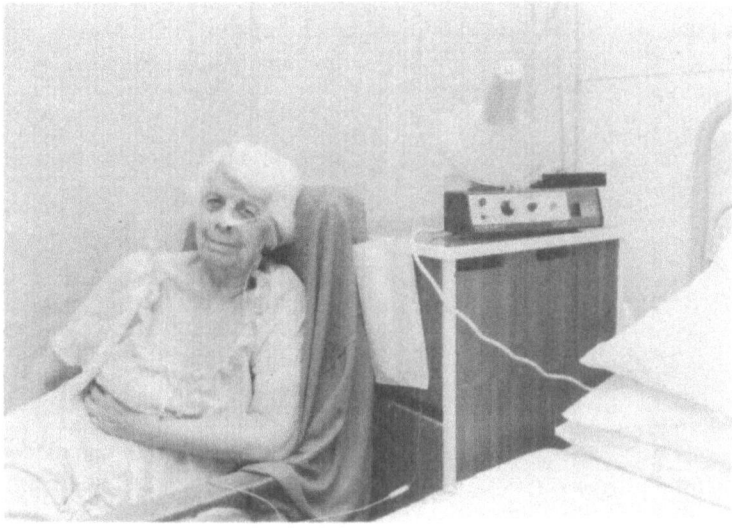

Figure 7.11   Mono-octanoin infusion via nasobiliary catheter

for treatment. Much of this has occurred in the complete absence of any comparative trials to aid decision-making and, indeed, there has been such enthusiasm for ES that the establishment of randomized trials has been difficult to organize. Nevertheless, they are essential to settle arguments about relative morbidity and mortality risks as different groups of patients are likely to be treated by either endoscopic or surgical means and these will not necessarily be comparable[32].

The endoscopist is now faced with the referral of a number of clearly defined groups of patients with confirmed or suspected bile duct stones for whom ES may be indicated (see Table 7.1) and these groups are described in detail later. Until such time that prospective trials are available to guide our decisions for ES or surgery it is the responsibility of endoscopists to review their own successes, failures and complications and, more importantly, for surgeons to do the same, in order to make representative comparisons possible and worthwhile and in order to offer our patients the best alternatives.

RESULTS AND COMPLICATIONS OF ENDOSCOPIC THERAPY

Short-term success of ES

Successful endoscopic treatment of bile duct stones requires an adequate ES and this is now achieved in over 90% of attempts in most reported series with noticeable improvement as experience increases[4,32-39]. Failure to achieve an ES or one of sufficient size is usually due to: (a) inaccessibility of the papilla, e.g. pyloric or duodenal stenosis, papilla within a duodenal diverticulum or in the afferent loop of a Billroth 2 partial gastrectomy, and occasionally difficulties due to a previous surgical duodenotomy or surgery to the papilla

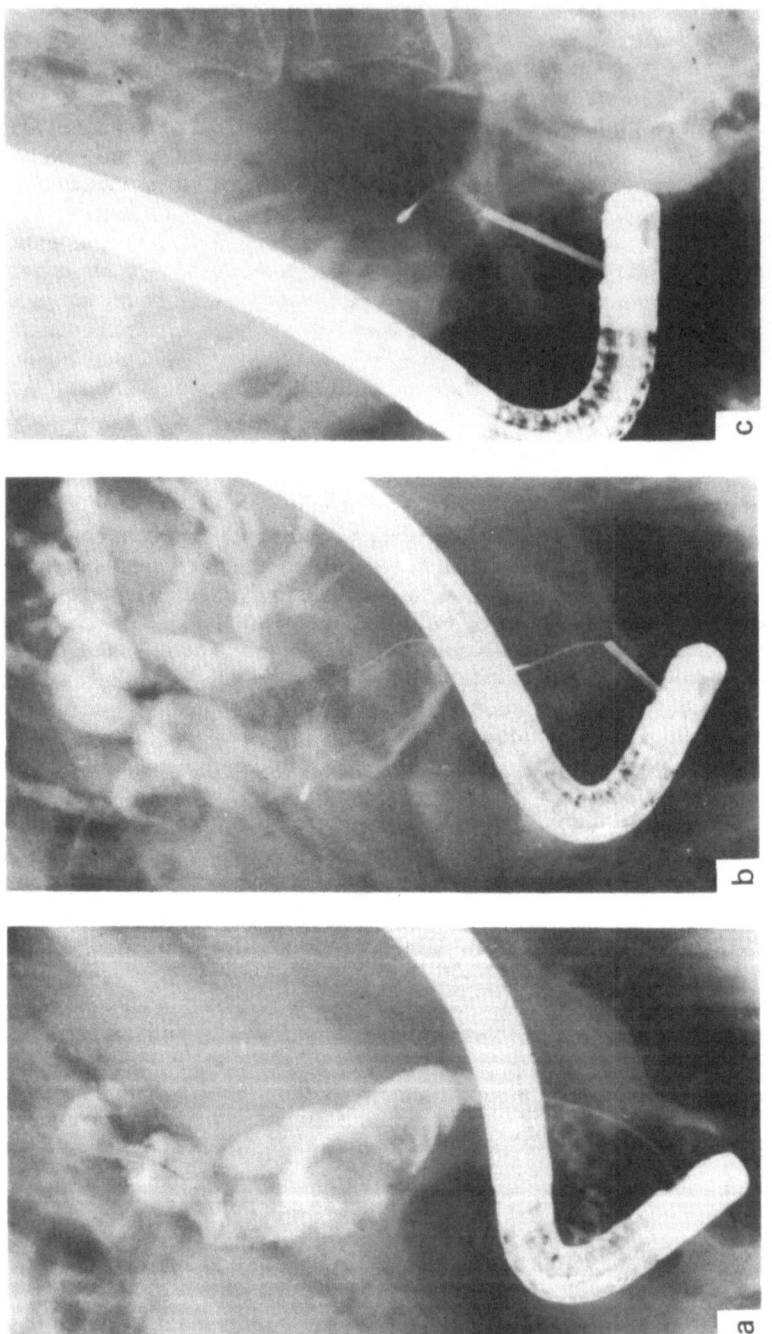

Figure 7.12 Radiograph in postcholecystectomy patient of (a) large stone above narrow lower CBD segment, (b) entrapped by basket of lithotriptor and (c) appearance after full closure of basket

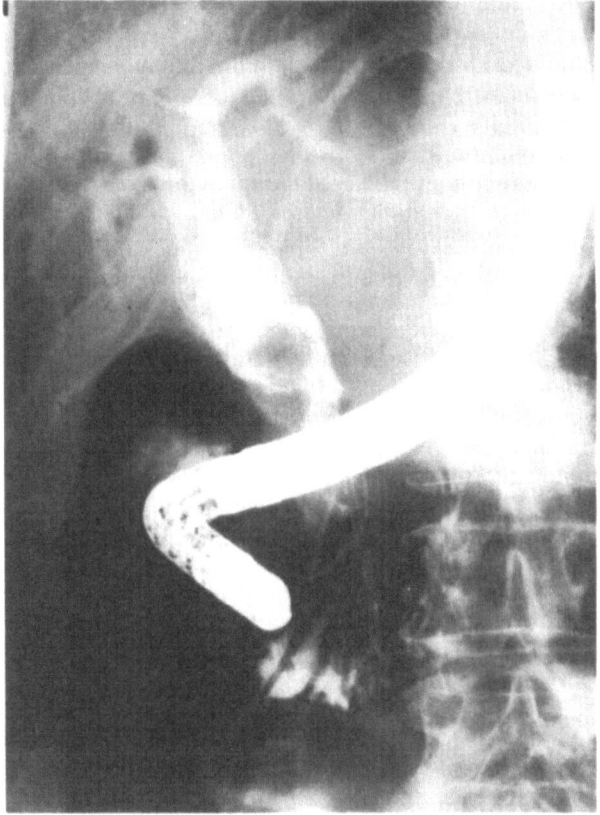

Figure 7.13 Radiograph showing double pigtail endoprosthesis *in situ* for large bile duct stone not removable after ES

Table 7.1 Clinical groupings of patients with bile duct stones amenable to endoscopic therapy

Recent biliary surgery, T-tube *in situ*, retained stone(s)
Remote biliary surgery, no T-tube, variable risk factors for surgical CBD (re)exploration
Recent cholecytostomy, CBD stone(s) shown on tubogram
Gallbladder in situ, variable risk factors for surgical management, variable need for subsequent cholecystectomy
Acute cholangitis irrespective of gallbladder status
Acute gallstone-associated pancreatitis irrespective of gallbladder status

itself; (b) technical failure resulting from cannulation difficulties; or (c) poor patient co-operation.

Although success rates for achieving ES are fairly uniform, rates for complete clearance of the CBD vary as not all endoscopists use extraction methods routinely and follow-up ERCP may be incomplete. Most experts would now expect to extract or confirm spontaneous passage of stones in at least 90% of successful sphincterotomies, making an overall successful therapeutic rate of over 80% and often over 90%. Failure to extract or pass stones may be due to size and/or number of stones within the duct or unfavourable duct diameter, usually in its retropancreatic segment (Figure 7.9). Stones up to 10 mm in diameter will rarely give rise to problems but with increasing size above 15–20 mm chance of retention rises.

Interpretation of success rates needs care as centres with greater expertise are more likely to be referred difficult cases who may be failures from attempts elsewhere and this will bias some results. Patient groups will also vary considerably from unit to unit and country to country reflecting different referral patterns, selection of patients and attitudes to endoscopic therapy.

In our own unit, over an 8-year period, of the 694 ES procedures performed by the author, 577 (83%) were for bile duct stones with a successful ES performance rate of 98%, extraction rate of 85% of the total group, with spontaneous passage in 5% and success in a further 2% after a period of nasobiliary drainage followed by infusion of Moctanin. This gives an overall successful therapeutic rate of 92% for all patients in whom a decision was taken to attempt ES but excludes those who were amenable to ES treatment but who were randomized to surgery as part of a comparative trial. In the earlier years of our experience some patients with unfavourable biliary anatomy or other potentially complicating problem were also excluded from analysis as there was no 'intention to treat' these endoscopically, but more recently with improvements in accessory instruments and expertise more of these difficult cases have been included. Results from other centres around the world[4,32–39] with individual and collected series of from 430 to 7585 patients range from 78% to 94% for duct clearance with a median value of 87%, figures very similar to our own. There does not appear to be any difference in technical success after ES in patients with and without gall-bladders.

An equivalent assessment of surgical success in the same terms is more difficult. In the first few years after the introduction of ES the majority of patients treated were those with bile duct stones following a previous cholecystectomy (with or without bile duct exploration). There was a predominance of elderly unfit cases but, with time, younger patients with less risk factors were treated. Endoscopic success rates of over 90%, and thus, conversely, a retained stone rate of less than 10% must, therefore, be put into the same context as secondary biliary operations and not primary duct procedures as these patients represent 'failures' of previous surgery. Reported results for retained stones after second bile duct explorations are as impressively low as 2.9%[40] but other series suggest that this is the exception rather than the rule and, despite the use of postexploration cholangiography and choledochoscopy, figures of 15%, 20%, and 33% may be more realistic[41,42] with even higher rates for third or subsequent operations[42]. With these results in mind many surgeons would now add a biliary drainage procedure to exploration in appropriate circumstances when the bile duct has not been completely cleared or when transpapillary bile flow is thought to be inadequate. This will presumably increase the success rate of bile duct clearance. In addition, secondary operations are potentially more difficult to perform and there must be a failure rate for exploration of the bile duct due, for example, to limitations of access in some patients but quantification of this is not possible. Non-comparability between endoscopically-treated and surgically-treated patients in this category is compounded by the selection of referrals to specialist centres when complicated biliary surgery is contemplated.

Most endoscopy centres are now referred increasing numbers of patients in whom the gallbladder is still *in situ* and in our unit the proportion has risen from under 50% in 1977 to 74% of all ES cases in 1985. It is in this group that primary bile duct surgery needs to be compared by randomized trial to define comparability. Surgical series suggest retained stone rates of from 4.3%[43] to 10% or higher[17] and, even with the use of choledochoscopy, figures of 6–8% are reported[44,45]. Some primary duct explorations may prove to be difficult or impossible and many surgeons in centres where alternative methods are available may now desist from further attempts and merely provide temporary biliary drainage by T-tube. This attitude is now common where surgeons and endoscopists work closely together and will add a further selection error to any retrospective analysis of surgical results.

Failures of ES

Management of failures of surgical bile duct exploration will depend on the availability of local expertise but many surgeons would now rather refer patients some distance for endoscopic treatment than carry out a second or subsequent biliary operation. Failures of ES, however, tend to be treated at the endoscopic centre as some patients will require emergency surgery for complications or the rapid relief of a pre-existing problem for which ES was undertaken but had been unsuccessful. A close liaison between the endoscopist and surgical teams is important in order that severe and potentially life-threatening complications are recognized and managed effectively with decisions, including early surgery where indicated, made jointly. From our series of 577 patients whose bile duct stones we attempted to treat endoscopically, there were 11 in whom ES was unsuccessful or incomplete (1.9%) and 35 in whom the bile duct could not be cleared (6.1%). Of these, five required urgent surgery, three for continuing cholangitis and retained stones of whom two elderly patients, aged 72 and 84, died, and two for impacted baskets although one was found to be lying free in the duodenal lumen and was removed by the anaesthetist! Six patients had no further treatment, four were moribund on admission and died before any intervention could be undertaken, and two elderly frail patients were left with biliary endoprostheses acting to prevent stone impaction at the papilla and both continue to be well. The remaining 35 were all operated upon successfully without complication and it is probable that many of these were rendered fitter by a period of preoperative bile drainage either through the ES or a nasobiliary catheter.

Early complications of ES

Early complications of ES have been well documented and, despite the disparate indications and selection of patients between centres, the incidence seems to be remarkably consistent at 8–10%[4,32–39]. The expected higher complication rate during early experience of the technique is reflected in a personal series comparing the results of the first 394 procedures in our unit[4] carrying an overall morbidity of 10.4% with a subsequent consecutive group of 300 sphincterotomies in which this rate has fallen to under 6%. The respective proportions of individual complications, however, remain similar in most reports with acute haemorrhage from the sphincterotomy site representing 2.3–2.9%, acute pancreatitis 1.5–3.3%, cholangitis 1.2–2.7% and retroperitoneal perforation about 1% with small numbers of other problems such as impacted basket, gallstone ileus and acute cholecystitis. Emergency surgery is required in 1–2.5% of cases for bleeding, cholangitis, perforation and pancreatitis in descending order of frequency. There must be reservations about some figures, however, as definitions of haemorrhage, acute pancreatitis, cholangitis and perforation are often not given. We have always included any episode of overt bleeding (haematemesis and/or melaena) and/or fall in haemoglobin of 2 g/dl or more following ES as significant haemorrhage while some reports have included only those requiring transfusion.

Pancreatitis and cholangitis must depend on the presence of clinically recognizable syndromes rather than asymptomatic hyperamylasaemia or transient elevation of temperature alone but these events may be underreported. There does not appear to be an influence on significant complication rate or type by the initial presentation of the bile duct stone event (pain alone, jaundice alone, pancreatitis, or a combination of these) except that cholangitis is more likely after ES if it pre-exists. Present evidence does not suggest that complications are more likely in older patients or after previous biliary surgery and duodenal diverticula, and although sometimes rendering ERCP and ES technically more difficult, do not seem to add any further risk. In addition, many series do not include non-endoscopic complications occurring after ES (cardiovascular, cerebrovascular or respiratory) and although surgery for the treatment of complications is usually documented, that for failed endoscopic therapy is often not and these factors are important if comparative data from surgical reports is to be interpreted correctly.

The management of complications by the centres performing ES will be clear and well standardized but many patients are referred from other hospitals and are returned there shortly after the procedure. It is therefore vital that appropriate advice be given and experience recorded[4]. Of all the complications, *haemorrhage* requires surgical intervention most commonly (in up to one third of cases) to control bleeding when the ES is usually converted to a formal surgical sphincteroplasty as the bleeding artery is nearly always at the apex of the endoscopic incision. Attempts to circumvent this feared event are being made by the development of Doppler probes which can be applied endoscopically to the intended sphincterotomy site in order to map the vascular anatomy. This may be particularly helpful when ES is contemplated after a previous ES or surgical sphincter procedure when aberrant vessels are more likely. Alternative methods for haemorrhage control have been tried with variable success and include direct diathermy coagulation, washing the area with adrenaline solution, application of laser coagulation, superselective arterial catheterization and embolization, and infiltration with sclerosant[46]. It should be emphasized, however, that the endoscopic view of the papillary area is often completely obscured by blood in these circumstances and further endoscopic therapy may not be possible.

Acute pancreatitis is managed along standard lines and, although many attacks will be mild and self-limiting, clinicians should not be complacent as some will be more severe and should therefore be graded and treated intensively as appropriate. There is no evidence that pre-ES or post-ES administration of aprotinin or glucagon influences the incidence or severity of pancreatitis. Unlike haemorrhage, the onset of pancreatitis may be delayed for several hours and, rarely, 1 or 2 days.

Cholangitis is almost completely confined to those patients in whom bile duct clearance has not been achieved and measures should be directed at providing adequate bile drainage, e.g. by nasobiliary catheter, as well as parenteral antibiotics in this context. Emergency surgery carries high risks when performed for cholangitis but will be indicated in those patients who do not improve within 24 hours.

Perforation may be asymptomatic and noticed only as retroperitoneal gas or extravasation of radiographic contrast but even in the symptomatic patient conservative treatment may be effective with spontaneous resolution and avoidance of potentially difficult surgery. Occasionally this complication presents late after ES with a retroperitoneal collection of bile or pus pointing in the flank or inguinal region[4,47] and will require surgical drainage.

Gallstone ileus should be treated along standard surgical lines but its recognition needs to be emphasized as symptoms may be obscure in elderly patients and present many days after ES and stone release. Although a complication of ES the operation required to treat it may be considerably more straightforward than the biliary procedure which has been avoided.

The *impaction* of an extraction basket now occurs rarely in experienced hands as many endoscopic manoeuvres have been learned by operators to prevent or save this embarrassing situation. Techniques available to help the endoscopist are:

(1) Non-closing of the basket during initial attempts to extract a large stone to avoid impaling the basket wires in the stone surface.

(2) Removal of the duodenoscope over an impacted basket catheter and reintroduction of it alongside the catheter to increase the ES incision.

(3) Introduction of a second duodenoscope to enlarge the ES.

(4) Passage of a sphincterotome down the same instrument channel as the impacted catheter when using large channel (3.7 or 4.2 mm) endoscopes in order to enlarge the ES.

(5) Conversion of the standard basket into a crushing type by replacement of the handle with a rachet device.

Complications affecting the gallbladder and the outcome of endoscopic failures are mentioned later.

Mortality after ES

Mortality after ES has not been reported in a standardized way by different centres. Those deaths directly attributable to the procedure are fairly constant at 0.8–1.5%[4,32–39] with almost equal causation distributed between haemorrhage, pancreatitis, cholangitis and perforation with many being postoperative. These deaths as a proportion of complications, however, range from 7 to 17%, which presumably reflects the comprehensive reporting of all complications by some but only more severe ones by others. The accepted method of reporting surgical mortality within 1 month of the operation should be applied to ES results also.

Treatment of our own data in this way[4] produces a mortality of 0.8% resulting from ES itself in 394 patients but an overall 3.3% within 1 month of ES. The additional deaths were due to a variety of vascular, respiratory, renal, infective and malignant conditions in a group whose mean age was 79 years. A further series of 59 elderly patients considered unfit for surgery underwent ES[48] with only one death (1.7%).

Early complications and mortality after bile duct surgery

It is relevant here to consider complications and mortality rates after bile duct surgery which have been well documented[17,40–43,49–55], with more recent interest in specific risk factors[50–52] allowing some prediction of likelihood of complications and perhaps the need for preoperative biliary drainage. Direct comparisons with endoscopic data are not scientifically accurate as it is clear that very different groups of patients are being treated by these modes of therapy. Mention must be given, however, to published surgical figures to enable some clinical judgements to be made in the absence of randomized trials. It is immediately apparent that, unlike endoscopic therapy, surgical morbidity and mortality are very much determined by patient age[50,53–55], presence of other medical conditions[53–55], both acute and chronic, certain haematological and biochemical factors[50–52], and whether or not the operation is elective[56,57] or an emergency[58,59]. Mortality rates range from 1% in relatively fit younger patients to 5%, 12% and 28% in the unfit and elderly, and 12–14% in younger patients undergoing emergency surgery for cholangitis. These practically all refer to primary bile duct operations which should only be compared with results of ES when the gallbladder is *in situ*. Equivalent results for secondary bile duct explorations are less well recorded but mortality rates of 0–2% are possible for elective surgery[40,49] presumably in relatively fit patients.

Consideration must also be given to biliary drainage operations which will avoid problems of stone retention but at the expense of an increased postoperative morbidity and mortality. Average mortality rates of 1–5% for choledochoduodenostomy (CDD) and transduodenal sphincteroplasty (TDS) are reported[60–65]. We have recently completed a review of 246 such operations

(Baker, A. R., Neoptolemos, J. P., Leese, T. and Fossard, D. P., unpublished observations) carried out between 1972 and 1981 in which one of these drainage procedures was employed and a mortality of 5.4% was found for each of the two types of operation with major morbidity of 12% for CDD and 21% for TDS.

Long-term morbidity after ES

Long-term morbidity after ES cannot be fully assessed until follow-up data extend well beyond 10 years. This will not be possible for some years in order to include sufficient numbers of younger patients as it is in this group that long-term results may eventually determine choice of therapy. Results in postcholecystectomy patients already available, with follow-up information from 1 to 7 years after ES[3,39], show in excess of 90% of patients to be well on symptomatic review alone and about 8% with significant symptoms found to be due to recurrent stones (5%) and/or stenosis of the ES (3%) site on investigation. Radiological review of all patients after ES by plain abdominal radiograph for detecting air cholangiograms, repeat ERCP, barium studies for duodenobiliary reflux, or radionuclide scanning does not seem justified outside clinical trials but a higher rate of asymptomatic stones and stenosis might be the result. The majority of these long-term complications are amenable to further endoscopic treatment. An air cholangiogram on plain radiography is present in half to two thirds of patients after ES but does not exclude recurrent bile duct stone formation.

Long-term morbidity after bile duct surgery

Long-term follow-up of surgically explored and re-explored bile ducts is surprisingly lacking. The wide variation in reported recurrent stone rates has been mentioned but morbidity and the need for further surgery has been found in 5% after 5 years[66], 10% after 12 years[67], and 21% after 6–11 years[68] when exploration without biliary drainage has been performed. Following CDD there may be no morbidity in a 6–11 year follow-up[68] with similar results for TDS[64]. Follow-up of 90% of the survivors of our series of 246 patients from 1 to 12 years postoperatively (mean 4.4 years) revealed that complications had been treated in 3% of the CDD group (mainly sump syndrome) and 6% of the TDS group (mainly cholangitis) with additional symptoms on interview in 8% of the CDD and 5% of the TDS groups.

ENDOSCOPIC THERAPY AFTER CHOLECYSTECTOMY

Recent biliary surgery, T-tube *in situ*, retained stone(s)

Bile duct stones detected in the early postoperative period on T-tube cholangiography occur in 4–15% of patients[69] and, although those less than 10 mm diameter may pass spontaneously or after flushing the T-tube, most

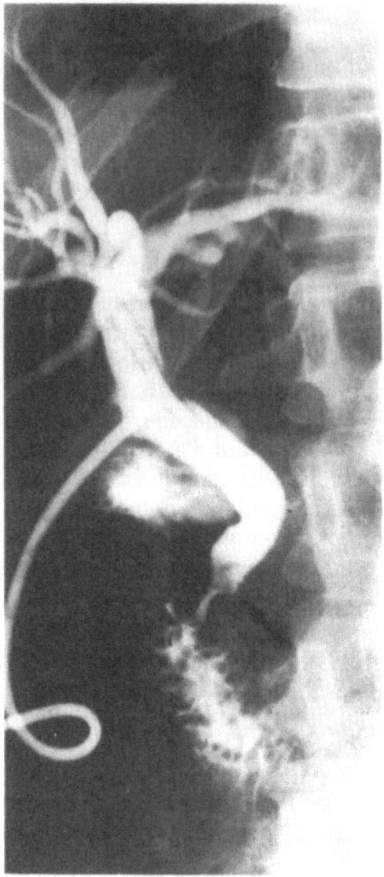

Figure 7.14   Radiograph showing retained stone below T-tube immediately prior to ES

will be retained and require mechanical removal (Figure 7.14). The increased morbidity, mortality and retained stone rate after secondary bile duct explorations has stimulated the development of alternative techniques such as hydraulic T-tube irrigation with or without pharmacological relaxation of the sphincter of Oddi with glucagon or ceruletide, T-tube infusion of cholesterol solvents, and percutaneous extraction via a mature T-tube track which requires a delay of 4–6 weeks to form. Advocates of this technique, pioneered by Burhenne[70] obtain extraction rates of 90% or more, although this has not been emulated in Britain where reports of 70–78% success are more usual, may require multiple sessions in a third of cases and be complicated by sepsis, biliary trauma and leakage in up to 12%[71,72]. We have recently reported[69] our results of ES in 39 patients with T-tubes in place in whom 76 stones were present, 53 distal and 23 proximal to the T-tube. Stones ranged in diameter from 5 to 15 mm and were single in 25, two to four in 11 and more than four in three patients (one with eight stones). Endoscopic sphincterotomy was successful in all and the bile duct was cleared in 38 (97.4%), requiring two attempts in two. Complications occurred in three (7.7%): an impacted basket in one, removed surgically, mild pancreatitis in one and transient cholangitis in another. Most patients were treated within 4 weeks of their operation but this reflected delays in referral as ES can be carried out immediately stones are demonstrated, usually on the tenth postoperative day allowing discharge from hospital the following day. There have been no long-term complications to date.

Remote biliary surgery, no T-tube, retained/recurrent stone(s)

For patients presenting from a few weeks to many years after cholecystectomy with bile duct stones, few would now question the use of ES in the treatment of elderly patients who are at high risk for further abdominal surgery, but there may remain doubts when surgeons are faced with younger and fitter patients. The successes, failures and complications of secondary bile duct operations have been discussed from which it may be deducted that, if endoscopic therapy can achieve the high success rates published by most established centres, this should be the treatment of first choice. It is most unlikely that any comparative trials of surgery against ES will be performed in postcholecystectomy patients in the light of current medical and surgical opinion but critical assessment of long-term morbidity following ES should be continued as this will determine whether or not the endoscopic approach should remain the correct one in this group.

ENDOSCOPIC THERAPY WITH GALLBLADDER *IN SITU*

Elderly patients with gallbladder

There has been an increasing trend over the last few years for patients who have not previously undergone biliary surgery to be referred for endoscopic therapy for bile duct stones. The reasoning behind this is twofold. Firstly, the elderly patient with pain, jaundice, cholangitis, pancreatitis or a combination of these may best be served by endoscopic clearance of the bile duct to relieve the acute biliary problem and not proceed to cholecystectomy unless symptoms dictate in view of the expected short life expectancy and the low possibility of gallbladder complications. Secondly, younger patients presenting with these acute biliary conditions may fare better with initial biliary decompression by ES followed by elective cholecystectomy when the acute problem has subsided. What is the present evidence that either of these propositions is justified?

The short- and long-term results and complications of ES in patients with gallbladders seems no different from those without[4,32-39,48]. The same arguments in favour of endoscopic bile duct clearance apply equally in these patients as to those who are postcholecystectomy. The difference in the elderly group, in whom a deliberate decision is made to leave the gallbladder in place, is thus the incidence of subsequent complications referrable to the residual gallbladder itself. Careful follow-up of 59 such patients for up to 4 years[48],

130 for up to 5 years[6] and 260 for up to 6 years[32] has shown that 4.6%, 6% and 10% respectively have developed gallbladder symptoms or complications sufficient to warrant cholecystectomy but nearly all were required within the first year. A small subgroup probably have empyema of the gallbladder at the time of presentation or develop it shortly after endoscopic treatment and all must be aware of this in view of the difficulty in diagnosis and high mortality connected with this condition if left untreated. One patient, aged 76 years, in our series[48] died from this condition 5 weeks after ES but all other late deaths were due to non-biliary causes as would be expected in this age group. These results suggest that the low risk of subsequent gallbladder complications after ES and bile duct clearance when patients are kept under supervision outweighs the known higher mortality for cholecystectomy in the elderly of up to 10%[56] and mitigates against routine cholecystectomy in this group. The low but definite risk of neoplastic change in the residual gallbladder becomes irrelevant in view of the short life expectancy in this elderly group of patients.

Younger patients with gallbladder

Emergency surgery in younger patients with acute biliary tract disease may carry a high risk although elective bile duct exploration is relatively safe. The place of preliminary ES in these patients can only be decided by controlled trial. We undertook a pilot study in 38 patients[48], with a mean age of 63 years, considered fit for surgery but presenting with combinations of jaundice in 95%, recent cholangitis in 45%, active cholangitis in 26%, and acute pancreatitis in 10%. Thirty-three (87%) were successfully treated by ES and extraction of stones with failure of performing ES in two and extraction in three. All were subsequently operated upon apart from one patient who felt well and refused further treatment. Of the remainder, all 37 had a cholecystectomy, three with negative bile duct explorations, owing to mis-interpretation of the peroperative cholangiogram from the presence of air in the duct, and five with positive explorations representing the five failures of endoscopic therapy. There were no postoperative deaths within 1 month and all are alive and well with no late complications.

With these encouraging results a prospective trial was established entering patients with bile duct stones shown on endoscopic or percutaneous chol-angiography who were considered treatable by either endoscopy or surgery and whose gallbladders were still intact. Clinicians were asked to offer patients for the study but could elect to exclude them and request one or other mode of therapy, usually ES, and the reasons for this were recorded. Trial patients were randomized either to preliminary ES followed by elective chole-cystectomy (Group I) or surgery (cholecystectomy, bile duct exploration and any additional procedure considered appropriate, Group II) with failures of either mode of therapy treated by the other or by an alternative method as indicated by the clinical situation. Preliminary analysis of the first 98 patients entered is available. The two groups are comparable in their demographic

Table 7.2 Preliminary results of prospective trial in patients with bile duct stones comparing initial ES and cholecystectomy (Group I) with cholecystectomy and bile duct exploration (Group II)

Groups	I	II
No. of patients	48	50
Failed endotherapy	4(8%)	—
Cholecysteomy	48	50
CBD exploration	4(8%)	50
Post-op. complication	16(33%)	25(50%)
Death	0	1(2%)
Wound infection	4(8%)	6(12%)
Burst abdomen	2(4%)	1(2%)
Chest infection	7(15%)	6(12%)
Septicaemia	1(2%)	1(2%)
Significant blood loss	2(4%)	4(8%)
Bile leak	1(2%)	2(4%)
Acute pancreatitis	0	1(2%)
Sump syndrome	0	1(2%)
Retained stone(s)	0	5(10%)

characteristics and results are summarized in Table 7.2. There were four failures of endoscopic treatment in Group I; two failed sphincterotomies and two failed duct clearances, all of whom underwent subsequent successful surgical duct exploration together with cholecystectomy. The remaining 44 (92%) in Group I underwent elective cholecystectomy after successful endoscopic clearance of bile ducts, usually within 1 month of ES and many during the same admission when jaundice had subsided. No unsuspected bile duct stones were detected at operation and there were no postoperative deaths. No serious complications of ES were encountered but two patients experienced exacerbations of their cholangitis after ES despite prophylactic antibiotics. In Group II, all patients had a positive bile duct exploration combined with cholecystectomy and there was one postoperative death in a patient with Nelson's syndrome following previous adrenalectomy for Cushing's disease. Thus the principal differences in early outcome between the two groups to date are the failures of endoscopic treatment (8%) in Group I and the failures of surgical bile duct clearance in Group II (12%, retained stones and sump syndrome), all of the latter being subsequently treated by ES. There does not appear to be a significant difference between the two groups in terms of other postoperative complications. Analysis of risk factors[50–52], however, reveals patients in the trial to be younger and fitter than a similar number referred specifically for ES at the clinicians' request during the trial period. This 'para-trial' group is being analysed separately as are patients who have undergone cholecystectomy with bile duct exploration for stones found unexpectedly on peroperative cholangiography during the trial period. It is hoped that comparison of these four groups will allow conclusions to be drawn concerning the risks and benefits of preoperative ES in younger patients.

Acute cholangitis

Acute cholangitis due to bile duct stones is traditionally treated by initial supportive measures with parenteral antibiotics followed by early surgery if improvement is slow or absent. The mortality from emergency surgery can be as high as 12–16% with higher rates for elderly patients[32,58,59]. We have analysed the results of treatment of 82 patients with severe acute cholangitis with bile duct stones admitted to our hospital over a 7-year period during which ES was available[73]. There were 28 males and 54 females with a mean age of 71 years (range 19–88). 87% were aged over 60 and 23% over 80 years. Overall 30-day mortality was 14.6% but varied considerably with different modes of therapy. Eleven received conservative treatment only. Of these, seven responded to antibiotics alone but four were moribund and died (36.4%) before any treatment could be instituted. Seventy-one underwent early biliary decompression surgically (28) or endoscopically (43). Of the eleven who were postcholecystectomy, four had early surgery with bilio-digestive bypass and two died within 30 days (50%) and seven had early ES with no mortality. Of the 60 with gallbladders, 24 were treated surgically (mean age 62 years) with a mortality of 16.7%, 13 had an ES followed by elective cholecystectomy (mean age 64 years) with no mortality and 23 had an ES with gallbladders left *in situ* (mean age 79 years) with a mortality of 8.7%. During follow-up of the 21 survivors with gallbladders, six have died from unrelated causes, two have required surgery for empyema of the gallbladder at 19 days post-ES in one and recurrence of cholangitis at 5 months in the other. Complications after ES occurred in 10: haemorrhage in five, exacerbation of cholangitis in three, mild acute pancreatitis in one and gallstone ileus in one with only the latter requiring surgical intervention. Bile duct clearance was achieved in 40 of 43 patients (93%). Of the three failures, one died without further therapy, one underwent surgery 4 weeks later and one remains asymptomatic having declined further treatment. Thus the 30-day mortality for patients treated by early surgery was 21.4% (six of 28) and that for early ES irrespective of subsequent treatment was 4.7% (two of 43). We have concluded that patients not responding to standard initial therapy within 24 hours or those who have already developed extrabiliary complications should be offered endoscopic biliary decompression and bile duct clearance if this is locally available.

Acute gallstone-associated pancreatitis

There have been advocates for early biliary surgery in acute gallstone-associated pancreatitis both to prevent progression of the current attack to one of more severity and to reduce the incidence of further attacks but this approach has been criticized as carrying too high a risk[74]. The application of ES seems logical although ERCP has long been regarded as contraindicated in the presence of active pancreatitis. After encouraging results in a pilot study involving 16 patients we implemented a prospective trial of ERCP and ES in acute pancreatitis with selection of those patients likely to have a biliary aetiology based on early ultrasound, biochemical criteria[75,76] or absence of other identifiable causes. Thus far, from a consecutive series of 112 patients, 70 have been included in the study with 35 randomized to urgent ERCP and ES if bile duct stones were present (Group I) and 35 to conventional treatment (Group II). Fifty were found to be gallstone-associated of whom 24 were in Group I and 26 in Group II. All but one in Group I had a successful ERCP and 11 an ES with bile duct clearance in all found to have bile duct stones. The proportion with bile duct stones was greater in those with severe attacks on prognostic grading (40%) compared to those with mild attacks (23%) and the overall complication rates were 35% and 10% respectively. The two deaths in the trial occurred in Group II (7.7%), one of whom had an impacted stone at the papilla at autopsy and may have been saved by early biliary intervention. There were no complications attributable to ERCP nor ES but three patients from each group developed pseudocyst or pancreatic abscess. Two patients with coexistent cholangitis made a dramatic recovery following ES and stone extraction. In the 42 excluded from trial entry, seven (16.7%) died of whom two had gallstones, making an overall mortality of 8% (9 of 112) but 6.8% (4 of 59) for gallstone-associated pancreatitis. No clear statistical difference has yet emerged between the two treatment groups but with larger numbers we hope that clear guidelines for predicting gallstone presence to enable selection for endoscopic therapy may be possible.

CONCLUSIONS

Endoscopic spincterotomy has matured rapidly with enthusiastic acceptance by physicians and surgeons for treating their patients with bile duct stones. Endoscopic technique is well established but supporting equipment will surely continue to develop and may improve the endoscopist's ability to remove stones successfully and safely. There would seem on current evidence to be little doubt that endoscopic therapy is the treatment of choice for elderly patients with bile duct stones whatever their presentation and gallbladder status and probably all patients presenting late after biliary surgery where a further operation is the only alternative. Our own studies have suggested that early postoperative patients with retained stones can safely be treated by ES without the need to await maturation of a T-tube track and discharge from hospital is usually expedited. In addition, cholangitis, when treated by ES, is likely to carry a much lower risk of morbidity and mortality. The case for endoscopic therapy in gallstone-associated pancreatitis and for those younger patients with bile duct stones presenting with other problems has yet to be clarified by trial results which are awaited. Integrated endoscopic and surgical management of gallstone disease is well advanced in those centres where endoscopist and surgeon work closely together and this provides the appropriate environment in which to evaluate available and new forms of treatment for the benefit of our patients.

References

1. Kawai. K., Akasaka, Y., Murakami, K., Taka, M., Kohli, Y. and Nakajima, M. (1974). Endoscopic sphincterotomy of the ampulla of Vater. *Gastrointest. Endosc.*, 20, 148–51
2. Classen, M. and Demling, L. (1974). Endoscopische Sphinkterotomie der papilla Vater.

Dtsch. Med. Wochschr., **99**, 496–7

3. Leese, T., Neoptolemos, J. P. and Carr-Locke, D. L. (1985). Successes, failures, early complications and their management following endoscopic sphincterotomy: results in 394 consecutive patients from a single centre. *Br. J. Surg.*, **72**, 215–9

4. Mustard, R., Mackenzie, R., Jamieson, C. and Haber, G. B. (1984). Surgical complications of endoscopic sphincterotomy. *Can. J. Surg.*, **27**, 215–7

5. Escourrou, J., Cordova, J. A., Lazorthes, F., Frexinos, J. and Ribet, A. (1984). Early and late complications after endoscopic sphincterotomy for biliary lithiasis with and without the gallbladder '*in situ*'. *Gut*, **25**, 598–602

6. Zimmon, D. (1984). Devices and techniques for endoscopic sphincterotomy. *Gastrointest. Endosc.*, **30**, 214–5

7. Siegel, J. H. (1980). Precut papillotomy: a method to improve success of ERCP and papillotomy. *Endoscopy*, **12**, 130

8. Osnes, M. (1979). Endoscopic choledocho-duodenostomy for common bile duct obstruction. *Lancet*, **1**, 1059

9. Forbes, A. and Cotton, P. B. (1984). ERCP and sphincterotomy after Billroth 2 gastrectomy. *Gut*, **25**, 971–4

10. Bedogni, G., Bertoni, G., Contini, S., Fabbian, F., Pedrazzoli, C. and Ricci, E. (1984). Endoscopic sphincterotomy in patients with Billroth II partial gastrectomy: comparison of three different techniques. *Gastrointest. Endosc.*, **30**, 300–5

11. Staritz, M., Poaralla, T., Dormeyer, H. H. and Meyer zum Buschenfelde, K. H. (1985). Endoscopic removal of common bile duct stones through the intact papilla after medical sphincter dilation. *Gastroenterology*, **88**, 1807–11

12. Staritz, M. (1983). Endoscopic papillary dilatation. *Endoscopy*, **15**, 197–8

13. Cotton, P. B., Burney, P. G. J. and Mason, R. R. (1979). Transnasal bile duct catherisation after endoscopic sphincterotomy. *Gut*, **20**, 285–7

14. Catt, P. B., Hogg, D. F., Clunie, G. J. A. and Hardie, I. R. (1974). Retained biliary calculi: removal by a simple, non-operative technique. *Ann. Surg.*, **180**, 247–51

15. Gardner, B. (1973). Experiences with the use of intracholedochal heparinized saline for the treatment of retained common bile duct stones. *Ann. Surg.*, **177**, 240–4

16. Walker, J. W. (1891). The removal of gallstones by ether solution. *Lancet*, **1**, 874–5

17. Way, L. W., Admirand, W. H. and Dunphy, J. E. (1972). Management of choledocholithiasis. *Ann. Surg.*, **176**, 347–59

18. Thistle, J. L., Carlson, G. L., Hofmann, A. F., LaRusso, N. F., MacCarty, R. L., Flynn, G. L., Higuchi, W. I. and Babayan, V. K. (1980). Mono-octanoin, a dissolution agent for retained cholesterol bile duct stones: physical properties and clinical application. *Gastroenterology*, **78**, 1016–22

19. Bogardus, J. B. (1984). Importance of viscosity in the dissolution of cholesterol in monooctanoin solutions. *J. Pharm. Sci.*, **73**, 906–10

20. Palmer, K. R. and Hofmann, A. F. (1876). Intraductal monooctanoin for the direct dissolution of bile duct stones: experience in 343 patients. *Gut*, **27**, 196–202

21. Leuschner, U., Wurbs, D., Baumgartel, H., Helm, E. B. and Classen, M. (1981). Alternating treatment of common bile duct stones with a modified glyceryl-1-mono-octanoate preparation and a bile salt-EDTA solution by nasobiliary tube. *Scand. J. Gastroenterol.*, **16**, 497–503

22. Leuschner, U. and Baumgartel, H. (1982). Gallstone dissolution in the biliary tract: *in vitro* investigations in inhibiting factors and special dissolution agents. *Am. J. Gastroenterol.*, **77**, 222–6

23. Allen, M. J., Borody, T. J., Bugliosi, T. F., May, G. R., LaRusso, N. F. and Thistle, J. L. (1985). Rapid dissolution of gallstones in humans using methyl tert butyl ether. *N. Engl. J. Med.*, **312**, 217–20

24. Riemann, J. F., Seuberth, K. and Demling, L. (1983). Mechanische Zertrummerung von Gallengangssteinen. *Dtsch. Med. Wochenschr.*, **108**, 373–5

25. Frimberger, E., Weingart, J., Kuhner, W. and Ottenjann, R. (1983). Eingeklemmter papillenstein: mechanische Lithotripsie moglich. *Dtsch. Med. Wochschr.*, **108**, 38

26. Staritz, M. (1983). Mechanical gallstone lithotripsy. *Endoscopy*, **15**, 316–18

27. Frimberger, E., Kuhner, W., Weingart, J. and Ottenjann, R. (1982). Eine neue Methode der elektrohydraulischen Cholelithotripsie (Lithokasie). *Dtsch. Med. Wochschr.*, **107**, 213–15

28. Sander, R. and Poesl, H. (1985). Endoscopic papillotomy with the Nd-YAG laser. *Endoscopy,* **17,** 115–16

29. Demling, L., Ermert, H., Riemann, J. F., Schmolke, G. and Heyder, N. (1984). Lithotripsy in the common bile duct using ultrasound: preliminary *in vitro* experiments. *Endoscopy,* **16,** 226–8

30. Ebbs, S. R., Beckly, D. E., Hammonds, J. C. and Teasdale, C. (1986). Percutaneous electrohydraulic lithotripsy of retained bile duct calculus. *Lancet,* **292,** 94

31. Blumgart, L. H. and Wood, C. B. (1978). Letter: Endoscopic treatment of biliary tract diseases. *Lancet,* **2,** 1249

32. Cotton, P. B. (1984). Endoscopic management of bile duct stones (apples and oranges). *Gut,* **25,** 587–97

33. Safrany, L. (1978). Endoscopic treatment of biliary tract diseases. *Lancet,* **2,** 983–5

34. Reiter, J. J., Bayer, H. P., Mennicken, C. and Manegold, B. C. (1978). Results of endoscopic papillotomy: a collective experience from nine endoscopic centers in West Germany. *World J. Surg.,* **2,** 505–11

35. Nakajima, M., Kizu, M., Akasaka, Y. and Kawai, K. (1979). Five years experience of endoscopic sphincterotomy in Japan: a collective study from 25 centres. *Endoscopy,* **2,** 138–41

36. Siegel, J. H. (1981). Endoscopic papillotomy in the treatment of biliary tract disease: 258 procedures and results. *Dig. Dis. Sci.,* **26,** 1057–64

37. Geenen, J. E., Vennes, J. A. and Silvis, S. E. (1981). Resumé of a seminar on endoscopic retrograde sphincterotomy (ERS). *Gastrointest. Endosc.,* **27,** 31–8

38. Cotton, P. B. and Vallon, A. G. (1981). British experience with duodenoscopic sphincterotomy for removal of bile duct stones. *Br. J. Surg.,* **68,** 373–5

39. Seifert, E., Gail, K. and Weismuller, J. (1982). Langzeitresultate nach endoskopischer Sphinkterotomie: follow-up-Studie aus 25 Zentren in der Bundesrepublik. *Dtsch. Med. Wochschr.,* **107,** 610–14

40. Girard, R. M. and Legros, G. (1981). Retained and recurrent bile duct stones: surgical or non-surgical removal? *Ann. Surg.,* **193,** 150–4

41. Kune, G. A. (1972). *Current Proceedings of Biliary Surgery.* pp. 221–3. (Boston: Little, Brown)

42. Allen, B., Shapiro, H. and Way, L. W. (1981). Management of recurrent and residual bile duct stones. *Ann. Surg.,* **142,** 41–7

43. Glenn, F. (1974). Retained calculi within the biliary ductal system. *Ann. Surg.,* **179,** 528–39

44. Rattner, D. W. and Warshaw, A. L. (1981). Impact of choledochoscopy in the management of choledocholithiasis. *Ann. Surg.,* **194,** 76–9

45. Feliciano, D. W., Mattox, K. L. and Jordan, G. L. (1980). The value of choledochoscopy in exploration of the common bile duct . *Ann. Surg.,* **191,** 649–53

46. Grimm, H. and Soehendra, N. (1983). Unterspritzung zur Behandlung der Papillotomie-Blutung. *Dtsch. Med. Wochschr.,* **108,** 1512–4

47. Neoptolemos, J. P., Harvey, M. H., Slater, N. D. and Carr-Locke, D. L. (1984). Abdominal wall staining and 'biliscrotum' after endoscopic sphincterotomy. *Br. J. Surg.,* **71,** 684

48. Neoptolemos, J. P., Carr-Locke, D. L., Fraser, I. and Fossard,, D. P. (1984). The management of common bile duct calculi by endoscopic sphincterotomy in patients with gallbladders *in situ. Br. J. Surg.,* **71,** 69–71

49. McSherry, C. K. and Glenn, F. (1980). The incidence and causes of death following surgery for non-malignant biliary tract disease. *Ann. Surg.,* **191,** 271–5

50. Pitt, H. A., Cameron, J. L., Postier, R. G. and Gadacz, T. R. (1981). Factors affecting mortality in biliary tract surgery. *Am. J. Surg.,* **141,** 66–72

51. Blamey, S. L., Fearon, K. C. H., Gilmore, W. H., Osborn, D. H. and Carter, D. C. (1983). Prediction of risk in biliary surgery. *Br. J. Surg.,* **70,** 535–8

52. Dixon, J. M., Armstrong, C. B., Duffy, S. W. and Davies, G. C. (1983). Factors affecting morbidity and mortality after surgery for obstructive jaundice; a review of 373 patients. *Gut,* **24,** 845–52

53. Glenn, F. (1975). Trends in surgical treatment of calculus disease of the biliary tract. *Surg. Gynecol. Obstet.,* **140,** 877–84

54. Vellacott, K. D. and Powell, P. H. (1979). Exploration of the common bile duct; a comparative study. *Br. J. Surg.,* **66,** 389–91

55. Doyle, P. J., Ward-McQuaid, J. N. and McEwen-Smith, A. (1982). The value of routine per-operative cholangiography – a report of 4000 cholecystectomies. *Br. J. Surg.*, **69**, 617–19
56. Sullivan, D. M., Ruffin Hood, T. and Griffen, W. O. (1982). Biliary tract surgery in the elderly. *Am. J. Surg.*, **143**, 28–220
57. Houghton, P. J. W. and Donaldson, L. A. (1983). Elective biliary surgery – a safe procedure. *Geriatr. Med.*, **13**, 814–16
58. Thompson, J. E., Tomkins, R. K. and Longmire, W. P. (1982). Factors in management of acute cholangitis. *Ann.Surg.*, **195**, 137–45
59. Boey, J. H. and Way, L. W. (1980). Acute cholangitis. *Ann. Surg.*, **190**, 264–70
60. Madden, J. L., Chun, J. Y., Kandalaft, S. and Parekh, M. (1970). Choledochoduodenostomy, an unjustly maligned surgical procedure? *Am. J. Surg.*, **119**, 45–54
61. Capper, W. M. (1961). External choledochoduodenostomy, an evaluation of 125 cases. *Br. J. Surg.*, **49**, 292–300
62. Jones, S. A. (1978). The prevention of and treatment of recurrent bile duct stones by transduodenal sphincteroplasty. *World J. Surg.*, **2**, 473–85
63. Lygidakis, N. J. (1981). Choledochoduodenostomy in calculous biliary tract disease. *Br. J. Surg.*, **68**, 762–5
64. Stuart, M. and Hoerr, S. O. (1972). Late results of side to side choledochoduodenostomy and of transduodenal sphincterotomy for benign disorders. *Am. J. Surg.*, **123**, 67–72
65. Speranza, V., Lezoche, E., Minervina, S., Carlei, F., Basso, N. and Simi, M. (1982). Trans-duodenal papillotomy as a routine procedure in managing choledocholithiasis. *Arch. Surg.*, **117**, 875–8
66. Larson, R. E., Hodgson, J. R. and Priestley, J. T. (1966). The early and long term results of 500 consecutive explorations of the common duct. *Surg. Gynecol. Obstet.*, **122**, 744–50
67. Peel, A. L. G., Bourke, J. B. and Hermon Taylor, J. (1975). How should the common bile duct be explored? *Ann. R. Coll. Surg.*, **56**, 124–34
68. Lygidakis, N. (1983). Surgical approaches to recurrent choledocho-lithiasis. *Am. J. Surg.*, **145**, 633–9
69. O'Doherty, D. P., Neoptolemos, J. P. and Carr-Locke, D. L. (1986). Endoscopic sphincter-otomy for retained common bile duct stones in patients with T-tube *in situ* in the early post-operative period. *Br. J. Surg.* (In press)
70. Burhenne, J. H. (1980). Percutaneous extraction of retained biliary tract stones. *Am. J. Roentgenol.*, **134**, 888–98
71. Mason, R. R. (1980). Percutaneous extraction of retained gallstones via the T-tube tract – British experience of 131 cases. *Clin. Radiol.*, **1**, 497–9
72. Mason, R. R. (1985). Percutaneous extraction of retained gallstones. *Clin. Gastroenterol.*, **14**, 403–19
73. Leese, T., Neoptolemos, J. P., Baker, A. R. and Carr-Locke, D. L. (1985). Management of acute cholangitis and the impact of endoscopic sphincterotomy. *Gut*, **26**, A553
74. Neoptolemos, J. P., London, N., Slater, N. D., Carr-Locke, D. L., Fossard, D. P. and Moossa, A. R. (1986). A prospective study of ERCP and endoscopic sphincterotomy in the diagnosis and treatment of gallstone acute pancreatitis. *Arch. Surg.* (In press)
75. Goodman, A. J., Neoptolemas, J. P., Carr-Locke, D. L., Finlay, D. B. L. and Fossard, D. P. (1985). Detection of gallstones after acute pancreatitis. *Gut*, **26**, 125–32
76. Neoptolemos, J. P., Hall, A. W., Finlay, D. B. L., Berry, J. M., Carr-Locke, D. L. and Fossard, D. P. (1984). The urgent diagnosis of gallstones in acute pancreatitis: a prospective study of three methods.. *Br. J. Surg.*, **71**, 230–3

8
Oral Medical Therapy

T. C. NORTHFIELD and D. P. MAUDGAL

INTRODUCTION

Until recently, cholecystectomy was the only treatment for gallstone disease. During the past 15 years, the discovery that gallstone patients have gallbladder bile that is supersaturated with cholesterol has led to the introduction of bile acid therapy aimed at desaturating bile and thus causing gallstone dissolution.

We plan to discuss all aspects of this subject, including practical recommendations for management. Emphasis will be placed on what are currently the two most important areas of controversy – the efficacy of oral litholytic therapy and the subsequent risk of gallstone recurrence, because doubts about these have been the main barriers to more widespread acceptance of this form of treatment. Concern over efficacy has been expressed in recent editorials from the UK[1] and USA[2], published under such titles as 'Dissolving hopes of gallstone dissolution' and 'Cholesterol gallstones: medical dissolution or disillusion?'. The immediate stimulus for these articles has come from the disappointing results for efficacy published in the American National Co-operative Gallstone Study[3] (NCGS), but this study used doses of chenodeoxycholic acid (CDCA) that were considerably lower than the previous dose recommendations based on studies published in both the UK[4] and the USA[5]. Concern has also been expressed about recurrence rate, the title for the best known article[6] on this subject being 'Is recurrence inevitable after gallstone dissolution by bile acid therapy?'. But this rhetorical question is based on the assessment of cumulative recurrence rate, which seriously overestimates the risk involved.

AVAILABLE COMPOUNDS

At present, only two compounds are generally accepted as capable of dissolving gallstones when given by mouth; both of them are bile acids. Discussion will therefore be limited mainly to these, although a third form of treatment will also be mentioned comprising a mixture of monoterpenes.

Chenodeoxycholic acid (CDCA)

Although first identified in goose bile (chenos, Greek for goose), cheno-deoxycholic acid (3α, 7α-dihydroxy-5β-cholan-24-oic acid) is one of the two primary bile acids synthesized by the human liver. Oral administration in man reduces the cholesterol saturation index (SI) of fasting gallbladder bile, and thus promotes dissolution of cholesterol gallstones. Its use was first described in 1972 in both the USA[7] and later in the UK[8]. It has since been licensed for clinical use in the USA, the UK and many other countries.

Ursodeoxycholic acid (UDCA)

UDCA is the 7β epimer of CDCA: it is similar in structure to CDCA, except that the hydroxyl group in the 7 position has a β configuration instead of an α configuration. UDCA is one of the major bile acids in the bear (ursus, Latin for bear), but only trace amounts are found in human bile. Long used as a folk remedy in Japan, it was not until 1975 in Japan[9] and 1977 in the West[10,11] that it was first reported to desaturate bile and to dissolve cholesterol gallstones. Although it is licensed for clinical use in the UK and most European countries, it has not yet received FDA approval for clinical use in the USA.

Monoterpenes

A mixture of compounds (marketed as Rowachol in the UK) has been reported to have a moderate effect in reducing SI of gallbladder bile, and to cause dissolution of a small proportion of cholesterol gallstones[12]. It may also be effective in dissolving stones with a calcified rim. At present, it is licensed in the UK only for use in conjunction with CDCA for treatment of common bile duct stones, and is not approved for clinical use in the USA.

MECHANISM OF ACTION

Chenodeoxycholic acid

Following oral administration of CDCA in the generally recommended dose of 15 mg/kg per day, 75–80% of the bile acid pool is converted to CDCA[13]. This has the effect of inhibiting endogenous cholesterol synthesis in the liver, as indicated by a reduction in the activity of the rate-limiting enzyme for cholesterol synthesis, hydroxymethyl-glutaryl-coenzyme A reductase[14,15] (HMG-CoA reductase). This in turn causes a decrease in cholesterol secretion from the liver[16], and a reduction in the cholesterol SI of fasting gallbladder bile. Desaturating the bile (reducing SI to less than unity) gives the micelles in bile the capacity to solubilize cholesterol from the surface of gallstones.

Ursodeoxycholic acid

UDCA has been reported to cause all the qualitative effects described above for CDCA. Quantitatively, only 50% of the bile acid pool is replaced with UDCA because it is less effective than CDCA in inhibiting endogenous bile acid synthesis[17,18]. Nevertheless, it has been consistently shown to desaturate gallbladder bile at a lower dose than CDCA. UDCA, but not CDCA, reduces cholesterol absorption from the small intestine in addition to reducing hepatic cholesterol secretion[17]. UDCA probably dissolves cholesterol gallstones by promoting the temporary formation of liquid crystals[19] at the gallstone surface. The cholesterol is subsequently transferred to micelles formed by the endogenous bile acids present in the bile. Whereas in micelles cholesterol is solubilized by both bile acid and phospholipid, in liquid crystals it is solubilized by phospholipid alone.

Monoterpenes

The monoterpenes have also been reported to reduce the activity of HMG-CoA reductase and to reduce cholesterol secretion[20].

PATIENT SELECTION

There is no point in considering medical treatment for a patient unless there is a good prospect that it will be successful in that individual. This depends on stone type and size and gallbladder function. If these criteria are satisfied, then a decision about the overall advisability of medical treatment can be considered in the light of other factors.

Gallstone type and size

One of the essential prerequisites for treatment with bile acids is that the stones should be rich in cholesterol[21] (more than 50%). This is highly likely if there are radiolucencies in an opacified gallbladder on oral cholecystography (Figure 8.1); about 80–85% of such stones are rich in cholesterol[22]. The remaining 15–20% are predominantly pigment stones, which contain less than 20% cholesterol and are therefore not amenable to bile acid therapy.

On oral cholecystography, 10–25% of radiolucent stones are seen to float[23]. Such stones are almost always rich in cholesterol, and respond very well to bile acid therapy. Using discriminant analysis, Dolgin and colleagues[24] have defined characteristics that differentiate between cholesterol and pigment stones: multiple, floating stones numbering more than 10 and measuring more than 6 mm in diameter are almost certain to be cholesterol rich, whereas stones with central calcification are likely to be pigment stones.

Most workers find that calcified stones do not dissolve with bile acid therapy and regard their presence as an absolute contraindication to bile acid therapy[13,25]. This may, however, be only a relative contraindication, since in the United States National Co-operative Gallstone Study (NCGS) complete gallstone dissolution was seen in a few patients who had stones with a small area of central calcification[3] (less than 3 mm in diameter).

Large gallstones respond poorly to bile acid therapy, and are therefore considered a contraindication to treatment. Dowling's group found that a diameter of 1.5 cm was the most appropriate cut-off point[25,26]. A greater size appears to prevent dissolution, rather than just slowing it up. This may relate

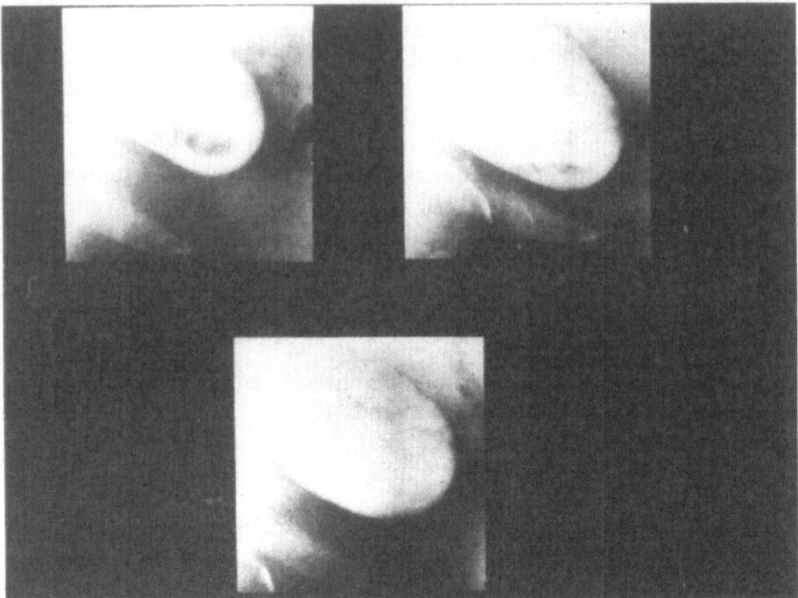

Figure 8.1. Partial dissolution (at 6 months) and complete dissolution (at 1 year) of small, radiolucent gallstones in a radiologically functioning gallbladder on full dose CDCA (15 mg per kg per day)

to the finding of Wolpers that large, mature gallstones have densely packed laminated outer layers, whereas small immature stones have loosely packed spoke-like crystalline radiations[27].

Gallbladder opacification

The second essential prerequisite for successful bile acid therapy is that the desaturated bile due to treatment should be able to enter the gallbladder via a patient cystic duct and bathe the gallstones. This is likely if oral cholecystography shows a well-opacified gallbladder (Figure 8.1). If the gallbladder opacifies poorly or not at all, and there has been a recent episode of biliary colic, oral cholecystography should be repeated 4–6 weeks later; it may then show opacification in up to 50% of cases. Persistent failure of the gallbladder to opacify prior to treatment precludes successful dissolution and is generally regarded as an absolute contraindication to bile acid therapy[28]. The development of non-opacification during treatment may also be transitory. In the NCGS, 60% of patients with a non-opacifying gallbladder at 9 months proceeded to show opacification again by the end of the 2-year study[3].

Medical contraindications to surgery

These include old age and the presence of serious concurrent disease. Obesity also increases the hazards of surgical treatment, unless the patient loses a lot of weight before operation. Obese patients are, however, relatively resistant to bile acid therapy[29] because of hypersecretion of biliary cholesterol, and may require a larger dose of bile acid than that usually recommended, or some other measure to improve efficacy.

Attitude of the patient

It is important to consider this carefully. Some patients prefer to deal with their problem once and for all by means of surgery. Others fear surgery and would prefer medical treatment, even if this is prolonged and followed by the risk of gallstone recurrence. It is important that the patient understands the disadvantages of bile acid therapy, and undertakes to co-operate fully before opting for this form of treatment.

Severity of symptoms

Patients with frequent biliary colic should not be given bile acid therapy; but this is a matter of judgement. If there are major contraindications to surgical treatment it is reasonable to give a trial of drug treatment for a limited period to assess its effect on symptoms. Although the main clinical indication for bile acid therapy is the presence of mild symptoms, several studies have reported an improvement in biliary colic during bile acid treatment[30]. The placebo-controlled NCGS showed no significant benefit from CDCA in biliary colic, although it confirmed earlier studies in dyspepsia by showing significantly more benefit than from placebo treatment[3]. The mechanism of this improvement is not known; Dowling and colleagues have reported that gallbladder emptying is slower during treatment with UCDA than before treatment[31].

Recent epidemiological studies indicate that 70% of gallstones detected by ultrasonography in the general population are 'silent' (asymptomatic) gallstones. They suggest that in these cases the probability of developing any biliary problem including biliary pain is only about 20% after 20 years[32]. It is therefore unnecessary to treat patients with gallstones until they develop symptoms.

Women of child-bearing age

CDCA has been shown to cross the placental barrier and to damage the fetal liver[33], and UDCA is toxic to some animal embryos[34]. The use of either bile acid in females of child-bearing age is therefore contraindicated unless contraception is being reliably practised by the patient or her partner, and pregnancy is not planned within 2 years.

ASSESSMENT OF RESPONSE TO TREATMENT

The ultimate goal of treatment is complete gallstone dissolution, but this may take a long time. It is therefore important to have methods of predicting whether treatment will prove successful. The two most important methods are the measurement of SI of gallbladder bile during treatment and the measurement of gallstone diameter after 6 months treatment. If the latter measurement indicates partial dissolution when compared with the diameter prior to treatment, then complete dissolution is likely to follow in due course[35]. If it does not, then continuation of the same treatment regimen is probably a waste of time; but a sample of gallbladder bile should be obtained to help decide on subsequent management. If the bile is supersaturated with cholesterol, then a more effective treatment regimen is necessary. If it is unsaturated, the patient probably has a radiolucent pigment stone and referral for surgical treatment should be considered.

Saturation index (SI) during treatment

Fasting gallbladder bile can be obtained by nasoduodenal intubation combined with a slow intravenous infusion of cholecystokinin. Before the infusion the aspirate is pale hepatic bile, but after the infusion starts this is replaced by dark green gallbladder bile. An aliquot of this is analysed for bile acid, phospholipid and cholesterol concentration. SI can then be calculated from a nomogram devised by Thomas and Hofmann[36]. In order to obtain a reliable answer, it is best to refer the patient to a specialized centre if measurement of SI is clinically indicated, or at least to send a sample of dark green fasting gallbladder bile to a specialized laboratory.

Since the presence of fasting gallbladder bile supersaturated with cholesterol is an essential prerequisite for cholesterol gallstone formation[37], early research studies aimed to desaturate bile. If the mechanism of dissolution is micellar solubilization of cholesterol from the gallstone surface, it can be predicted that treatment would have to reduce the SI to a value below the solubility line at thermodynamic equilibrium, which corresponds to the solubility line described by Hegardt and Dam[38] and by Holzbach and others[39]. Using CDCA, Iser and colleagues showed that the patients in whom gallstones dissolved usually achieved desaturation of bile by these criteria, whereas nonresponders did not. The mean fasting SI was 0.8 in those achieving gallstone dissolution[25].

The conventional policy is to measure the SI of gallbladder bile taken in the morning following an overnight fast[30], when the bile is most saturated. There is a diurnal variation in SI of gallbladder bile[40], and it would be predicted that SI of the most unsaturated sample would determine gallstone dissolution. The SI of a postprandial evening sample may therefore be a better predictor of gallstone dissolution than a fasting morning sample, and this warrants further investigation.

Partial gallstone dissolution

In most clinical trials partial gallstone dissolution, usually defined as more than 50% reduction in gallstone size on an oral cholecystogram, has been used to assess the response to treatment. Kupfer and colleagues have validated a method of quantitatively measuring reduction in gallstone size over a 6-

month period as an index of dissolution rate, based on carefully standardized oral cholecystography[41].

Complete gallstone dissolution

Complete gallstone dissolution was originally defined as the absence of gallstones on two consecutive oral cholecystograms performed at least 3 months apart during continuing treatment. A reliable alternative to cholecystography is now provided by real-time ultrasonography. This has the advantage of avoiding radiation exposure and of being more sensitive in detecting small stones[42,43].

FACTORS INFLUENCING EFFICACY

Assessments of partial and of complete gallstone dissolution give two different methods of expressing efficacy:

(1) As response rate, which is defined here as the proportion of patients showing evidence of partial or complete gallstone dissolution in a defined period of time.

(2) As dissolution rate, which is defined as percentage reduction in gallstone size over a 6-month period.

Tangedahl has pointed out the difference between drug failure, where failure is attributable to the drug itself; and treatment failure, where it is due to other factors such as inappropriate selection or poor compliance[44]. Compliance can be improved by regular follow-up appointment, by avoidance of unwanted effects and by a convenient regimen, e.g. bedtime administration. Drug efficacy is influenced by two major factors – initial gallstone size and SI of fasting gallbladder bile during therapy.

Gallstone size

Carey and colleagues[45] have demonstrated *in vitro* a linear relationship between gallstone dissolution rate and the surface area of the stone. Thus, the reason why multiple small stones dissolve faster than a single large stone is that their surface area per unit mass of cholesterol is much greater[46]. The same relationship has been shown to hold *in vivo*; gallstone dissolution rate during bile acid therapy is inversely related to initial diameter[47,48].

SI of gallbladder bile during treatment

Bell and colleagues demonstrated[49], using human cholesterol gallstones and monkey bile *in vitro*, that dissolution rate is dependent upon the degree of desaturation of bile. Using model bile solutions, Carey and colleagues[45] demonstrated that, even though UDCA micelles are poor cholesterol solubilizers, the dissolution of cholesterol monohydrate discs is greater when cholesterol SI is lowered. A similar relationship between SI during treatment and gallstone dissolution rate has been demonstrated *in vivo* in patients with cholesterol gallstones taking either CDCA or UDCA[47,48]. The existence of such a relationship *in vitro* and *in vivo* for UDCA does not necessarily contradict the theory that liquid crystals rather than micelles form the most important vehicle for cholesterol gallstone dissolution using this bile acid. It does indicate that measurement of SI during treatment with UDCA is a useful predictor of efficacy as with CDCA.

METHODS OF IMPROVING EFFICACY

Patient selection and dose

Efficacy was disappointingly poor in the American NCGS, the response rate being 13% in terms of those achieving complete gallstone dissolution within 2 years in the 'high dose group' and 5% in the low dose group (compared with 1% on placebo); but when expressed in terms of body weight, both these doses (10 mg/kg per day and 5 mg/kg per day respectively) are lower than the generally recommended dose (15 mg/kg daily). Dowling's group have reported a final efficacy rate of 38% in a retrospective study[27] of 125 patients studied during the period 1971–1977 till they had either achieved complete dissolution or been withdrawn from treatment for some reason. All patients were preselected as having radiolucent gallstones in opacifying gallbladders, but they were treated with differing doses of CDCA for differing periods of time. They found that if they considered only patients who had completed 12 months treatment and who had developed desaturated gallbladder bile, the 'corrected' efficacy rate was 76%. This is close to the theoretical maximum of 80–85% (the rest being radiolucent pigment stones). When they took account of complications, dropouts and biological resistance, then the 'corrected' efficacy figure dropped by 10–20% to an overall maximum of 60–70%.

In a prospective study of 40 patients, all with radiolucent stones in an opacifying gallbladder, and all treated with CDCA in a fixed dose of 15 mg/kg per day for $3\frac{1}{2}$ years, or until complete dissolution occurred, Kupfer and colleagues[41] found an efficacy rate of 50% by intention to treat. When analysis was limited to a subgroup of 26 patients having stones less than 1.5 cm in diameter, the efficacy rate rose to 77%, again close to the theoretical maximum (Figure 8.2); on an intention to treat basis, the figure was 70%. The actual time taken to achieve dissolution depended on dose timing and diet. These two studies emphasize that, with appropriate selection of patients and dosage, efficacy can be much better than is generally assumed.

Choice of bile acid, dose and duration of treatment

In view of the relationship between SI and dissolution rate during both CDCA and UDCA, any measure that enhances the effect of treatment on gallbladder bile SI should improve efficacy. SI during treatment is related to dose for both CDCA and UDCA, but UDCA has a greater effect on SI than has CDCA. Figure 8.3 shows the results for two similar dose–response studies carried out by Dowling's group using CDCA[4] and UDCA[11]. They found a significant cor-

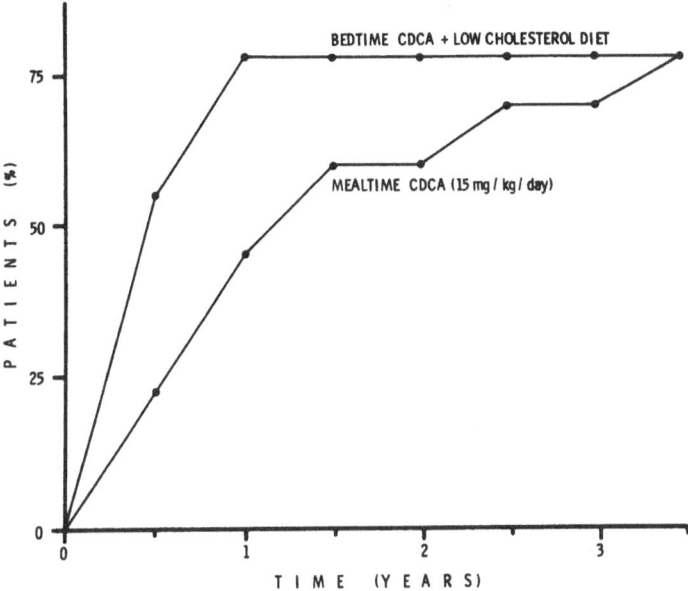

Figure 8.2 Percentage of patients achieving complete dissolution of small gallstones (< 15 mm diameter) at different time intervals on bedtime CDCA (15 mg/kg per day) plus a low cholesterol diet or on mealtime CDCA plus an unrestricted diet (based on Kupfer *et al.*, 1982)[41]

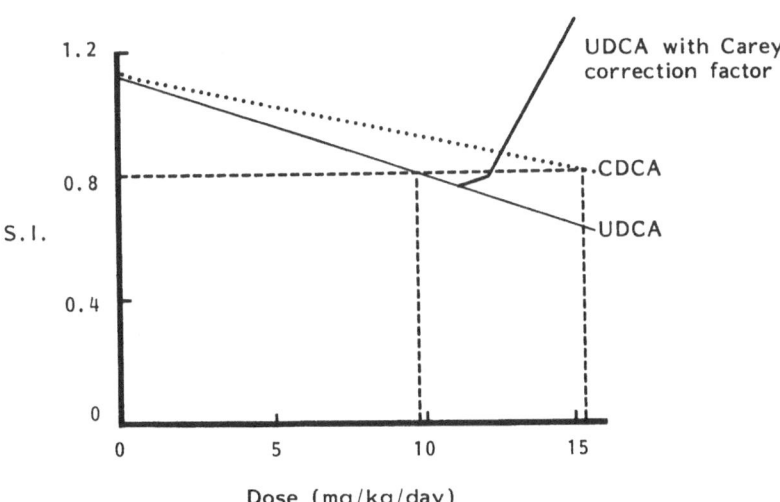

Figure 8.3 Dose–response relationship for gallbladder SI during CDCA (dotted line, from Mok *et al.*, 1974)[4] and UDCA (continuous line, from Maton *et al.*, 1977)[11]. At doses above 12 mg/kg per day), the regression line for UDCA deviates sharply upward if the Carey correction factor is applied to SI (second continuous line, Stiehl *et al.*, 1980)[52]. The dashed lines indicate the recommended dose, necessary to achieve mean SI of 0.8

211

relation between dose and SI for both bile acids. The calculated regression lines indicated a recommended dose (or minimum effective dose) of 15 mg/kg per day for CDCA, based on the fact that this dose gave a mean SI of 0.8, which had previously been demonstrated to be associated with consistent evidence of gallstone dissolution during CDCA treatment[25]. The corresponding minimum effective dose for UDCA was about 10 mg/kg per day[11]. In a subsequent study they confirmed that this dose gave consistent gallstone dissolution during UDCA treatment. The Mayo Clinic group studies have yielded similar dosage recommendations[5,50].

Carey and Ko[51] have argued from *in vitro* studies that a correction factor should be applied to SI in the presence of UDCA-rich bile. This Carey correction factor takes into account the fact that UDCA conjugates are poor solubilizers of cholesterol in micellar solution; UDCA therefore has to be subtracted from the total solvent (bile acid plus phospholipid) available for micellar solubilization of cholesterol. At higher UDCA doses (more than 12 mg/kg per day), the Carey correction factor has the effect of markedly increasing the SI of bile by comparison with the value obtained without the correction factor[52]. Figure 8.3 shows the declining regression line of Dowling and colleagues for UDCA without application of the correction factor, and the sharply rising regression line obtained at doses above 12 mg/kg per day with application of the Carey correction factor by Stiehl and colleagues[52].

A dose–response relationship for CDCA has been confirmed for gallstone dissolution rate. The American NCGS reported faster gallstone dissolution with CDCA at an average dose of 10 mg/kg per day than at 5 mg/kg per day[3]. Using CDCA 14 mg/kg per day, Barbara and colleagues[53,54] showed that this dose dissolved gallstones in a significantly higher proportion of patients than a dose of 7 mg/kg per day. By contrast, they did not find a difference between these two doses for UDCA. The dose–response relationship for UDCA has been examined in more detail by Erlinger and colleagues[55] in a Franco–Belgian multicentre study (Figure 8.4). The proportion of patients achieving complete dissolution increased with dosage increases up to 8 mg/kg per day, but was then halved (from 29 to 15%) when the dose was doubled from 8 to 16 mg/kg per day. This diminution in efficacy with high doses is in keeping with the results for SI if the Carey correction factor is applied, and suggests that the Carey correction factor may indeed provide a better way of predicting gallstone dissolution during UDCA than the conventional method of measuring SI.

When gallstone dissolution rate is considered, the greater efficacy of UDCA at doses 12 mg/kg per day or less, predicted from SI measurements, has been confirmed for gallstone dissolution rate over the first 6 months[48]. Barbara's group[53,54] have demonstrated that this is also true when assessed in terms of the proportion of patients achieving complete dissolution during the first 6 months (Figure 8.5); but in their study the difference between CDCA and UDCA at 6 months was lost by 12 months due to a slowing of the dissolution rate on UDCA. Fromm and colleagues[56] have also demonstrated significant differences in gallstone dissolution (partial or complete) during the early stages of therapy which are lost later on. Since gallstone calcification is one of the complications of UDCA therapy, it is tempting to speculate that this

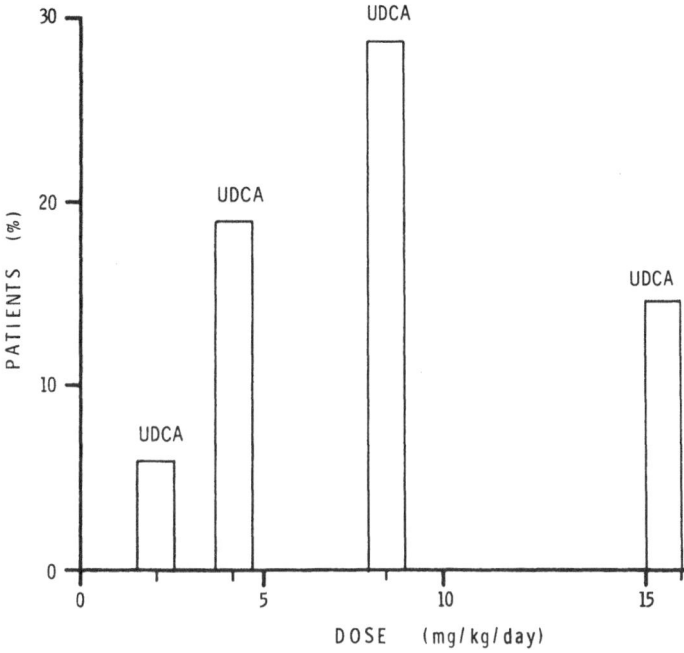

Figure 8.4 Percentage of patients having complete gallstone dissolution at 6 months for different doses of UDCA (based on Erlinger *et al.*, 1984)[55]

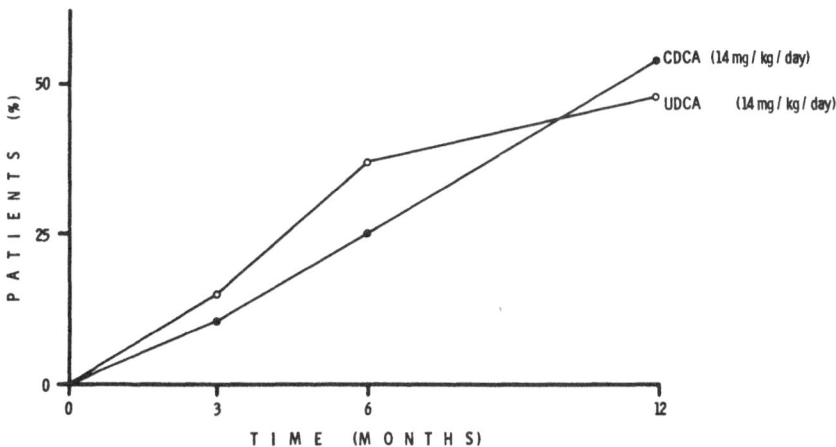

Figure 8.5 Percentage of patients having complete dissolution of small gallstones following administration of CDCA or UDCA for periods up to 1 year (based on Barbara *et al.*, 1982)[54]

213

slowing may be due to subradiological calcifications of the gallstones during UDCA, but this needs confirmation.

Dose timing

Clinical trials have shown that with bedtime administration of either CDCA or UDCA, the SI of fasting gallbladder is lower than with mealtime administration of the same total daily dose[57,48]. This is because bedtime administration of exogenous bile acid prevents nocturnal interruption of the enterohepatic circulation[58], and thus prevents the secretion of super-saturated hepatic bile at night. Bedtime administration enables a lower dose of CDCA to be given in those with diarrhoea on full dose treatment. The minimum effective dose for gallstone dissolution is reduced from 15 to 10 mg/kg per day[59].

Alternatively, a more rapid dissolution rate can be achieved if the full dose of CDCA is given all at bedtime[41]. By contrast, bedtime administration does not enhance the effect of UDCA 12 mg/kg per day on gallstone dissolution rate[48]. This may be because a maximum effect has already been achieved, as suggested by Erlinger's dose–response study (Figure 8.4). Bedtime admin-istration does enhance dissolution rate on a lower dose of UDCA (3–5 mg/kg per day, unpublished observations).

Diet

A low cholesterol diet enhances the effect of CDCA therapy of gallbladder bile SI[60] and causes a further reduction in the minimum effective dose of CDCA from 10 to 7 mg/kg per day at bedtime[59]. It does not enhance the effect of UDCA on SI[48]. This difference may be explained by the recent observation that UDCA, unlike CDCA, can reduce biliary cholesterol secretion without suppressing hepatic cholesterol synthesis, possibly by enhancing conversion of cholesterol to bile acid[61].

A low cholesterol diet in combination with bedtime CDCA 15 mg/kg per day achieved complete gallstone dissolution within 1 year in 77% of patients (Figure 8.2) with radiolucent gallstones that were less than 1.5 cm in diameter, whereas the conventional regimen (mealtime CDCA, plus an unre-stricted diet) did not achieve the same efficacy until given for a total period of 3 years[41]. No further patients on the bedtime regimen achieved complete dissolution after the first year, supporting the concept that this is the maximum response rate. These results indicate that the effect of bedtime administration is to improve the dissolution rate rather than the total response rate. It is not clear at present how much the lower cholesterol diet contributed to this improvement in efficacy.

Combination therapy

A combination of CDCA and UDCA has been advocated on the basis that this should combine the advantages of both forms of therapy, while reducing the dose (and the adverse effects) of each bile acid individually. The advantages of CDCA are that it suppresses primary bile acid synthesis more effectively than UDCA[18], so that greater conversion of the bile acid pool to litholytic bile acids is possible. The advantage of UDCA is that it has a greater effect of SI than CDCA. Furthermore, the evidence that CDCA acts mainly by micellar solubilization of cholesterol, whereas UDCA acts mainly by liquid crystal formation, raises the possibility of potentiation. The disadvantages of CDCA (diarrhoea and raised transaminase levels) and of UDCA (gallstone calcification) should be reduced when a lower dose of the individual bile acids is used in combination. It is not yet known whether a combination UDCA and CDCA achieves faster dissolution than either bile acid given alone.

The combination of monoterpenes with CDCA has been studied by Bell and colleagues[62]. They have reported a significant enhancement of the effect of CDCA on SI. They have also reported partial dissolution of radio-opaque stones using the same combination, but it is not clear whether this effect is greater than with CDCA alone.

ADVERSE EFFECTS OF BILE ACID THERAPY

The main benefit of the American NCGS is that it has provided a large amount of controlled data on the adverse effects of CDCA, the bile acid reported to cause the most frequent adverse effects. It should be remembered that UDCA has been introduced more recently, and that no similar large controlled trial has been published.

Diarrhoea

Diarrhoea is a frequent unwanted effect during treatment with CDCA, but not with UDCA[4,13,25,28,63]. It is dose-related, and affects 30–60% of patients treated with CDCA in the conventional dose of 15 mg/kg per day[4]. It usually occurs within weeks of starting treatment, and tends to settle spontaneously even with continued full dose therapy. A temporary reduction in bile acid dose is beneficial. Up to 25% of patients have diarrhoea troublesome enough to prevent them taking the conventional dose of CDCA. In the NCGS[3], clinically significant diarrhoea (defined as an average of at least two episodes of diarrhoea per month during a 3-month period) occurred in 41% of patients on 750 mg daily, in 23% of patients on 375 mg daily, and in 26% of patients in the placebo group. The exact mechanism underlying the diarrhoea is unknown.

Hypertransaminaemia

Treatment with CDCA, but not UDCA, has been associated with modest but transient increases in serum transaminase levels in approximately one third of patients[28]. In the NCGS, 17% of those treated with 750 mg daily had a major rise (more than threefold) in serum glutamate pyruvate transaminase (SGPT) and a further 14% had a minor rise. When present the enzyme abnormalities always began during the first 3 months of treatment, and usually resolved within 6–9 months of continued treatment. Treatment was terminated because of clinically significant liver abnormalities in only eight patients (3%) on CDCA 750 mg daily, in one patient on 375 mg daily and in one patient on placebo. Only three of these patients had liver biopsies: two showed chronic active hepatitis (one on 750 mg CDCA daily and one on 375 mg daily) and the third showed fatty change (on placebo). Liver biopsy was performed in a random subset of 126 patients from the CDCA-treated groups. These showed no severe dose-related changes in morphology by light microscopy over the 2 years of the study. Previous light and electron-microscopic studies in smaller groups of CDCA-treated patients had shown no significant change[64,66].

The underlying mechanism for the raised serum transaminase levels during CDCA therapy is not clear, although the favoured hypothesis concerns litho-cholic acid, a bacterial breakdown product of CDCA present in large amounts in the human colon. In animals, feeding of CDCA causes accumulation of lithocholate in the enterohepatic circulation, where it is known to be capable of causing cholestatic liver damage[67,68]. Most clinical investigators, however, have found only very small changes in lithocholate content of human bile during CDCA treatment, probably because the human liver sulphates litho-cholic acid very efficiently and sulphation prevents the absorption of litho-cholate from the colon[69]. Marks and colleagues have reported a lower sul-phation fraction for lithocholate in patients having a rise in serum transaminase level on CDCA than in those not having a rise[70].

Effects on lipid metabolism

Despite the prediction of an effect by Small[71] in 1971, early clinical studies using CDCA showed no change in fasting serum cholesterol levels[7,8] or in cholesterol kinetics and pool size[72,73]. In the NCGS[3], mean cholesterol levels rose by 20 mg/dl over a 2 year period in patients treated with CDCA 750 mg daily, compared with a rise of 10 mg/dl in the placebo group. This small rise was confined to LDL cholesterol. Any increased risk of ischaemic heart disease must be very small, since CDCA is only given for gallstone dissolution over a period of 1-2 years. UDCA has not been reported to cause any effect on LDL cholesterol, but it should be noted that UDCA has not been studied in such large numbers of patients as has CDCA, and the effect of CDCA itself did not emerge until large numbers had been studied.

Several investigations have reported a 20–30% fall in fasting serum tri-glyceride levels during CDCA treatment[74-76]. This is thought to be due to a reduction in triglyceride synthesis[77,78].

Risk of colon cancer

Animal experiments suggest that bile acids are a risk factor in colon cancer[79,80], and an increase in the faecal output of bile acids during treatment with CDCA or UDCA could therefore be of concern[81,82]. There is no clinical evidence yet of an increase in the incidence of colonic cancer in patients treated with CDCA or UDCA during the past 15 years. On the other hand, there is evidence that cholecystectomy may predispose to the development of right-sided colonic cancer[83,84].

Acquired gallstone calcification

Calcification of gallstones during UDCA treatment has been reported in about 10% of patients during UDCA treatment[85]. The underlying mechanism is not clearly understood, and information about the chemical composition and distribution of calcium in such stones is limited. Igimi and Carey[86] have shown that the glycine conjugate of UDCA is relatively insoluble, with a high precipitation pH and a tendency to form gels, thus facilitating calcium precipitation. Hofmann[87] has suggested that calcium carbonate crystals may form in a mesophase composed of phosphatidylcholine and cholesterol, which is observed on the surface of cholesterol gallstones in patients taking UDCA. In animals, ingestion of UDCA increases biliary output of calcium and bicarbonate[88,89]. Whether this is true in man is not known, but the solubility of calcium carbonate in UDCA-rich bile is less than in CDCA-rich bile.

Since calcified stones tend not to respond to bile acid therapy, acquired calcification might delay or even prevent gallstone dissolution. In the NCGS, however, calcification acquired during the study period in 61 patients did not prevent gallstone dissolution[3].

GALLSTONE RECURRENCE

On cessation of bile acid therapy, the bile reverts to its supersaturated state in 1–3 weeks[90]. As formation of bile supersaturated with cholesterol is a prerequisite for formation of cholesterol gallstones[37], this may put patients at risk of forming further stones.

Diagnosis

In most published studies, the diagnosis of complete gallstone dissolution has been based on two consecutive negative oral cholecystograms during continued bile acid therapy. Similarly, gallstone recurrence has been diagnosed by oral cholecystography. With the advent of sensitive real-time ultrasonography and with growing operator experience, several reports have questioned the reliability of oral cholecystography in the diagnosis both of gallstone dissolution and of gallstone recurrence[42,43]. In the NCGS[3], Schoenfield and colleagues found that complete gallstone dissolution diagnosed by oral cholecystogram was not confirmed by follow-up X-ray 3 months later in 19% of patients. Gleeson and Ruppin[91] have reported marked discrepancies between ultrasonography and cholecystography and also between successive ultrasonographies. Their study involved different types of ultrasonographic apparatus and different operators, and ultrasonography is notoriously operator-dependent. A surgically validated study by Jazrawi and colleagues[92] has suggested that ultrasound is more sensitive than cholecystography in detecting gallstones if a single experienced operator uses a real-time machine. The ability to detect small gallstones is particularly important in the diagnosis of complete gallstone dissolution and of gallstone recurrence; but even ultra-sonography in the best hands cannot detect stones smaller than 1 mm in diameter. Therefore therapy should be continued for at least 3 months after the initial diagnosis of dissolution.

Frequency of gallstone recurrence

In most reported studies, gallstone recurrence rate has been calculated in terms of cumulative recurrence. This method overestimates the recurrence rate, because all patients who have had a recurrence within a set time interval will contribute to the numerator, whereas those having no recurrence will contribute to the denominator only if they have been followed for the des-ignated time period. The 100% cumulative recurrence rate at 5 years reported by Ruppin and Dowling[6] was based on only two subjects followed up for the full length of time, whilst the rate of 88% at 6 years reported by Toulet and colleagues[93] was also based on two subjects only.

An actuarial method (life table analysis) gives the best estimate of the risk of gallstone recurrence, as it takes into account different lengths of follow-up. The method was originally introduced to calculate survival rates following operations for gastric cancer, and was first applied to the risk of gallstone recurrence by Lanzini and colleagues[94]. They have now followed 42 patients for up to 7 years after complete gallstone dissolution on ultrasound and oral cholecystogram; recurrence was also diagnosed by both techniques[95]. They found that the corrected recurrence rate using the actuarial method reached a plateau of 45% at 5–7 years (Figure 8.6), whereas the cumulative recur-rence rate was double this figure, reaching a peak of 92% similar to that reported by previous authors.

A third method of expressing recurrence rate is as an overall recurrence rate, also shown for comparison in Figure 8.6. By contrast with cumulative recurrence rate, this gives an underestimate, because most of the patients have not reached the longest time of observation, and some of the gallstone-free are likely to develop recurrence if followed for longer. In the study of Lanzini and colleagues[95], the overall recurrence rate was 26% at 5 years. This is lower than previous studies, which have given figures of 40–50%[6,93,96]. These higher figures may be due to the fact that earlier studies relied on oral cholecystography to diagnose complete gallstone dissolution, and may therefore have included some patients whose stones had not completely dissolved. Incompletely dissolved gallstones will figure as recurrences. If ultra-sound examination had not been carried out in the study of Lanzini and colleagues, six patients with a probable residual stone not shown on chole-cystography would have been admitted to the postdissolution study with the likely consequence of being counted as having a recurrence if their stones increased in size. This fact alone would have raised the overall recurrence rate to 45%. Another possible explanation is provided by the fact that these earlier studies included patients who had received a second or even a third course of bile acid therapy to redissolve recurrent gallstones (secondary dissolutions), as well as primary dissolutions. The former group of patients is at high risk for gallstone recurrence; all five patients in this group had

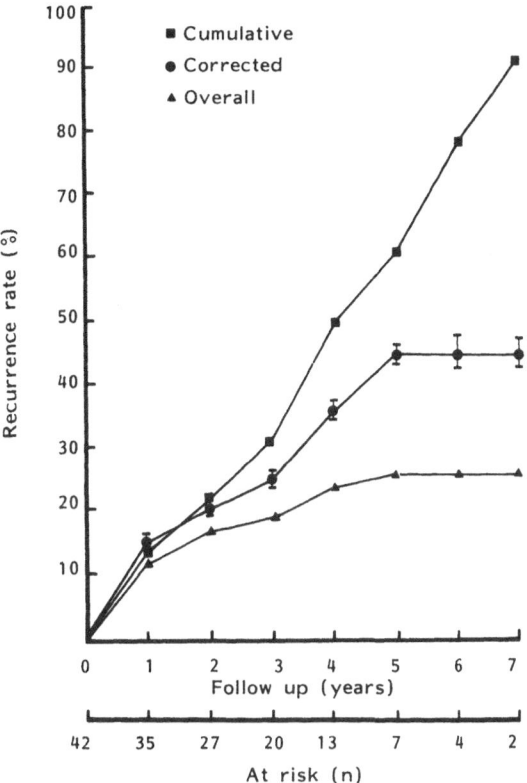

Figure 8.6 Gallstone recurrence rate (cumulative, actuarially corrected and overall) over a 7-year period (based on Lanzini *et al.*, 1986)[95]. The 95% confidence limits are shown for corrected recurrence rate (reproduced from Lanzini *et al.*, 1986[95.] by kind permission of the publishers of *J. Hepatol.*)

recurrence in the series of Toulet and colleagues[93], as did five of the six followed for longer than 6 months in the study of Ruppin and Dowling[6].

Prevention of recurrence

Research on this very important subject has so far been limited mainly to finding methods of reducing the SI of fasting gallbladder bile, such as a small bedtime dose of bile acid, or dietary measures, including a high fibre[97], low carbohydrate diet[98], or a bedtime drink of milk[94]. A sustained reduction in body weight should prevent recurrence in some obese patients, since it has been shown to be associated with a reduction in SI once weight reduction has been achieved. The period of weight reduction itself is accompanied by a rise in SI, probably due to mobilization of cholesterol stores, so that bile acid therapy should be continued during this period. Although all these measures reduce SI of gallbladder bile, none of them given alone consistently desaturates fasting gallbladder bile, which is necessary for gallstone dissolution; but in theory the prevention of gallstone recurrence should require a smaller reduction in SI than does gallstone dissolution.

Preliminary results from the American NCGS[91] show that low dose CDCA at bedtime does not prevent gallstone recurrence. It has been suggested that low dose UDCA might be more effective than CDCA, because it acts by liquid crystal formation. The British and Belgian Gallstone Study Group is carrying out a multicentre controlled trial, comparing the effect of low dose bedtime UDCA with that of a diet containing a low refined carbohydrate intake plus added bran and with that of placebo treatment. No differences between groups were found in preliminary analysis of this trial (in press). Full dose bile acid therapy might be effective, but has not been tested.

Treatment of recurrence

If prevention of gallstone recurrence is not feasible, a repeat course of bile acid therapy should prove rapidly effective. If a recurrence is treated at an early stage, the stones are small and being immature are likely to be composed mainly of cholesterol. Follow-up ultrasound examinations at yearly intervals, with reinstitution of bile acid therapy if recurrence is detected, may prove the best approach to managing those patients (about half) in whom early recurrence (within 5 years) is a problem. The resulting cycle of dissolution→recurrence→dissolution is shown in Figure 8.7, which gives a clinical algorithm that summarises the recommendations given in this chapter for oral medical therapy of gallbladder stones.

DEMOGRAPHIC AND ECONOMIC PERSPECTIVES

Proportion of patients suitable for oral medical therapy

This varies markedly, according to the population being studied. Physicians with a special interest in this subject will see patients who have been largely preselected as preferring medical therapy to surgery, and as being suitable for medical therapy. By contrast, surgeons will see a higher proportion of patients with complications of gallstones, e.g. cholecystitis and pancreatitis. This difference in patient populations is emphasized by a recent study from physicians in Frankfurt[99], which concluded that about 60% of patients with gallstones were suitable for medical treatment; and by a study from surgeons in Stockholm[100], which concluded that 6% were suitable.

As far as the general population is concerned, the best information can be obtained from epidemiological studies carried out in Italy[101,102]. On oral cholecystography, 30% of patients could be excluded from oral therapy because their gallstones were calcified, an additional 10% because their gallbladder did not opacify and 35% of the remainder because their gallstones were more than 2 cm in diameter. On this basis, the authors regarded about 30% of patients with gallstones as potentially suitable for medical therapy; but they found that only about one third of their gallstone subjects had symptoms, so that if only symptomatic patients were considered the pro-

ORAL MEDICAL THERAPY

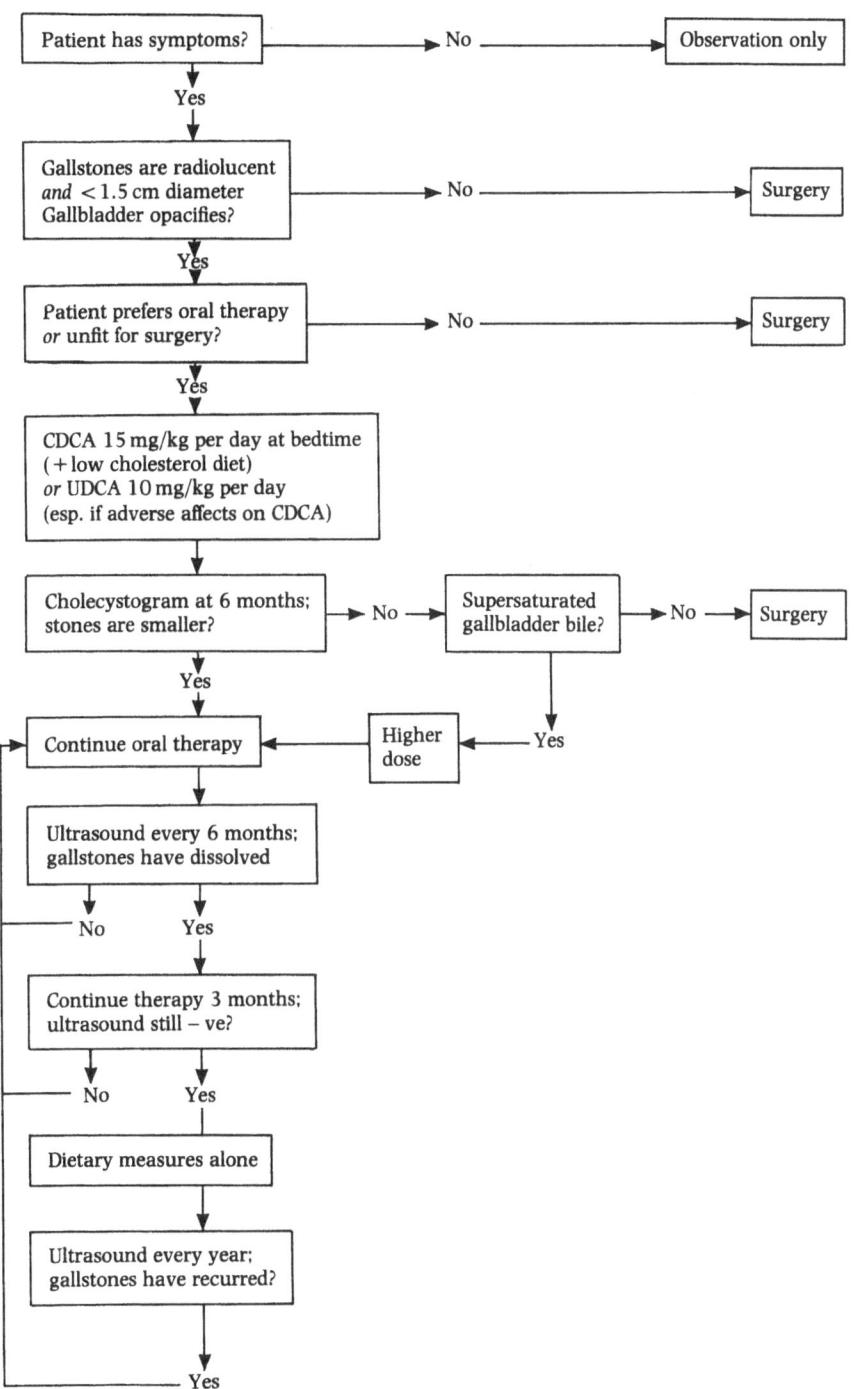

Figure 8.7   Clinical algorithm for management

portion would drop further to a maximum of 10% of the total gallstone population. Since the overall prevalence of gallstones in adults was 11% (7% in males, 15% in females), this means that about 1% of the population (i.e. approximately 500 000 people in the UK) is potentially suitable for medical therapy.

Only 1300 patients are currently receiving oral therapy in the UK (700 patients on UDCA, 400 on CDCA and 150 on monoterpenes) according to figures based on a record of prescriptions issued. These figures assume that the average weight of the patients is 75 kg, and that they are receiving oral therapy in the conventionally recommended dose. A major reason for this small proportion (about 0.3% of the total) is that general practitioners traditionally consider gallstones as a 'surgical' disease, and therefore automatically refer gallstone patients to surgeons, without considering the possibility of medical therapy and regardless of the patient preference. If the surgeon is prepared to consider medical therapy at all, he is likely to consider it only if there is a strong contraindication to surgery or if the patient is strongly opposed to surgery.

Cost effectiveness

The current trade price in the UK for 1 year's supply of CDCA in the recommended dose of 15 mg/kg per day for a 75 kg patient is £490 or £550, depending on the supplier. The corresponding price for UDCA in the recommended dose of 10 mg/kg per day is £510–£590. It is difficult to obtain a reliable figure for the total cost of cholecystectomy within the NHS, but in private practice with standard BUPA rates it amounts to £2100, including 7 day's stay in hospital, the services of a consultant surgeon and anaesthetist, theatre costs and other miscellaneous costs. Thus, in appropriately selected patients receiving optimum bile acid therapy for 1–2 years to achieve complete gallstone dissolution the cost of oral therapy for gallstones is far less than surgical treatment, even allowing for 6-monthly oral cholecystograms and outpatient attendances. In the case of surgery, there will be the additional cost to the economy, if not to the patient, of about 6 weeks off work following operation. These is also the human cost of the very small but definite mortality rate following surgical treatment[103,104] (no death has been reported during oral bile acid therapy). On the other hand, with medical treatment there is the subsequent cost of yearly ultrasonography to check that the stones have not recurred, and repeat courses of bile acid therapy if they do occur; and the possibility of final resort to surgical treatment if complications occur or if the patient becomes disillusioned with continuing medical supervision and opts for surgery after all.

References

1. Dissolving hopes for gallstone dissolution (Editorial) (1981). *Lancet*, **2**, 905–6
2. Isselbacher, K. J. (1981). Chenodiol for gallstones: dissolution or disillusion? (Editorial). *Ann. Intern. Med.*, **95**, 377–9
3. Schoenfield, L. J., Lachin, J. M., The Steering Committee and the National Co-operative

Gallstone Study Group (1981). Chenodiol (chenodeoxycholic acid) for dissolution of gall-stones: the National Co-operative Gallstone Study. *Ann. Intern. Med.*, **95**, 257–82

4. Mok, H. Y. I., Bell, G. D. and Dowling, R. H. (1974). Effect of differing doses of cheno-deoxycholic acid of bile lipid composition and frequency of side effects in patients with gallstones. *Lancet*, **2**, 253–7

5. Thistle, J. L., Hofmann, A. F., Yu, P. Y. S. *et al.* (1977). Effect of varying doses of chenodeoxycholic acid on bile lipid and biliary bile acid composition in gallstone patients: a dose–response study. *Dig. Dis.*, **22**, 1–6

6. Ruppin, D. C. and Dowling, R. H. (1982). Is recurrence inevitable after gallstone dissolution by bile acid treatment? *Lancet*, **1**, 181–5

7. Danzinger, R. G., Hofmann, A. F., Schoenfield, L. J. and Thistle, J. L. (1972). Dissolution of cholesterol gallstones by chenodeoxycholic acid. *N. Engl. J. Med.*, **286**, 1–8

8. Bell, G. D., Whitney, B. and Dowling, R. H. (1972). Gallstone dissolution in man using chenodeoxycholic acid. *Lancet*, **2**, 1213–6

9. Makino, I., Hashimoto, H., Shinozaki, K. *et al.* (1975). Dissolution of cholesterol gallstones by ursodeoxycholic acid. *Jap. J. Gastroenterol.*, **72**, 690–702

10. Kutz, C. and Schulte, A. (1977). Effectiveness of ursodeoxycholic acid in gallstone dissolution. *Gastroenterology*, **83**, 632–3

11. Maton, P. M., Murphy, G. M. and Dowling, R. H. (1977). Ursodeoxycholic acid treatment of gallstones. Dose–response study and possible mechanism of action. *Lancet*, **2**, 1297–1301

12. Doran, J., Keighley, M. R. B. and Bell, G. D. (1979). Rowachol – a possible treatment for cholesterol gallstones! *Gut*, **20**, 312–17

13. Hofmann, A. F., Thistle, J. L., Klein, P. D. *et al.* (1978). Chenotherapy for gallstone dissolution. II. Induced changes in bile composition and gallstone response. *J. Am. Med. Assoc.*, **239**, 1138–44

14. Salen, G., Nicolau, G. and Shefer, S. (1973). Chenodeoxycholic acid inhibits elevated hepatic HMG-CoA reductase activity in subjects with gallstones. *Clin. Res.*, **21**, 523

15. Coyne, M. J., Bonnoris, G. G., Goldstein, L. I. and Schoenfield, L. J. (1976). Effect of chenodeoxycholic acid and phenobarbital on the rate-limiting enzymes of hepatic chol-esterol and bile acid synthesis in patients with gallstones. *J. Lab. Clin. Med.*, **87**, 281–91

16. Northfield, T. C., LaRusso, N. F., Hofmann, A. F. and Thistle, J. L. (1975). Biliary lipid output during three meals and an overnight fast. II. Effect of chenodeoxycholic acid treatment in gallstone subjects. *Gut*, **16**, 12–17

17. Hardison, W. G. and Grundy, S. M. (1984). Effect of ursodeoxycholate and its taurine conjugate on bile acid synthesis and cholesterol absorption. *Gastroenterology*, **87**, 130–5

18. Von Bergmann, K., Epple-Gutsfeld, M. and Leiss, O. (1984). Differences in the effects of chenodeoxycholic and ursodeoxycholic acid on biliary lipid secretion and bile acid synthesis in patients with gallstones. *Gastroenterology*, **87**, 136–43

19. Corrigan, O. I., Su, C., Higuchi, W. and Hofmann, A. F. (1980). Mesophase formation during cholesterol dissolution in ursodeoxycholic-lecithin solutions: new mechanism for gallstone dissolution in humans. *J. Pharmaceut. Sci.*, **69**, 869–71

20. Ellis, W. R., Bell, G. D. and Clegg, R. J. (1981). Mechanisms for adjuvant cholelitholytic properties of the monoterpene mixture Rowachol. *Gastroenterology*, **80**, 1141

21. Thistle, J. L. and Hofmann, A. F. (1973). Efficacy and safety of chenodeoxycholic acid for dissolving gallstones. *N. Engl. J. Med.*, **289**, 655–9

22. Bell, G. D., Dowling, R. H., Whitney, B. and Sutor, D. J. (1975). The value of radiology in predicting gallstone type when selecting patients for medical treatment. *Gut*, **16**, 359–64

23. Wolpers, C. (1976). Auswahl der gallensteintrager zue litholyse. *Leber Magen Darm*, **6**, 43–6

24. Dolgin, S. M., Schwartz, J. S., Kressel, H. Y. *et al. (1981).* Identification of patients with cholesterol or pigment gallstones by discriminant analysis of radiographic features. *N. Engl. J. Med.*, **304**, 808–11

25. Iser, J. H., Dowling, R. H., Mok, H. Y. I. and Bell, G. D. (1975). Chenodeoxycholic acid treatment of gallstones – a follow-up report and analysis of factors influencing response to therapy. *N. Engl. J. Med.*, **293**, 378–83

26. Maton, P. N., Iser, J. H., Reuben, A. *et al.* (1982). The final outcome of CDCA-treatment in 125 patients with radiolucent gallstones: factors influencing efficacy, withdrawal, symp-toms and side effects and post-dissolution recurrence. *Medicine*, **61**, 85–96

27. Wolpers, C. (1974). Morphologie der gallensteime. *Leber Magen Darm*, 4, 43–57

28. Dowling, R. H. (1983). Cholelithiasis: medical treatment. *Clin. Gastroenterol.*, 12, 125–78

29. Iser, J. H., Maton, P. N., Murphy, G. M. and Dowling, R. H. (1978). Resistance to cheno-deoxycholic acid therapy. Treatment in obese patients with gallstones. *Br. Med. J.*, 1, 1509–12

30. Dowling, R. H., Ruppin, D. C., Meredith, T., Myszor, M., Forgacs, I. and Murphy, G. M. (1983). Efficacy of bile acid treatment in dissolving gallstones: colateral benefits of CDCA and UDCA therapy; gallstone recurrence and post-dissolution management. In Paumgartner, G., Stiehl, A. and Gerok, W. (eds.) *Bile Acids and Cholesterol in Health and Disease.* pp. 345–62. (Lancaster: MTP Press)

31. Forgacs, I. C., Maisey, M. N., Murphy, G. M. and Dowling, R. H. (1984). Influence of gallstones and ursodeoxycholic acid therapy on gallbladder emptying. *Gastroenterology*, 87, 299–307

32. Ransohoff, D. F. (1985). Natural history of silent gallstones. In Paumgartner, G., Stiehl, A. and Gerok, W. (eds.) *Enterohepatic Circulation of Bile Acids and Sterol Metabolism.* pp. 277–84. (Lancaster: MTP Press)

33. Palmer, A. K. and Heywood, R. (1974). Pathological changes in the rhesus fetus associated with the oral administration of chenodeoxycholic acid. *Toxicology*, 2, 239–46

34. Sarva, R. P., Fromm, H., Farivar, S. *et al.* (1980). Comparison of the effects between ursodeoxycholic and chenodeoxycholic acid on liver function and structure and on bile acid composition in the rhesus monkey. *Gastroenterology*, 79, 629

35. Bateson, M. C., Trash, D. B. and Bouchier, I. A. D. (1980). Can a 6-month cholecystogram predict eventual response to gallstone dissolution therapy? *Gut*, 21, 433 (abstract)

36. Thomas, P. J. and Hofmann, A. F. (1973). A simple calculation of lithogenic index of bile. Experimental biliary lipid composition on rectangular coordinates. *Gastroenterology*, 65, 698–700

37. Admirand, W. H. and Small, D. M. (1968). The physico-chemical basis of cholesterol gallstone formation in man. *J. Clin. Invest.*, 47, 1045–52

38. Hegardt, F. G. and Dam, H. (1971). The solubility of cholesterol in aqueous solution of bile salts and lecithin. *Z. Ernahrungswiss.*, 10, 223–33

39. Holzbach, R. T., Marsh, M., Olszewski, M. and Holan, K. (1973). Cholesterol solubility in bile: evidence that supersaturated bile is frequent in healthy man. *J. Clin. Invest.*, 52, 1467–79

40. Kupfer, R. M. and Northfield, T. C. (1983). Diurnal variation in cholesterol saturation of gallbladder bile. *Gut*, 24, 950–3

41. Kupfer, R. M., Maudgal, D. P. and Northfield, T. C. (1982). Gallstone dissolution rate during chenic acid therapy. Effect of bedtime administration plus low cholesterol diet. *Dig. Dis. Sci.*, 27, 1025–9

42. Somerville, K. W., Rose, D. H., Bell, G. D. *et al.* (1983). Gallstone dissolution and recurrence: are we being misled? *Br. Med. J.*, 284, 1295–7

43. Shapero, T. F., Rosem, I. E., Milson, S. R. and Fisher, M. M. (1982). Discrepancy between ultrasound and oral cholecystography in the assessment of gallstone dissolution. *Hepatology*, 2, 587–90

44. Tangedahl, T. (1979). Dissolution of gallstones – when and how? *Surg. Clin. N. Am.*, 59, 797–809

45. Carey, M. C., Park, Y.-H., Igimi, H. and Salvioli, G. (1985). Factors affecting speed of gallstone dissolution during litholytic therapy. In Paumgartner, G., Stiehl, A. and Gerok, W. (eds.) *Enterohepatic Circulation of Bile Acid and Sterol Metabolism.* (Lancaster: MTP Press)

46. Park, Y.-H., Igimi, H. and Carey, M. C. (1982). The 'mirroring' of gallstones: description of a novel silvering method to determine the surface area of an irregular object: *in vitro* demonstration that multiple gallstones from the same gallbladder dissolve in unsaturated 'bile' at the same rato. *Gastroenterology*, 83, 1071–8

47. Maudgal, D. P., Kupfer, R. M. and Northfield, T. C. (1983). Factors affecting gallstone dissolution rate during chenic acid therapy. *Gut*, 24, 7–10

48. Northfield, T. C., Lanzini, A., Jazrawi, R., Maudgal, D. P. and Kupfer, R. (1985). Methods of improving the efficacy of litholytic therapy. In Paumgartner, G., Stiehl, A. and Gerok, W. (eds.) *Enterohepatic Circulation of Bile Acids and Sterol Metabolism.* pp. 335–50. (Lancaster: MTP Press)

49. Bell, G. D., Sutor, D. J., Whitney, B. and Dowling, R. H. (1972). Factors influencing human gallstone dissolution in monkey, dog and human bile. *Gut*, 13, A856

50. Thistle, J. L., LaRusso, N. F., Hofmann, A. F., Turcotte, J., Carlson, G. L. and Ott, B. J. (1982). Differing effects of ursodeoxycholic or chenodeoxycholic acid on biliary cholesterol saturation and bile acid metabolism in man: a dose response study. *Dig. Dis. Sci.*, 27, 161–8

51. Carey, M. C. and Ko, G. (1979). The importance of total lipid concentration in determining cholesterol solubility in bile and the development of critical tables for calculating % cholesterol saturation with a correction factor for ursodeoxycholate-rich bile. In Paumgartner, G., Stiehl, A. and Gerok, W. (eds.) *Biological Effects of Bile Acids*. pp. 299–308. (Lancaster: MTP Press)

52. Stiehl, A., Raedsch, R., Czygan, P., Gotz, R., Manner, C. H. and Walker, S. (1980). Effects of biliary bile acid composition on biliary cholesterol saturation in gallstone patients treated with chenodeoxycholic acid and/or ursodeoxycholic acid. *Gastroenterology*, 79, 1192–8

53. Barbara, L., Bazzoli, F., Festi, D., Marselli, A. M. L. and Roda, E. (1983). A comparative study of chenodeoxycholic acid and ursodeoxycholic acid as cholesterol gallstone dissolving agents. In Paumgartner, G., Stiehl, A. and Gerok, W. (eds.) *Bile Acids and Cholesterol in Health and Disease*. pp. 367–70. (Lancaster: MTP Press)

54. Roda, E., Bazzoli, F., Labate, A. M. N., Mazzella, G., Roda, A., Sama, C., Festi, D., Aldini, R., Taroni, F. and Barbara, L. (1982). Ursodeoxycholic acid vs chenodeoxycholic acid as cholesterol gallstone-dissolving agents: a comparative randomised study. *Hepatology*, 2, 804–10

55 Erlinger, S., Go, A. L., Hussen, J. M. and Fervery, J. (1984). Franco–Belgium co-operative study of ursodeoxycholic acid in the medical dissolution of gallstones: a double blind randomised, dose–response study, and comparison with chenodeoxycholic acid. *Hepatology*, 4, 308–14

56. Fromm, H., Roat, J. N., Gonzalev, V., Sarva, R. J. and Farivar, S. (1983). Comparative efficacy and side effects of ursodeoxycholic acid and chenodeoxycholic acid in dissolving gallstones. *Gastroenterology*, 85, 1257–64

57. Maudgal, D. P., Bird, R. and Northfield, T. C. (1979). Optimal timing of doses of chenic acid in patients with gallstones. *Br. Med. J.*, 1, 922–3

58. Lanzini, A., Facchinetti, D. and Northfield, T. C. (1984). Therapeutic manipulation of the enterohepatic circulation in cholesterol cholelithiasis. *Clin. Sci.*, 66, 11P

59. Maudgal, D. P., Kupfer, R. M. and Northfield, T. C. (1982). Minimum effective dose of chenic acid for gallstone patients: reduction with bedtime administration and a low cholesterol diet. *Gut*, 23, 280–4

60. Maudgal, D. P., Bird, R., Blackwood, W. S. and Northfield, T.C. (1978). Low cholesterol diet: enhancement of effect of CDCA in patients with gallstones. *Br. Med. J.*, 2, 851–3

61. Nilsell, K., Angelin, B., Leijd, B. and Einarsson, K. (1983). Comparative effects of ursodeoxycholic acid and chenodeoxycholic acid on bile and kinetics and biliary lipid secretion in humans. Evidence for different modes of action on bile acid synthesis. *Gastroenterology*, 85, 1248–56

62. Ellis, W. R., Bell, G. D., Middleton, B. and White, D. (1981). Adjunct to bile acid treatment for gallstone dissolution: low dose chenodeoxycholic acid combined with terpene preparation. *Br. Med. J.*, 282, 611–12

63. Bachrach, W. H. and Hofmann, A. K. (1982). Ursodeoxycholic acid in the treatment of cholesterol cholelithiasis: a review. *Dig. Dis. Sci.*, 27, 833–56

64. Bateson, M. C., Hopwood, D. and Bouchier, I. A. D. (1977). Effect of gallstone dissolution therapy on human liver structure. *Am. J. Dig. Dis.*, 22, 293–9

65. Bell, G. D., Mok, H. Y. I., Thwe, M. *et al*. (1974). Liver structure and function in cholelithiasis: effect of chenodeoxycholic acid. *Gut*, 15, 165–72

66. Koch, M. M., Giamperi, M. P., Lorenzini, I. *et al*. (1980). Effect of chenodeoxycholic acid on liver structure and function in man: a serological and biochemical study. *Dig. Dis. Sci.* 27, 1025–9

67. Carey, J. B., Hoffbauer, F. W., Zaxi, F. G. and Nwokolo, C. (1965). Cholelithiasis and hepatic ductular proliferation induced in rats by lithocholic acid (a bile acid occurring naturally in man). *Gastroenterology*, 48, 809–10

68. Palmer, R. H. (1969). Toxic effect of lithocholic acid and related 5-H steroids. In Schiff, L.,

Carey, J. B. and Dietschy, J. M. (eds.) *Bile Salt Metabolism*. pp. 184–204. (Illinois: Springfield)

69. Low-Beer, T. S., Tyor, M. P. and Lack, L. (1969). Effects of sulfation of taurolithocholic acid and glycolithocholic acids on their intestinal transport. *Gastroenterology*, **56**, 721–5

70. Marks, J. W., Sue, S. O., Pearlman, B. J. *et al.* (1981). Sulfation of lithocholate as a possible modifier of chenodeoxycholic acid-induced elevations of serum transaminase in patients with gallstones. *J. Clin. Invest.*, **68**, 1190–6

71. Small, D. M. (1971). Gallstone disease – is therapy safe? (Editorial). *N. Engl. J. Med.*, **284**, 214–6

72. Pedersen, L., Arnfred, T. and Hess-Thaysem, E. (1974). Cholesterol kinetics in patients with cholesterol gallstones before and during chenodeoxycholic acid treatment. *Scand. J. Gastroenterol.*, **9**, 787–91

73. Hoffman, N. E., Hofmann, A. F. and Thistle, J. L. (1974). Effect of bile acid feeding on cholesterol metabolisn in gallstone patients. *Mayo Clin. Proc.*, **49**, 236–9

74. Bell, G. D., Lewis, B., Petrie, A. and Dowling, R. H. (1973). Serum lipids in cholelithiasis: effect of chenodeoxycholic acid therapy. *Br. Med. J.*, **3**, 520–3

75. Bateson, M. C., MacLean, D., Evans, J. R. and Bouchier, I. A. D. (1978). Chenodeoxycholic acid therapy for hypertriglyceridaemia in man. *Br. J. Clin. Pharm.*, **5**, 249–54

76. Albers, J. I., Grundy, J. M., Clearly, P. A. *et al.* (1982). For the National Co-operative Gallstone Study Group (NCGS): the effect of chenodeoxycholic acid on lipoproteins and apoproteins. *Gastroenterology*, **82**, 638–46

77. Angelin, B., Einarsson, K., Hellstrom, K. and Leijd, B. (1978). Effects of cholestyramine and chenodeoxycholic acid on the metabolism of endogenous triglyceride in hyper-lipoproteinaemia. *J. Lip. Res.*, **19**, 1017–24

78. Begemann, F. (1978). Influence of chenodeoxycholic acid on the kinetics of endogenous triglyceride transport in man. *Eur. J. Clin. Invest.*, **8**, 283–99

79. Narisawa, T., Sato, T., Hayakawa, M., Sukuma, A. and Nakano, H. (1971). Carcinoma of the colon and rectum and rats by rectal infusion of MNNG. *Gut*, **62**, 231

80. Sarwal, A. M., Cohen, B. I. and Raicht, R. F. (1979). Effects of dietary administration of chenodeoxycholic acid on N-methyl-nitrosurea-induced cancer in rats. *Biochem. Biophys. Acta.*, **574**, 423

81. Salvioli, G. and Salati, R. (1979). Faecal bile acid loss and bile acid pool size during short-term treatment with ursodeoxycholic and chenodeoxycholic acid in patients with radiolucent gallstones. *Gut*, **20**, 698

82. Stiehl, A. (1983). Side-effects of chenodeoxycholic and ursodeoxycholic acid. In Paumgartner, G., Stiehl, A. and Gerok, W. (eds.) *Bile Acids and Cholesterol Metabolism in Health and Disease*. pp. 387–92. (Lancaster: MTP Press)

83. Linos, D. A., Beard, L., O'Fallon, W. M. *et al.* (1981). Cholecystectomy and carcinoma of the colon. *Lancet*, **2**, 379

84. Vernick, L. J. and Kuller, L. H. (1971). Cholecystectomy and right-sided colon cancer: an epidemiological study. *Lancet*, **2**, 381

85. Bateson, M. C., Bouchier, I. A. D., Trash, D. B., Maudgal, D. P. and Northfield, T. C. (1981). Calcification of radiolucent gallstones during treatment with ursodeoxycholic acid. *Br. Med. J.*, **283**, 645–6

86. Igimi, H. and Carey, M. C. (1980). pH-solubility relation of chenodeoxycholic and urso-deoxycholic acids: physical–chemical basis for dissimilar solution and membrane phenomena. *J. Lip. Res.*, **21**, 72–89

87. Hofmann, A. F. (1985). Secretion and precipitation of calcium in bile. In Paumgartner, G., Stiehl, A. and Gerok, W. (eds.) *Enterohepatic Circulation of Bile Acids and Sterol Metabolism*. pp. 305–19. (Lancaster: MTP Press)

88. Cummings, S. A. and Hoffman, A. F. (1984). Physiological determinants of biliary calcium secretion in the dog. *Gastroenterology*, **87**, 664–73

89. Dumont, M., Erlinger, S. and Uchman, S. (1980). Hypercholeresis induced by urso-deoxycholic acid and 7-ketolithocholic acid in the rat. Possible role of bicarbonate transport. *Gastroenterology*, **79**, 82–9

90. Iser, J. H., Murphy, G. M. and Dowling, R. H. (1977). Speed of change in biliary lipids and bile acids with chenodeoxycholic acid – is intermittent therapy feasible? *Gut*, **18**, 7–15

91. Gleeson, D. and Ruppin, D. C. (1985). Discrepancies between cholecystocraphy and ultra-sonography in the detection of recurrent gallstones. *J. Hepatol.*, **1**, 597–607

92. Jazrawi, R. P., Joseph, A. E. A., Wilson, A. G. and Northfield, T. C. (1984). Comparison of cholecystography and ultrasonography for detection of gallstones. *Gut*, **25**, A561

93. Toulet, J., Rousset, J., Viteau, J. M., Douchon, Y. *et al.* (1983). Recidives et prevention des recidives apres dissolution de la lithiasis vesiculaire par lacide chenodeoxyclique chez 22 patients. *Gastroenterol. Clin. Biol.*, **7**, 605

94. Northfield, T. C., Maudgal, D. P., Kupfer, R. M. and Lanzini, A. (1983). Gallstone dissolution and recurrence. In Paumgartner, G., Stiehl, A. and Gerok, W. (eds.) *Bile Acids in Health and Disease*. pp. 371–9. (Lancaster: MTP Press)

95. Lanzini, A., Jazrawi, R. P., Kupfer, R. M., Maudgal, D. P., Joseph, A. E. A. and Northfield, T. C. (1986). Gallstone recurrence after medical dissolution: an overestimated threat? *Hepatology*. (In press)

96. Marks, J. W., Lan, S. and the Steering Committee for the NCGS. (1984). Low dose chenodiol for the prevention of gallstone recurrence following dissolution therapy. *Arch. Intern. Med.*, **100**, 976–81

97. Pomare, E. W., Heaton, K. W., Low-Beer, T. S. and Espiner, H. J. (1976). The effect of wheat bran upon bile salt metabolism and upon the lipid composition of bile in gallstone patients. *Am. J. Dig. Dis.*, **21**, 521–6

98. Thornton, J. R., Emmett, P. M. and Heaton, K. W. (1983). Diet and gallstones: effects of refined and unrefined carbohydrate diets on bile cholesterol saturation and bile acid metabolism. *Gut*, **24**, 2–6

99. Leuschner, M., Leuschner, U., Strohm, W. D., Trube, E., Fuchs, H. and Classen, M. (1984). Radiological and ultrasonographic investigations with respect to patient selection and monitoring for chemical gallstone dissolution. *Hepato-gastroenterology*, **31**, 140–3

100. Johansson, G. (1984). A prospective study of the clinical significance of the treatment of gallstones with chenodeoxycholic acid. *Surg. Gynaecol. Obstet.*, **159**, 127–9

101. Lalloni, L. and the GREPCO Study (1984). Gallbladder ultrasonography as a diagnostic tool in epidemiological screenings. In Capocaccia *et al.* (eds.) *Epidemiology and Prevention of Gallstone Disease*. pp. 111–15. (Lancaster: MTP Press)

102. Ricci, G. (1986). Prevalence of gallbladder disease (The GREPCO and Sirmione studies). Presented at the *9th International Symposium on Bile Acids*, Cortina, Italy, March

103. Glenn, F., McSherry, C. K. and Dineen, P. (1968). The morbidity of surgical treatment for non malignant biliary tract disease. *Surg. Gynaecol. Obstet.*, **126**, 15–26

104. McSherry, C. K. and Glenn, F. (1980). The incidence and causes of death following surgery for non-malignant biliary tract disease. *Ann. Surg.*, **191**, 271–5

9
Future Trends

M. C. BATESON

INTRODUCTION

Predictions of developments in diseases and health care are fun to make, if only for the retrospective pleasure spectators derive when they prove wrong, as with Aneurin Bevan's famous forecast that expenditure on health care would fall as the British welfare state improved health generally. Demand for health care services is apparently insatiable, but there are signs that containment of money spent will be practised in the future even in wealthy economies. It is necessary to estimate changes so that finite resources may be used to best advantage. In the absence of a time machine to transmit information back from the 21st century we must base our expectations on the current position and the recent past. Over the last 15 years striking developments in gallstone disease have been the advent of ultrasonography, the introduction of treatments without the need for formal laparotomy, and the better evaluation of the natural history of gallstones. Stimulated by these there has been a more critical approach to the overall requirement for a surgical approach to gallbladder disease, interestingly coupled with policies of much earlier surgery, both in acute cholecystitis and in gallstone-associated pancreatitis. What will be the pattern of gallstone disease and how will patients be cared for in the year 2000 and after? This chapter will succeed if it stimulates thought, though it will take some time to know how much of the informed speculation will prove to be on target.

AETIOLOGY

Alteration of biliary lipid metabolism has been extensively investigated as offering clues to the reason why cholesterol gallstones form, and it is accepted that hepatic oversecretion of cholesterol relative to bile acids is a necessary but not sufficient explanation[1]. Cholesterol oversaturation of bile is frequent in the healthy population and tends to increase with age even in non-obese subjects with no evidence of predisposition to stone formation[2]. Studies of biliary lipids have suggested that various factors may be important in stone formation; for example, moderate alcohol consumption may be preventive[3],

229

even though alcoholism predisposes to stones via cirrhosis. The picture is less clear with dietary bran which seems to reduce biliary cholesterol saturation in gallstone patients but not in healthy controls, and with dietary sucrose which does not affect bile adversely in the short-term even though it may induce undesirable obesity. Biliary lipid analysis after oral contraceptive usage clearly indicated that this might cause gallstone formation, but this was discounted by subsequent ultrasonic surveys and other epidemiological work[4-6]. By contrast clofibrate (and probably all the other fibric acid derivatives) acts by increasing cholesterol content of bile, and this was shown to be associated with an unacceptably high rate of gallstone disease[7,8]. This will probably continue to be a major limitation on the use of these drugs except in highly selected patients such as Fredrickson type III disease; severe hypertriglyceridaemia; and refractory hypercholesterolaemia, when used in combination with bile acid-binding resins.

Interest in the concept of nucleation of bile as a crucial factor in stone formation has grown rapidly since its proposal[9]. It seems that there is a heat-labile gallbladder protein[10,11] which initiates the process of stone formation, and no effective antinucleating factors are present to counteract this[12]. This may explain some of the inconsistencies of prior work focused on biliary lipid solubility[13], though the picture is not completely clear as biliary sludge is not necessarily a prestone condition[14].

Abnormalities of gallbladder emptying, which is slow in gallstone disease, may be another important aetiological factor[15], though there is as always a suspicion that this may be a secondary rather than primary phenomenon.

Animal models for gallstone disease are likely to fall out of favour[16] since they can give misleading answers. For instance, cholestyramine reliably causes gallstones in guinea pigs but does not seem to in people. Future work on aetiology may well be concentrated more on epidemiology, which has already yielded important new information about vegetarian diets[17] and alcohol[18].

EPIDEMIOLOGY

The principal and probably causative associations of gallstone disease are increasing age, female sex, race and obesity. Clofibrate therapy and cirrhosis are important but minor factors, and there is a whole host of others such as hypertriglyceridaemia and diet where the link is not so certain.

Past prevalence studies have been largely based on autopsies or iodine cholecystography surveys of selected groups. More recent cross-sectional studies with ultrasonography have yielded important information on symptoms. In future longitudinal studies with repeated real-time ultrasonography in the same patients will probably be undertaken to give an even clearer picture of the natural history of gallstones and changes in prevalence, though these will almost certainly be confined to the detection of gallbladder stones in developed societies.

Other developing societies are likely to experience the rapid increase in gallstone prevalence seen in Japan, simultaneously with the adoption of western lifestyles. In addition, it is certain that gallstones will become commoner in developed societies because of trends already identified. Autopsy surveys have already shown increases in gallstone prevalence over the last 40 years for men (but not women) in Ohio, USA[19] and for both men and women in Dundee, Scotland[20]. The reasons for these changes are not clear but affect all ages of patients. The predicted increasing proportion of the very aged in society[21] will itself lead to an increased overall frequency of gallstones, as the elderly are especially prone to the disease, which increases in prevalence with succeeding decades of age. In addition there has been a clear tendency for obesity to become commoner[22,23] and this would be likely to further increase the number of gallstones seen in the future[24]. Not only are the morbidly obese at high risk from gallstones, but operative treatment designed to reduce body mass may actually increase the tendency to cholelithiasis[25]. Whether the health consciousness of modern society will lead to a reduction in the fatness of the community remains to be seen, but some of the cholelithiasis yet to be diagnosed will result from the increasing obesity of the past and present.

NATURAL HISTORY

Important recent work has shown that gallstones are usually asymptomatic and remain so[26-28]. However, when symptoms do occur they are likely to persist and worsen so that treatment is required[28]. It is interesting that women with gallstones seem more prone to develop symptoms than men. Also gallstones are much more commonly treated by cholecystectomy in Italy and the United States (one in three) than in the United Kingdom or Spain (one in seven to ten). The mortality attributable to gallstone disease and cholecystitis is not high, but has fallen markedly in various countries between 1950 and 1980[29]. This could reflect a continuing change in the natural history of gallstone disease rather than medical treatment, and does not seem to be explained by cholecystectomy rates. A 66% fall in mortality between 1956 and 1978 in England and Wales was simultaneous with a rise in cholecystectomy rates[30] (K. W. Heaton, personal communication), whereas an 83% fall in mortality in Sweden during the same period was associated with a steeply declining cholecystectomy rate[31].

A novel technique of carbon-14 dating has indicated that symptoms only occur after an interval of at least 2 years from gallstone formation (average time 8 years)[32]. This will require validation.

PROPHYLAXIS

The population is currently bombarded by streams of propaganda aimed at making it more healthy. It is always difficult to recommend changes in lifestyle to normal people in the hope of preventing diseases which they may not consider themselves likely to develop. However, gallstone disease is so common that the community is well aware of it. Unexceptionable but not necessarily acceptable advice which would prevent some gallstones developing is the avoidance of obesity. Since this condition is exceedingly difficult to treat once it has developed, efforts are required to encourage people to stay slim.

This has become an even more difficult issue with the current controversies as to what represents a desirable weight at different ages[22]. There is suggestive evidence that an increased amount of fibre in the diet and a decreased intake of both sugar and animal products will protect from gallstones. Nutritional advice offered at present tends to encourage these and there is some evidence that the population is changing its eating habits along these lines. Although there is an increased alcohol intake in countries such as Britain and this has caused concern because of its association with various alcohol-related diseases, the average level of intake in developed societies is more likely to protect from gallstones and heart disease than to cause health problems. In practice no specific recommendations about alcohol are likely to be useful. In patients who have had gallstones successfully treated or in subgroups who are especially prone to develop gallstones there may be a role for specific drug therapy. Chenodeoxycholic acid, ursodeoxycholic acid and dehydrocholic acid have all been recommended for use in this way, but the doses required and the effectiveness and safety of prolonged therapy are in doubt. In any event this could only apply to very small and highly selected groups such as those with recurrent stone formation after cholecystectomy.

There are no clues as to any techniques which might prevent the development of pigment or mineral gallstones, and this is likely to be an area of continuing research into bilirubin and calcium metabolism for some time, rather than a field for clinical recommendations. Similarly the intriguing recent work on the importance of nucleation of bile in the development of stones might provide a technique of prophylaxis if safe, and effective antinucleating manoeuvres can be identified. Restriction of the use of clofibrate should avoid gallstone problems for a few patients.

DIAGNOSIS

Real-time cholecystosonography is likely to remain the procedure of choice for diagnosing gallbladder stones[33]. Oral cholecystography can yield results which are almost as good and the two techniques should probably be regarded as complementary in the detection of very small stones[34]. It seems unlikely that there will be any further use for refinement in the standard double-dose oral cholecystogram, though digital processing of images has been proposed to improve results[35]. The pace of change in ultrasonography is rapid, and more sophisticated machines, perhaps with computer-assisted operation, may further increase what is an exceptionally good performance for diagnosing gallbladder stones. Detection of calcification not apparent on plain radiographs may be usefully assessed by high resolution ultrasonography[36] or computed X-ray tomography. An even more exciting possibility is that the advent of nuclear magnetic resonance may permit *in vivo* chemical analysis of stones. NMR is too costly to be envisaged as more than a research procedure for the biliary tract in the foreseeable future[37]. Ultrasonography is ideally suited for population surveys of gallstone disease, but is relatively ineffective in diagnosing bile duct stones, which are clinically much more important than those in the gallbladder. Endoscopic retrograde cholangiopancreatography and percutaneous transhepatic cholangiography are likely to remain the diagnostic procedures of choice in those patients not yet submitted to surgery. If it is accepted that bile duct dilatation is itself a hallmark of choledocholithiasis then ultrasonography may have a more useful role in diagnosis here[38,39], though its value will probably be the negative one of excluding biliary duct stones when normal.

A diagnosis of acute cholecystitis continues to cause problems, with 20–25% of clinical diagnoses proving incorrect[40,41]. Though ultrasonography can confirm or refute the presence of gallstones in these patients, it may still continue to be necessary to perform isotope scanning with compounds such as HIDA in addition before proceeding to early cholecystectomy[42].

The patient with right upper quadrant abdominal pain who definitely does not have gallstones will continue to be a problem. Two procedures which may be helpful in diagnosing these patients in the future are pressure studies of the gastrointestinal tract and gallbladder motility assessment. Many patients with no gallstones but 'biliary symptoms' can be shown to have irritable bowel syndrome by inflation of balloons in the small or large bowel[43]. Though an invasive and troublesome procedure, this may be useful in evaluation and management of a difficult problem. Much more contentious is the use of cholecystokinetic agents such as sincalide and caerulein (or CCK itself) to demonstrate 'abnormal' gallbladder motility and to reproduce abdominal symptoms[44]. It is known that CCK itself can produce various symptoms including abdominal pain and vomiting in completely healthy individuals[45] and even more puzzling it is reported that caerulein can actually relieve biliary pain[46]. With the important but uncommon exceptions of emphysematous cholecystitis or gallbladder carcinoma it is likely to remain the dogma of the future that patients without gallstones do not have gallbladder disease.

A special application of ultrasonography is the use of special ultrasound probes at laparotomy (or passed via endoscopes) to diagnose bile duct and also gallbladder stones. Current techniques of flexible and rigid chole-dochoscopy and peroperative cholangiography may in the future usefully be supplemented or replaced by direct ultrasonic probe scanning of the bile ducts, which has the attraction of being less invasive.

CHOLECYSTECTOMY

Since 1882 removal of the gallbladder has become established as the standard treatment for cholecystolithiasis. There is no reason to suppose that this will change, though ideas about the requirement for any treatment in gallstone disease are under scrutiny. For instance, the rate of cholecystectomy in the United States is several times higher than in the United Kingdom, without any clear advantage to the patients[47]. There is indeed an indication that higher surgical rates may worsen the overall mortality of patients with gallstone disease [47,48]. It is of great interest that the cholecystectomy rate in Stockholm has fallen continuously since 1969[31], since Sweden may be regarded as having the best developed health service in the world. It is likely that other developed countries will follow suit and that, though gallstones become commoner, operations will be less often performed.

Though cholecystectomy rates in the United States still seem to be increasing, there was a 20% fall in rates in Canada between 1970 and 1976[49]. Cholecystectomy rates in Scotland and Bristol, England seem to have risen to a peak in about 1978 and subsequently to have reached a plateau or even a decline[20] (K. W. Heaton, personal communication). Though the reasonable suggestion has been made that cholecystectomy rates do correlate with the prevalence of gallstones[50], changes in surgical rates cannot be explained by the prevalence of gallstones and they are probably almost entirely governed by surgical resources and organization of health services[51].

In those patients who are judged to require cholecystectomy in the future early surgery is likely to be increasingly practised. Overall there may be some increase in operative mortality, but the prevention of recurrent cholecystitis and improved symptom relief are worthwhile benefits[52-54]. In the particular case of acute pancreatitis associated with gallstones, early cholecystectomy and/or exploration of the common bile duct are clearly desirable and will probably be the main indication for operative intervention in the future[55,56].

Figures for mortality following cholecystectomy vary, depending upon the technique of analysis used, but there is some evidence of a reduction in deaths in recent years[54,57]. It would be hard to improve further in the claim of no deaths at all after elective cholecystectomy[57]! However, the overall mortality rate following gallstone surgery $(0.7-1.2\%)$[57,58] may actually apparently deteriorate in the future because of an increasing workload in the elderly, who are more prone to have bile duct stones requiring choledochotomy[59]. In addition the overall mortality in patients over 64 is appreciably increased at 3.3%[60].

Though unusual groups such as Pima Indians may have a high risk of gallbladder carcinoma and benefit from an energetic cholecystectomy policy in gallbladder disease[61], this does not apply to other racial groups where cancer risks should not influence the decision about surgery[62]. The conclusion of a long debate about the relationship between gallstones, bowel carcinoma and cholecystectomy will probably be that there is a small increase in carcinomas of the large bowel in patients over 60 years who had a cholecystectomy more than 10 years before[63] and that this relates to the results of surgery rather than an association between bowel carcinoma and gallstone disease. It does not seem likely that this risk will influence decisions on surgical management.

Is there scope for improvement in operative mortality? Experimental procedures such as preoperative stenting or nasobiliary draining in obstructive jaundice may be an improvement, but have yet to be fully evaluated. In elective cholecystectomy without any other procedure in younger patients, mortality is currently very close to the risk of the general anaesthetic. Prophylaxis of pulmonary embolism with low dose heparin and antibiotic prophylaxis of wound infections appear attractive and safe options for improving results further.

MEDICAL TREATMENT OF GALLBLADDER STONES

In the 15 years since gallstone dissolution was first described following treatment with chenodeoxycholic acid there has been a wealth of information published on the non-operative management of gallstones. Only a minority of patients with gallstone disease will be suitable for attempts at dissolution treatment even though three-quarters of gallstones in western societies are cholesterol-rich[64]. Severe symptoms, large stones and non-functioning gallbladders all make successful dissolution therapy unlikely. Studies on pigment gallstones reveal the presence of polymer networks which makes dissolution very unlikely with any agent[65], though EDTA has been used by direct infusion. The current concept is that gallstone dissolution with bile acids is achieved by reduction of cholesterol content of bile, and during ursodeoxycholic acid treatment also by the formation of a surface mesophase around the stone[66]. Efforts to predict the outcome of treatment for individuals by analysis of biliary lipids have been disappointing and it is likely that future assessments will be based entirely on careful selection of suitable patients and a trial of therapy assessed by serial ultrasonography or cholecystography[67]. The overall results of treatment with chenodeoxycholic acid and urso-deoxycholic acid appear comparable. There is still confusion about optimal dosage[68-70]. The best recommendation that can be given at present is for chenodeoxycholic acid to use a dose of 1000 mg daily or 15 mg/kg daily, or the biggest dose which avoids diarrhoea if less than these. For ursodeoxycholic acid there is even less impressive evidence that larger doses are more effective and none at all that body weight is important, so the author's rec-ommendation is to use 750 mg daily as 250 mg in the morning and 500 mg at night in all cases. Though successful dissolution therapy normally requires 6-24 months' treatment, more prolonged therapy is often successful where a partial response has been seen by 2 years[71]. Ursodeoxycholic acid is prone to cause calcification of radiolucent gallstones though this may not necessarily interfere with successful dissolution therapy[72,73]. Efforts to explain acquired calcification of stones during bile acid therapy have been unsuccessful to date[74] but further research in this field will be undertaken. Though cheno-deoxycholic acid may also sometimes induce gallstone calcification[75] and may reduce HDL cholesterol concentration in the serum[76], diarrhoea is the principal drawback of this agent. Combinations of chenodeoxycholic acid and ursodeoxycholic acid, or use of the trihydroxy bile acid ursocholic acid[77,78] show promise and may become standard treatments in the future. Response to chenodeoxycholic acid may be enhanced by bedtime dosage and treatment with a low animal fat low cholesterol diet[79]. Diet therapy does not improve response to ursodeoxycholic acid, but dosage at bedtime may prove to be useful[80]. One way of improving results is to ensure patient compliance, which during ursodeoxycholic acid may simply be done by estimating serum ursodeoxycholic acid levels[81-83]. Serum chenodeoxycholic acid is much less useful in monitoring compliance during treatment with this agent as there is such a wide overlap of results with normal and untreated levels.

Prevention of gallstone recurrence is ripe for some advance. The rate of recurrence of stones after dissolution is high[84]. The British Gallstone Study

Group has shown that advising patients to take a high fibre low sugar diet is ineffective in preventing relapse. This group has also shown that urso-deoxycholic acid 3mg/kg a day does not absolutely prevent recurrence, though there could be some delaying effect. Treatment with full dose bile acid therapy may prove to be effective if cumbersome. Alternate-month full dose chenodeoxycholic acid therapy has certainly been proposed[85]. Low dose chenodeoxycholic acid is known to be ineffective and will probably not be further investigated in the future[86]. Though treatment with ursodeoxycholic acid is very effective in relieving symptoms associated with gallstones and also those of bile reflux gastritis[87], it remains to be seen whether these will prove to be of practical use in maintenance therapy. By contrast, long-term treatment with chenodeoxycholic acid 750 mg daily in the rare condition cerebrotendinous xanthomatosis (CTX) looks extremely promising[88]. Use of the terpene mixture Rowachol has been proposed as adjuvant treatment with chenodeoxycholic acid for gallstones[89]. Much more extensive experience with this agent is required before it can be recommended for general use, and scepticism about its value has been caused by the failure of one study to show any useful effect on biliary lipids in normal volunteers[90].

The search for new agents for gallstone dissolution will continue and it could be that other bile acids or their analogues are shown to be more effective or even safer[91] than current treatment.

BILE DUCT STONES

Although choledochotomy is always likely to have an important place in the management of bile duct stones, an important advance is that standard treatment is now by endoscopic stone removal which carries a lower mortality[92]. Anxiety about the long-term consequences of endoscopic papillotomy may mean that at least the smaller duct stones are removed after medical sphincter dilatation with or without glycerin trinitrate[93,94].

Where expertise exists percutaneous extraction of retained bile duct stones through T-tube drain tracts[15] will continue to be useful. A further development of percutaneous treatment is direct puncture of biliary tract to assist duodenoscopic sphincterotomy in difficult cases[96].

Various bile duct infusions have been tested and discarded in the past for dissolving bile duct stones. Dextro-limonene, heparin, EDTA and sodium cholate seem unlikely to have much future in management of bile duct stones. The standard current treatment is mono-octanoin infusion which has a good success rate with smaller stones after prolonged treatment[97,98]. An interesting powerful cholesterol solvent currently under evaluation is methyl tertiary butyl ether[99,100]. If the safety of this agent is proved then infusion combined with bile aspiration may become the local dissolution treatment of choice for choledocholithiasis. Where oral treatment must be used ursodeoxycholic acid 750 mg daily or 12 mg/kg a day is standard therapy[101]. Results might be improved by the addition of Rowachol. Oral preparations of the ethers are available and could have a place in both gallbladder and bile duct stone dissolution[102].

NEW TREATMENT MODES

Several recently described techniques may come to have general application. The technique of cholecystectomy has been refined so that stones can be retrieved percutaneously both from the gallbladder and bile ducts in patients who have a high risk for general anaesthesia[103]. Even where stones are not removed, percutaneous ultrasonically guided cholecystectomy may have a useful role in management with acute cholecystitis or obstructive jaundice[104,105]. Obliteration of the gallbladder by use of acrylate has been proposed as an alternative for cholecystectomy[106]. Experience with animals was encouraging though this is not yet known to be a safe technique for humans. Perhaps the most interesting recent development which could change our approach to gallstones is the use of ultrasound or mechanical shock waves to fragment stones which can then be passed or dissolved[107-110]. These procedures may require snaring of stones by basket. If external shock lithotripsy can be developed as successfully as with urinary calculi, then the need for cholecystectomy might well reduce further, though the overall applicability may be only about 10%, and adjuvant bile acid therapy may be required.

SUMMARY

A more critical approach to requirement for operative treatment in gall-stone disease, combined with endoscopic treatment, dissolution and litho-tripsy seems likely to lead to a decline in the cholecystectomy rates, even in the face of increased frequency of gallstone disease.

References

1. Nilsell, K., Angelin, B., Liljequist, L. and Einarsson, K. (1985). Biliary lipid output and bile acid kinetics in cholesterol gallstone disease. Evidence for an increased hepatic secretion of cholesterol in Swedish patients. *Gastroenterology*, **98**, 287–93
2. Einarsson, K., Nilsell, K., Leijd, B. and Angelin, B. (1985). Influence of age on secretion of cholesterol and synthesis of bile acids by the liver. *N. Engl. J. Med.*, **313**, 277–82
3. Thornton, J., Symes, C. and Heaton, K. (1983). Moderate alcohol intake reduces bile cholesterol saturation and raised HDL cholesterol. *Lancet*, **2**, 819–22
4. Scragg, R. K. R., McMichael, A. J. and Seamark, R. F. (1984). Oral contraceptives, pregnancy, and endogenous oestrogen in gallstone disease – a case–control study. *Br. Med. J.*, **2**, 1795–9
5. Royal College of General Practitioners' Oral Contraceptive Study (1982). Oral contraceptives and gallbladder disease. *Lancet*, **2**, 957–9
6. Everson, R. B., Byar, D. P. and Bischoff, A. J. (1982). Estrogen predisposes to cholecystectomy but not to stones. *Gastroenterology*, **82**, 4–8
7. Coronary Drug Project Research Group (1977). Gallbladder disease as a side-effect of drugs influencing lipid metabolism. *N. Engl. J. Med.*, **296**, 1185–7
8. Bateson, M. C., Maclean, D., Ross, P. E. and Bouchier, I. A. D. (1978). Clofibrate therapy and gallstone induction. *Am. J. Dig. Dis.*, **23**, 623–8
9. Holan, K. R., Holzbach, R. T., Hermann, R. E., Cooperman, A. M. and Claffey, W. J. (1979). Nucleation time: a key factor in the pathogenesis of cholesterol gallstone disease. *Gastroenterology*, **77**, 611–17
10. Gollish, S. H., Burnstein, M. J., Ilson, R. G., Petrunka, C. N. and Strasberg, S. M. (1983). Nucleation of cholesterol monohydrate crystals from hepatic and gallbladder bile of patients with cholesterol gallstones. *Gut*, **24**, 836–44
11. Gallinger, S., Taylor, R. D., Harvey, P. R. C., Petrunka, C. N. and Strasberg, S. M. (1985). Effect of mucous glycoprotein on nucleation time of human bile. *Gastroenterology*, **89**, 648–58

12. Burnstein, M. J., Ilson, R. G., Petrunka, C. N., Taylor, R. D. and Strasberg, S. M. (1983). Evidence for a potent nucleating factor in gallbladder bile of patients with cholesterol gallstones. *Gastroenterology*, **85**, 801–7

13. Whiting, M. J. and Watts, J. McK. (1984). Supersaturated bile from obese patients without gallstones supports cholesterol crystal growth but not nucleation. *Gastroenterology*, **86**, 243–8

14. Bolondi, L., Gaini, S., Testa, S. and Labo, G. (1985). Gallbladder sludge formation during prolonged fasting after gastrointestinal surgery. *Gut*, **26**, 734–8

15. Pomeranz, I. S. and Schaffer, E. A. (1985). Abnormal gallbladder emptying in a subgroup of patients with gallstones. *Gastroenterology*, **88**, 787–91

16. Holzbach, R. T. (1984). Animal models of cholesterol gallstone disease. *Hepatology*, **4**, 1915–85 (suppl.)

17. Pixley, F., Wilson, D., McPherson, K. and Mann, J. (1985). Effect of vegetarianism on development of gallstones in women. *Br. Med. J.*, **291**, 11–12

18. Scragg, R. K. R., McMichael, A. J. and Baghurst, P. A. (1984). Diet, alcohol, and relative weight in gallstone disease: a case control study. *Br. Med. J.*, **288**, 1113–18

19. Gutierrez, Y., Ransohoff, D. F. and Gracie, W. A. (1984). Frequency of gallstone disease: trends over time at autopsy. *Gastroenterology*, **86**, 1103 (abstract)

20. Bateson, M. C. (1984). Gallstone prevalence and cholecystectomy rates are independently variable. *Lancet*, **2**, 621–5

21. Editorial (1986). Geriatrics and the U.S.A. *Lancet*, **1**, 133–4

22. Andres, R., Elahi, D., Tobin, J. D., Muller, D. C. and Brant, L. (1985). Impact of age on weight goals. *Ann. Intern. Med.*,, **103**, 1030–3

23. Feinlieb, M. (1985). Epidemiology of obesity in relation to health hazards. *Ann. Intern. Med.*, **103**, 1019–24

24. Rimm, A. A., Werner, L. H., Van Yserloo, B. and Bernstein, R. A. (1975). Relationship of obesity and disease in 73,532 weight-conscious women. *Pub. Health Rep.*, **90**, 44–51

25. Amaral, J. F. and Thompson, W. R. (1985). Gallbladder disease in the morbidly obese. *Am. J. Surg.*, **149**, 551–7

26. Gracie, W. A. and Ransohoff, D. F. (1982). The natural history of gallstones. The innocent gallstone is not a myth. *N. Engl. J. Med.*, **307**, 798–800

27. Thistle, J. L., Cleary, P. A., Lachin, J. M. *et al.* (1984). The natural history of cholelithiasis: the national co-operative gallstone study. *Ann. Intern. Med.*, **101**, 171–5

28. McSherry, C. K., Ferstenberg, H., Calhoun, W. F., Lahman, E. and Virshup, M. (1985). The natural history of diagnosed gallstone disease in symptomatic and asymptomatic patients. *Ann. Surg.*, **302**, 59–63

29. Charlton, J. R. H. and Velez, R. (1986). Some international comparisons of mortality amenable to medical intervention. *Br. Med. J.*, **292**, 295–301

30. Holland, C. and Heaton, K. W. (1972). Increasing frequency of gallbladder operations in the Bristol clinical area. *Br. Med. J.*, **3**, 672–5

31. Ahlberg, J., Bergstrand, L. O. and Sahlin, S. (1984). Changes in gallstone morbidity in a community with a decreasing frequency of cholecystectomy. *Acta Chir. Scand.*, **520**, 53–8 (suppl.)

32. Mok, H. Y. I., Druffel, E. R. M. and Rampone, W. M. (1986). Chronology of cholelithiasis. *N. Engl. J. Med.*, **314**, 1075–7

33. Cooperberg, P. L. and Burhenne, H. J. (1980). Real-time ultrasonography: diagnostic technique of choice in calculous gallbladder disease. *N. Engl. J. Med.*, **302**, 1277–9

34. Gleeson, D., Ruppin, D. C. and the British Gallstone Study Group (1985). Discrepancies between cholecystography and ultrasonography in the detection of recurrent gallstones. *J. Hepatol.*, **1**, 597–607

35. Taenzer, V. (1983). Conventional cholecystography. In Lutz, H. and Remling, L. (eds.) *Diagnostic Methods in Hepatology*. pp. 73–7. (Lancaster: MTP Press)

36. Parulekar, S. G. (1984). Ultrasonic detection of calcification in gallstones; the reverberation shadow. *J. Ultrasound Med.*, **3**, 123–9

37. Cherryman, G. R. (1985). Cost of operating a nuclear magnetic resonance imaging system. *Br. Med. J.*, **291**, 1437–8

38. Lygidakis, N. J. (1984). The incidence and significance of common bile duct dilatation in biliary calculous diseases. *World J. Surg.*, **8**, 327–34

39. Niederay, C., Sonnenberg, A. and Mueller, J. (1984). Comparison of the extra-hepatic bile duct size measured by ultrasound and by different radiographic techniques. *Gastroenterology*, **87**, 615–21

40. Halasz, N. A. (1975). Counterfeit cholecystitis: a common diagnostic dilemma. *Am. J. Surg.*, **130**, 189–93

41. Gunn, A. A. (1982). The management of gallstones. In Russell, R. C. G. (ed.) *Recent Advances in Surgery*. pp. 183–96. (Edinburgh: Churchill Livingstone)

42. Stephens, R. B., Keane, F. B., Freyne, P. and Hennessy, T. P. J. (1982). HIDA scanning without ultrasonography is insufficient for early diagnosis of acute gallbladder disease. *Gut*, **23**, A455

43. Kingham, J. G. C. and Dawson, A. M. (1984). Origin of chronic right upper quadrant pain. *Gut*, **25**, A550

44. Pickleman, J., Peiss, R. L., Henkin, R., Salo, B. and Nagel, P. (1985). The role of sincalide cholescintigraphy in the evaluation of patients with acalculus gallbladder disease. *Arch. Surg.*, **120**, 693–7

45. Hopman, W. P. M., Jansen, J. B. M. J., Grosenbusch, G. and Lamers, C. B. H. W. (1986). Gallbladder contraction induced by cholecystokinin: bolus injection or infusion? *Br. Med. J.*, **292**, 375–6

46. Basso, N., Bagarani, M., Materia, A. *et al.* (1985). Effect of caerulein in patients with biliary colic pain. *Gastroenterology*, **89**, 605–9

47. Bates, T., Godfrey, P. J., Harrison, M., Walsh, B. and Levien, D. H. (1984). Cholecystectomy rates in the U.S. and the U.K. compared: does the difference matter? *Gut*, **25**, A1147–8

48. Ransohoff, D. F., Gracie, W. A., Wolfenson, L. B. and Neuhauser, D. (1983). Prophylactic cholecystectomy or expectant management for silent gallstones. *Ann. Intern. Med.*, **99**, 199–204

49. Vayda, E. and Mindell, W. R. (1982). Variations in operative rates: what do they mean? *Surg. Clin. N. Am.*, **62**, 627–39

50. McPherson, K., Strong, P. M., Jones, L. and Britton, B. J. (1985). Do cholecystectomy rates correlate with geographic variations in the prevalence of gallstones? *J. Epidemiol. Commun. Health*, **39**, 179–82

51. Fowkes, F. G. R. (1980). Cholecystectomy and surgical resources in Scotland. *Health Bull.*, May, 126–32

52. Hoey, J. and Psihramis, K. (1979). Cholelithiasis: a comparison of surgical and non-surgical management strategies based on available evidence. *Clin. Invest. Med.*, **2**, 75–81

53. Lahtinen, J., Alhava, E. M. and Aukee, S. (1978). Acute cholecystitis treated by early and delayed surgery. A controlled clinical trial. *Scand. J. Gastroenterol.*, **13**, 673–8

54. Mitchell, A. and Morris, P. J. (1982). Trends in management of acute cholecystitis. *Br. Med. J.*, **284**, 27–30

55. Mayer, D. and McMahon, M. J. (1982). Operations for gallstones in patients with acute pancreatitis. *Gut*, **23**, A440

56. Imrie, C. W. and Shearer, M. G. (1986). Diagnosis and management of severe acute pancreatitis. In Russell, R. C. G. (ed.) *Recent Advances of Surgery*. pp. 143–54. (Edinburgh: Churchill Livingstone)

57. Crumplin, M. K. H., Jenkinson, L. R., Kassab, J. Y., Whittaker, C. M. and Al-Boutiahi, F. H. (1985). Management of gallstones in a district general hospital. *Br. J. Surg.*, **72**, 428–32

58. Godfrey, P. J., Bates, T., Harrison, M., King, M. B. and Padley, N. R. (1984). Gallstones and mortality: a study of all gallstone related deaths in a single health district. *Gut*, **25**, 1029–33

59. Hermann, R. E. (1983). Biliary disease in the aging patient. In Texter, E. C. (ed.) *The Aging Gut*. Ch. 5. (Cleveland, Ohio: Masson Publishing)

60. Houghton, P. W. J., Jenkinson, L. R. and Donaldson, L. A. (1985). Cholecystectomy in the elderly: a prospective study. *Br. J. Surg.*, **72**, 220–2

61. Carraher, M. J., Wilson, D. L. and Knowler, W. C. (1984). Biliary carcinoma and mortality in Pima Indians: 15 year follow-up after oral cholecystography survey. *Gastroenterology*, **86**, 1041 (abstract)

62. Stubbs, R. S., McLoy, R. F. and Blumgart, L. H. (1983). Cholelithiasis and cholecystitis: surgical treatment. *Clin. Gastroenterol.*, **12**, 179–201

63. Mannes, A. G., Weinzierl, M., Stellard, F., Thieme, C., Wiebecke, B. and Paumgartner, G.

(1984). Adenomas of the large intestine after cholecystectomy. *Gut*, **25**, 863–6

64. Whiting, M. J., Bradley, B. M. and Watts, J. McK. (1983). Chemical and physical properties of gallstones in south Australia: implications for dissolution treatment. *Gut*, **24**, 11–15

65. Ohkybo, H., Ostrow, J. D., Carr, S. H. and Rege, R. V. (1984). Polymer networks in pigment and cholesterol gallstones assessed by equilibrium swelling and infrared spectroscopy. *Gastroenterology*, **87**, 805–14

66. Su, C. C., Higuchi, W. I., Gilmore, I. T., Danzinger, R. G. and Hofmann, A. F. (1984). Mesophase formation during cholesterol gallstone dissolution in human bile: effect of bile acid composition. *J. Pharmaceut. Sci.*, **73**, 1160–1

67. Bateson, M. C., Trash, D. B. and Bouchier, I. A. D. (1980). Can a six month cholecystogram predict eventual response to gallstone dissolution therapy? *Gut*, **21**, A443

68. Erlinger, S., Lego, A., Husson, J. M. and Fevery, J. (1984). Franco–Belgian co-operative study of ursodeoxycholic acid in the medical dissolution of gallstones: a double-blind, randomised, dose–response study and comparison with chenodeoxycholic acid. *Hepatology*, **4**, 308–14

69. Fisher, M. M., Roberts, E. A., Rocen, I. E. *et al.* (1985). The Sunnybrook gallstone study: a double-blind controlled trial of chenodeoxycholic acid for gallstone dissolution. *Hepatology*, **5**, 102–7

70. Lachin, J. M., Schoenfield, L. J. and the National Co-operative Gallstone Study Group (1983). Effects of dose relative to body weight in the national co-operative gallstone study: a fixed-dose trial. *Controlled Clin. Trials*, **4**, 125–31

71. Marks, J. W., Baum, R. A., Hanson, R. F. *et al.* (1984). Additional chenodiol therapy after partial dissolution of gallstones with two years of treatment. *Ann. Intern. Med.*, **100**, 382–4

72. Bateson, M. C., Maudgal, D. P., Trash, D. B., Northfield, T. C. and Bouchier, I. A. D. (1981). Gallstone calcification caused by ursodeoxycholic acid. *Br. Med. J.*, **283**, 645–6

73. Bouchier, I. A. D. and Neligan, P. (1983). Calcification of radiolucent gallstones during ursodeoxycholic acid therapy. In Parmgartner, G., Stiehl, A. and Gerok, W. (eds.) *Bile Acids and Cholesterol in Health and Disease.* (Lancaster: MTP Press)

74. Marteau, C., Portugal, H., Pauli, A. M. and Gerolami, A. (1985). Effect of glycoursodeoxycholate on precipitation of calcium carbonate. *Hepatology*, **5**, 1209–12

75. Schoenfield, L. J., Lachin, J. M., the Steering Committee and the National Co-operative Gallstone Study Group (1981). Chenodiol for dissolution of gallstones. *Ann. Intern. Med.*, **95**, 257–82

76. Leiss, O. and von Bergmann, K. (1982). Different effects of chenodeoxycholic acid and ursodeoxycholic acid on serum lipoprotein concentrations in patients with radiolucent gallstones. *Scand. J. Gastroenterol.*, **17**, 587–92

77. Loria, P., Carulli, N., Medici, G. *et al.* (1986). Effect of ursocholic acid on biliary lipid secretion and composition. *Gastroenterology*, **90**, 865–74

78. Zuin, M. and Podda, M. (1984). Ursocholic acid: a new litholytic agent. *Hepatology*, **4**, 1060 (abstract)

79. Kupfer, R. M., Maudgal, D. P. and Northfield, T. C. (1982). Gallstone dissolution rate during chenodeoxycholic acid therapy. Effect of bedtime administration and low cholesterol diet. *Dig. Dis. Sci.*, **27**, 1025–9

80. Conte, D., Bozzani, A., Sironi, L., Rocca, F., Camassa, L. and Bianchi, P. A. (1981). Radiolucent gallstone dissolution with bedtime ursodeoxycholic acid administration. *Digestion*, **22**, 302–4

81. Ewerth, S., Angelin, B., Einarsson, K., Nilsell, K. and Björkmeim, I. (1985). Serum concentrations of ursodeoxycholic acid in portal venous and systemic venous blood of fasting humans as determined by isotope dilution: mass spectrometry. *Gastroenterology*, **88**, 126–33

82. Bazzoli, F., Roda, A., Fromm, H. *et al.* (1983). Predictive value of serum ursodeoxycholic acid and chenodeoxycholic acid measurements for evaluating patient compliance with the respective bile acid treatment. *Gastroenterology*, **84**, 1101

83. Bateson, M. C., Hill, A. and Bouchier, I. A. D. (1980). Analysis of response to ursodeoxycholic acid for gallstone dissolution. *Digestion*, **20**, 358–64

84. Ruppin, D. C. and Dowling, R. H. (1982). Is recurrence inevitable after gallstone dissolution by bile acid treatment? *Lancet*, **1**, 181–5

85. Toulet, J., Rousselet, J., Viteau, J. M. *et al.* (1983). Relapses and preventive treatment of relapses after dissolution of gallstones in 22 patients. *Gastroenterol Clin. Biol.*, **7**, 605–9

86. Marks, J. W., Lan, S. P., The Steering Committee and the National Co-operative Gallstone Study Group. (1984). Low-dose chenodiol to prevent gallstone recurrence after dissolution therapy. *Ann. Intern. Med.*, **100**, 376–81

87. Stefaniwsky, A. B., Tint, G. S., Speck, J., Shefer, S. and Salen, G. (1985). Ursodeoxycholic acid in the treatment of bile reflux gastritis. *Gastroenterology*, **89**, 1000–4

88. Berginer, V. M., Salen, G. and Shefer, S. (1984). Long-term treatment of CTX with cheno-deoxycholic acid. *N. Engl. J. Med.*, **311**, 1649–52

89. Ellis, W. R., Somerville, K. W., Whitten, B. H. and Bell, G. D. (1984). Pilot study of combination treatment for gallstones with medium dose chenodeoxycholic acid and a terpene preparation. *Br. Med. J.*, **289**, 153–6

90. Leiss, O. and von Bergman, K. (1985). Effect of Rowachol on biliary lipid secretion and serum lipids in normal volunteers. *Gut*, **26**, 32–7

91. Kurokis, U. M. and Mosbach, E. H. (1985). Synthesis of potential cholelitholytic agents. *J. Lipid. Res.*, **26**, 1205–11

92. Safrany, L. (1978). Endoscopic treatment of biliary tract diseases. *Lancet*, **2**, 983–5

93. Staritz, M., Poralla, T., Dormeyer, K-H. and Zum Buschenfeld, M. K. H. (1985). Endoscopic removal of common bile duct stones through the intact papilla after medical sphincter dilation. *Gastroenterology*, **88**, 1807–11

94. Stave, R. and Osnes, M. (1985). Endoscopic gallstone extraction following hydrostatic balloon dilatation of stricture in the common bile duct. *Endoscopy*, **17**, 159–60

95. Burhenne, H. J. (1976). Complications of non-operative extraction of retained common bile duct stones. *Am. J. Surg.*, **131**, 260–2

96. Shorvon, P. J., Cotton, P. B., Mason, R. R., Siegel, J. H. and Hatfield, A. R. W. (1985). Percutaneous transhepatic assistance for duodenoscopic sphincterotomy. *Gut*, **26**, 1373–6

97. Jarrett, L. N., Balfour, T. W., Bell, G. D., Knapp, D. R. and Rose, D. H. (1981). Intraductal infusion of mono-octanoin: experience in 24 patients with retained common duct stones. *Lancet*, **1**, 68–70

98. Palmer, K. R. and Hofmann, A. F. (1986). Intraductal mono-octanoin for the direct dissolution of bile duct stones: experience in 343 patients. *Gut*, **27**, 196–202

99. Allen, M. J., Borody, T. J., Bugliosi, T. F., May, G. R., Larusso, N. F. and Thistle, J. L. (1985). Rapid dissolution of gallstones with methyl-tert-butyl ether. *N. Engl. J. Med.*, **312**, 217–20

100. Allen, M. J., Borody, T. J. and Thistle, J. L. (1985). *In vitro* dissolution of cholesterol gallstones. *Gastroenterology*, **89**, 1097–103

101. Salvioli, G., Salati, R., Lugli, R. and Zanni, C. (1983). Medical treatment of biliary duct stones: effect of ursodeoxycholic acid administration. *Gut*, **24**, 609–14

102. Sama, C., Petronelli, A., Malavolti, M., Mastroroberto, G. and Roda, E. (1983). A double-blind comparative trial of dihydroxydibutrylether in patients with cholesterol gallstones. *Int. J. Clin. Pharmacol. Ther. Toxicol.*, **21**, 95–7

103. Burhenne, H. J. and Stoller, J. L. (1985). Minicholecystostomy and radiologic stone extraction in high-risk cholelithiasis patients. Preliminary experience. *Am. J. Surg.*, **149**, 632–5

104. Akiyama, H., Nagusa, Y., Fujita, T. *et al.* (1985). A new method for non-surgical chole-cystolithotomy. *Surg. Gynaecol. Obstet.*, **161**, 73–4

105. Dunham, F., Marliere, P., Mortier, C. and Gulbis, A. (1985). Ultrasound-guided per-cutaneous and transhepatic cholecystostomy: a complementary procedure to therapeutic endoscopy. *Endoscopy*, **17**, 153–6

106. Salomonowitz, E., Frick, M. P., Simmons, R. L. *et al.* (1984). Obliteration of the gallbladder without femoral cholecystectomy. *Arch. Surg.*, **119**, 725–9

107. Delius, M., Enders, G. and Brendel, W. (1986). Passage of stone fragments from canine gallbladders. *Gut* (In press)

108. Riemann, J. F., Sueberth, K. and Demling, L. (1982). Clinical application of new mechanical lithotriptor for smashing common bile duct stones. *Endoscopy*, **14**, 226–30

109. Ebbs, S. R., Beckly, D. E., Hammonds, J. C. and Teasdale, C. (1986). Percutaneous elec-trohydraulic lithotripsy of retained bile duct calculus. *Br. Med. J.*, **292**, 94

110. Gadacz, T. R. (1985). Ultrasonic fragmentation of gallstones *in vitro*. *Surgery*, **97**, 511–13

111. Sauerbruch, T., Delius, M., Paumgartner, G. *et al.* (1986). Fragmentation of gallstones by extracorporeal shock waves. *N. Engl. J. Med.*, **314**, 818–22

Index